Issues in
Abnormal
Child
Psychology

Issues in Abnormal Child Psychology

Edited by

Anthony Davids
Brown University

Brooks/Cole Publishing Company
Monterey, California
A Division of Wadsworth Publishing Company, Inc.

ISBN: 0-8185-0095-6
L.C. Catalog Card No.: 73-76924
Printed in the United States of America
1 2 3 4 5 6 7 8 9 10—77 76 75 74 73

35376

Production Editor: Mara Robezgruntnieks-Niels
Interior & Cover Design: Linda Marcetti
Typesetting: Holmes Composition Service, San Jose, California
Printing & Binding: Kingsport Press, Kingsport, Tennessee

Preface

Issues in Abnormal Child Psychology presents the most significant issues and problems that face clinicians, educators, and researchers who are concerned with childhood psychopathology. It will acquaint the reader with the many perplexing issues that need much further study and research attention. No directly comparable book of readings covers the topics included in this volume, which presents articles from several areas of the social and behavioral sciences. This book serves a valuable heuristic function for both students and teachers in contemporary psychology, psychiatry, education, and the social services by bringing together much of the most relevant, significant material about childhood psychopathology.

The impetus for preparing this book came from my experience in teaching an abnormal child psychology course for undergraduates. After several years of following a conventional approach, I began to structure the course around controversial issues and unresolved problems in this field. Students who completed this course evaluated the issues approach as highly successful. Many of the topics and readings that they found particularly interesting are included in this book.

While most of the important areas covered in abnormal child psychology textbooks are included here, this book is not an exhaustive review of the literature in each area or a comprehensive book in terms of conventional textbook scope; the topical coverage is somewhat more limited, and the choice of material is much more selective than in a standard text. Although the reader is assumed to have the background of psychological theory and basic concepts that an elementary course would provide, the chapter introductions present the essential information and proper setting for considering each issue.

The conventional basic textbook usually presents material in keeping with the author's beliefs and theoretical orientation. This book's approach to studying childhood psychopathology, with its focus on controversial issues, presents theoretical views and empirical evidence pertinent to both sides of each topic. Only a few of the chapters offer solutions. This book is not meant to provide ready answers or factual material to be memorized; instead, it should stimulate readers to think critically about these issues, to formulate their own views, and perhaps even to dedicate at least part of their lives to helping troubled children. While the primary goal is educational, this material is also intended to make interesting reading.

This book consists of twelve chapters, each of which focuses on a specific issue or problem. Each chapter begins with a discussion of the topic and an introduction to the articles that follow. Where there are opposing schools of thought, conflicting theoretical viewpoints, or contradictory data from independent investigations, the articles have been selected to present different sides of the controversy. Some chapter introductions or articles attempt to resolve the problem or provide integrative reviews of relevant literature. A concluding chapter discusses the most critical issues and challenges for the decade ahead.

Throughout this book, the term "myth" appears frequently. A major purpose is to make students and professional workers aware of the myths that are being perpetuated in some areas of this field. Wherever we discover a myth, an important issue is usually involved. Since we are here concerned with significant issues and problems whenever we encounter myths, we must strive to understand them and to correct the misconceptions that undoubtedly have important influences on diagnosis and treatment of children in various psychiatric and educational settings.

We will see myths about diagnosis and classification of various types of childhood abnormalities, aspects of psychological testing, mental retardation, and special education. Myths and stereotypes are often related, although they are not identical. They both involve uncritical acceptance of commonly held beliefs about people, places, and practices. A stereotype could be valid and serve some useful purpose, but myths by definition are fictitious and unverified and can lead only to confusion and misunderstanding. In some instances, myths may even encourage what should rightfully be viewed as malpractice.

Myths are an important concern in this volume because I hope that making the reader aware of them will contribute to dispelling them. Of course, a theorist or practitioner who protests against what he terms a myth may be incorrect in his criticism. Therefore, this book presents the so-called myth and the issues related to it, leaving the reader, himself, to grapple with the problem of what is right and to decide what action seems necessary to resolve the controversy.

The issues discussed here are of grave concern to anyone seriously interested in the helping professions, including college undergraduates, graduate students, and workers in the field. The issues and problems are timely, with enormous significance for the understanding and treatment of childhood psychopathology and for programs of education and child development.

I would like to thank the following reviewers for their critical evaluation of the manuscript: Wayne R. Carroll, The University of Arizona; Eugene S. Cherry, Iowa State University; John J. Conger, University of Colorado Medical School; Lucy R. Ferguson, Michigan State University; Alfred B. Heilbrun, Jr., Emory University; William C. Morse, The University of Michigan; and Jeanne S. Phillips, University of Denver.

Anthony Davids

Contents

Part IV. Ethical Considerations and General Conclusions 383

Issues in Abnormal Child Psychology

Part I

Some General Issues

Chapter One

Current Status of the Field of Childhood Psychopathology

This chapter introduces the field of childhood psychopathology, the kinds of disorders that are subsumed under this broad heading, and some of the most significant issues and challenges according to major figures working on the contemporary front of psychology and psychiatry.

Classification and Categorization

In recent years there has been considerable controversy concerning problems of diagnosis or labeling of childhood disorders. It has been found that classification schemes traditionally used with adult mental patients tend to be inadequate for diagnosis of childhood disorders. In view of this, some clinicians and investigators have attempted to modify existing classification schemes or have devised entirely different diagnostic categories for children.

In 1968, the American Psychiatric Association published a major revision of the Diagnostic and Statistical Manual of Mental Disorders (APA, 1968). Known as DSM-II, it was an attempt to develop a diagnostic scheme that could be used throughout the world, thereby facilitating universal understanding of the kinds and prevalence of mental disorders. The earlier edition of the manual, originally published in 1952, was used in all psychiatric facilities in this country and thus formed the basis for statistics concerning various categories and classifications of mental disorders.

The current manual, like its predecessor, was compiled by a committee of physicians and, according to the requirements of the APA, must be used in classifying every patient treated in psychiatric institutions. In the area of child treatment, these diagnostic manuals and the requirement of assigning diagnostic labels have been disconcerting to many non-medical professionals who work with disturbed children. The APA requires that exact statistics be kept in terms of the established categories of mental disorder. At times, the staff in a child treatment facility must assign a label that does not fit well; nevertheless, the regulations require classification according to one of the diagnostic categories in DSM-II.

In favor of this procedure, the diagnoses described in the manual often seem perfectly appropriate for a given child patient, and all staff members concerned with the case agree on the classification assigned. An accurate diagnosis contributes to formulation of a proper plan of treatment and can help all personnel working with the child to communicate with a minimum of ambiguity and misunderstanding. Also, statistics on the incidence of different types of psychopathology can contribute to increased understanding of the nature and degree of prevalence of the disorder. This knowledge can influence both research and practical issues, which are often determined by the magnitude of the problem behavior revealed through statistical analyses.

DSM-II contains 10 major diagnostic categories, including "Behavior Disorders of Childhood and Adolescence." This category was not in the first edition of the manual; it contains diagnoses of disorders "occurring in childhood and adolescence that are more stable, internalized, and resistant to treatment than transient situational disturbances, but less so than psychoses, neuroses, and personality disorders. This intermediate stability is attributed to greater fluidity of all behavior at this age."

The specific diagnoses within this overall category are: (1) hyperkinetic reaction—characterized by overactivity, restlessness, distractibility; (2) withdrawing reaction—characterized by shyness and timidity; (3) overanxious reaction—characterized by chronic anxiety and fears; (4) runaway reaction—characterized by feeling inadequate and rejected at home and escaping from threat by running away; (5) unsocialized aggressive reaction—characterized by hostile disobedience, physical and verbal aggression, and destructiveness; (6) group delinquent reaction (typical of individuals who have acquired the values, behavior, and skills of a delinquent group to whom they are loyal)—characterized by stealing, truancy, and staying out late at night.

While the category of "Behavior Disorders of Childhood and Adolescence" is the only one devoted exclusively to children, certain other types of childhood disorders are located under the categories of transient situational disturbances, psychoses, neuroses, and personality disorders.

The category of transient situational disturbances refers to disorders that are subdivided into adjustment reactions of infancy, childhood, and adolescence. Examples from each of these three developmental stages would be, respectively, severe grief following separation from mother; extreme jealousy following birth of younger sibling; and depression following school failure. If the symptoms persist after the stress is removed, the diagnosis must be changed to another category.

Under the major category "psychoses," there is a subdivision termed "schizophrenia, childhood type," which is used when schizophrenic symptoms appear before puberty. This condition may be manifested by autistic, atypical, and withdrawn behavior; failure to form separate identity from the mother's; or general unevenness, gross immaturity, and inadequacy in development. In describing these characteristics, the manual points out that these developmental defects may result in mental retardation, which should also be diagnosed.

Under the category of neuroses, in which anxiety is the chief characteristic, the sub-type most often found in children is phobic neurosis. In this condition, the child is intensely afraid of an object or situation that possesses no real danger for him. Phobias are generally attributed to fears displaced onto the phobic object from some other situation or object that the patient is unaware of or unable to face.

Among the personality disorders, the one found most frequently in children and adolescents is "passive-aggressive personality." This behavior pattern is characterized by both passivity and aggression, with the aggressive aspect being expressed passively. For example, the child reveals his hostility and resentment through such maneuvers as pouting, procrastination, intentional inefficiency, or stubbornness. It is believed that this behavior commonly reflects hostility that the person is afraid to express openly. Often it is attributed to resentment at failing to find gratification in relationships with people on whom he is overly dependent.

Symptom Typologies

While most child treatment centers use the APA classifications, some clinicians and researchers have employed different systems for viewing childhood disorders. Recently, Garmezy (1970) has emphasized two major types of disturbance that form the core of psychopathology in children. Some children tend to internalize their conflicts, resulting in symptoms such as excessive inhibition, withdrawal, avoidance, fearfulness, and physical complaints. In contrast to these internalizing types of children are those who externalize their conflicts, showing aggressive, destructive, anti-social behaviors.

This internalizing-externalizing symptom dimension (Achenbach, 1966) bears a certain similarity to other classifications that have been proposed in the psychiatric and psychological literature. For example, Horney (1945) described two very different neurotic types—those who "move away" from others, and those who "move against" other people. Similarly, Rosenzweig (1945) described opposite modes of handling aggression in the face of frustration. Some people react in a manner Rosenzweig termed "extrapunitive"—tending to blame and strike out against others when confronted with frustration. On the other hand, some people show a very different type of response to frustration, termed "intropunitive"—blaming themselves and turning their aggression inward.

Focusing on childhood disorders, Jenkins (1966) has reported that the majority of psychiatric syndromes can be dichotomized into the categories of "inhibited" versus "aggressive." Studies of behavior problems in middle childhood (Peterson, 1961) and in early adolescence (Quay & Quay, 1965) have led to the typologies "personality disorder" versus "conduct disorder." Other investigators who have studied abnormal children (for example, Bennett, 1960) have categorized them into two broad groups labeled "neurotic children" and "delinquent children." As Garmezy (1970) has indicated, most of these classification schemes can be viewed as varieties of the internalizing-externalizing dimension of disturbed behavior.

Treatment

Regardless of which specific diagnostic classifications are used, these are the kinds of personality and behavioral abnormalities that often lead to a child being institutionalized in a psychiatric hospital, residential treatment center, training school for delinquents, or facility for the mentally retarded. If not sufficiently severe to warrant institutionalization, childhood psychopathology may be treated on an outpatient basis by a pediatrician, psychiatrist, psychologist, social worker, or special educator. The specific type of treatment is determined both by the nature of the child's problems and the professional orientation of the therapist.

Models for Viewing Psychopathology

Just as there is considerable disagreement regarding diagnostic classifications, there are opposing models for understanding and treating disordered behavior. One viewpoint is known as the "mental illness model" and the other as the "psychosocial model" of abnormal behavior. Some believe that emotional upsets, neuroses, and psychoses are actually forms of mental illness and should be regarded as such when it comes to treatment of and theorizing about them. However, others feel that abnormal behaviors, similar to most behaviors, are acquired through the process of psychosocial development. The first orientation assumes that unhealthy hereditary factors or some form of disease has been inflicted on the individual, causing him to suffer from an illness that requires treatment administered by members of the medical professions. The second orientation assumes that deviant or aberrant behaviors merely provide evidence of misguided learning or traumatic interpersonal experiences during the developmental years; consequently, the disorder is not viewed as requiring medical treatment but instead calling for some form of re-education, psychotherapy, guidance, or behavior modification.

From the historical perspective, it seems quite natural that when physicians first attempted to treat behavioral disorders they did so in a conceptual framework emphasizing physical malfunction and disease. "Mental disease" became the province of psychiatry, a medical specialty. Recently, however, the adequacy of this disease model (Ausubel, 1961) has been seriously questioned. One of the most outspoken critics of this view is Szasz (1961), himself a physician and psychiatrist, who has written extensively on what he terms "the myth of mental illness." He has been joined by other psychologists (including Albee, whose paper is reprinted in this chapter) who cite accumulating evidence in support of their contention that most abnormal behaviors result from learning and social interactions, not from affliction or infection.

The Issues

This chapter contains three papers concerned with significant, comprehensive issues in this broad field. The opening paper, prepared by the Joint Commission on Mental Health of Children, describes present shortcomings in treatment of children in this country; it highlights the challenges confronting parents, educators, professionals, and legislators in the decade ahead. This call for a genuine commitment to our children and youth is followed by Leon Eisenberg's scholarly review of important psychological and psychiatric research conducted with children during the past quarter century. This distinguished professor of child psychiatry at Harvard Medical School also discusses some of the most pressing issues awaiting future attention.

In the closing paper, George W. Albee, a former president of the American Psychological Association, discusses some of the more prevalent myths that he feels have had a detrimental effect on the entire mental health movement. He maintains that traditional approaches to treatment of troubled children and adults have been completely misguided and are in need of major changes. He recommends alternative models for coping with psychosocial problems and suggests how manpower available in this country could be used much more effectively in this undertaking. These three papers discuss significant accomplishments in the recent past, the most pressing challenges for the future, and some suggested approaches for coping with them.

References

American Psychiatric Association. *Diagnostic and statistical manual: Mental disorders* (DSM-II). Washington, D.C.: American Psychiatric Association, 1968.

Achenbach, T. M. The classification of children's psychiatric symptoms: A factor analytic study. *Psychological Monographs*, 1966, **80**, 6.

Ausubel, D. P. Personality disorder is disease. *American Psychologist*, 1961, **16**, 69–74.

Bennett, I. *Delinquent and neurotic children*. New York: Basic Books, 1960.

Garmezy, N. Vulnerable children: Implications derived from studies of an internalizing-externalizing symptom dimension. In J. Zubin & A. M. Freedman (Eds.), *Psychopathology of adolescence*. New York: Grune & Stratton, 1970.

Horney, K. *Our inner conflicts*. New York: Norton, 1945.

Jenkins, R. L. Psychiatric syndromes in children and their relation to family background. *American Journal of Orthopsychiatry*, 1966, **36**, 450–457.

Peterson, D. R. Behavior problems of middle childhood. *Journal of Consulting Psychology*, 1961, **25**, 205–209.

Quay, H. C., & Quay, L. C. Behavior problems in early adolescence. *Child Development*, 1965, **36**, 215–220.

Rosenzweig, S. An outline of frustration theory. In J. McV. Hunt (Ed.), *Personality and the behavior disorders*. Vol. 1. New York: Ronald, 1945.

Szasz, T. S. *The myth of mental illness*. New York: Hoeber-Harper, 1961.

1. Digest of Crisis in Child Mental Health: Challenge for the 1970s

The Joint Commission on Mental Health of Children

We proclaim that we are a Nation devoted to its young. We believe that we have made great strides toward recognizing the needs of children and youth. We have enacted child labor laws, established a public education system, created treatment services for our disturbed and handicapped, and devised imaginative programs such as Head Start for our disadvantaged young. Yet, we find ourselves dismayed by the violence, frustration, and discontent among our youth and by the sheer number of emotionally, mentally, physically and socially handicapped youngsters in our midst. It is shocking to know that thousands of children are still excluded from our schools, that millions in need go untreated, and that many still suffer from hunger and malnutrition. We recognize in these ills some of the sources and symptoms of poverty and racism in which all of us, as a Nation, take part. Poverty, in this the richest of world powers, is still our heritage. Racism, in a country dedicated to its peoples' inalienable rights, speaks as clearly of ''man's inhumanity to man'' as did slavery.

In spite of our best intentions, our programs are insufficient; they are piecemeal, fragmented and do not serve all those in need. Unwittingly, we have failed to commit our vast resources to promote the healthy development of our young. We have yet to devise a strategy which will maximize the development of our human resources. Congress gave national recognition to this need in issuing a mandate to establish the Joint Commission on Mental Health of Children. In fulfillment of its task, the Commission declares:

—This Nation, the richest of all world powers, has no unified national commitment to its children and youth. The claim that we are a child-centered society, that we look to our young as tomorrow's leaders, is a myth. Our words are made meaningless by our actions—by our lack of national, community, and personal investment in maintaining the healthy development of our young, by the minuscule amount of economic resources spent in developing our young, by our tendency to rely on a proliferation of simple, one-factor, short-term and inexpensive remedies and services. As a tragic consequence, we have in our midst millions of ill-fed, ill-housed, ill-educated and discontented youngsters and almost ten million under age 25 who are in need of help from mental health workers. Some means must be devised to delegate clear responsibility and authority to insure the well-being of our young.

—This Nation, which looks to the family to nurture its young, gives no real help with child-rearing until a child is badly disturbed or disruptive to the community. The discontent, apathy, and violence today are a warning that society has not assumed its responsibility to insure an environment which will provide optimum care for its children. The family cannot be allowed to withstand alone the enormous pressures of an increasingly technological world. Within the community some mechanism must be created which will assume the responsibility for insuring the necessary supports for the child and family.

—This Nation, which prides itself on democratic values and equal opportunity, still imposes on its young the psychological repercussions of poverty and racism. No one is effectively empowered to intercede.

—This Nation, richly endowed with the knowledge to develop its youthful resources, has yet to fill the gap between knowledge and action. We know, for example, that preventive measures are most essential and effective if taken in the earliest years of life; that during this period there are critical stages of development which, if neglected or mishandled, may result in irreversible damage. Yet, our services are nowhere more deficient than in the area of prenatal and infant care.

—This Nation, highly sophisticated and knowledgeable about mental health and child development, continues its planning and programming largely around the concept of treating, rather than preventing, mental illness. But no agency has the task and responsibility for assuring that treatment is, in fact, received by those who need it.

—This Nation, despite its emphasis on treatment, has yet to develop adequate mental health services and facilities for all children and youth, regardless of race and economic circumstances. Many receive no attention. The number of young, particularly adolescents, who are committed to mental institutions continues to rise markedly. Yet, we have not provided the resources and manpower to assist those who are devoted to caring for these children. As a result, any possible benefits of confinement are lost in the tragic waste of the back ward. Even less effort is made to develop coordinated community services so these children can be kept as closely as possible within their normal, routine setting.

The Commission strongly urges better treatment for the mentally ill, the handicapped, the retarded, the delinquent, and the emotionally disturbed. We join forces with those who propose a broader but more meaningful concept of mental health, one which is based on the developmental view with prevention and optimum mental health as the major goal. We contend that the mentally healthy life is one in which self-direction and satisfying interdependent relationships prevail, one in which there is meaning, purpose, and opportunity. We believe that lives which are uprooted, thwarted, and denied the growth of their inherent capacities are mentally unhealthy, as are those determined by rigidity, conformity, deprivation, impulsivity, and hostility. Unfulfilled lives cost us twice—once in the loss of human resources, in the apathetic, unhappy, frustrated, and violent souls in our midst, and again in the loss of productivity to our society, and the economic costs of dependency. We believe that, if we are to optimize the mental health of our young and if we are to develop our human resources, every infant must be granted:

—*the right to be wanted* yet, millions of unwanted children continue to be born—often with tragic consequences—largely because their parents have not had access to or knowledge of the benefits of birth control information and devices.

—*the right to be born healthy* yet, approximately one million children will be born this year to women who get no medical aid during their pregnancy or no adequate obstetrical care for delivery; thus many will be born with brain damage from disorders of pregnancy. For some, protein and vitamin supplements might have prevented such tragedy.

—*the right to live in a healthy environment* yet, thousands of children and youth become physically handicapped or acquire chronic damage to their health from preventable accidents and diseases, largely because of impoverished environments. Even greater numbers living in poverty will become psychologically handicapped and damaged, unable to compete in school or on a job or to fulfill their inherent capabilities—they will become dependents of, rather than contributors to, our society.

—*the right to satisfaction of basic needs* yet, approximately one-fourth of our children face the probability of malnutrition, inadequate housing, untreated physical and mental disorders, educational handicaps, and indoctrination into a life of marginal work and opportunity.

—*the right to continuous loving care* yet, millions of our young never acquire the necessary motivation or intellectual and emotional skills required to cope effectively in our society because they do not receive consistent emotionally satisfying care. Society does little to help parents. There are few programs which provide good day care, which aid in developing more adequate child-rearing techniques, or which assist in times of temporary family crisis or where children are neglected or abused.

—*the right to acquire the intellectual and emotional skills necessary to achieve individual aspirations and to cope effectively in our society* yet, each year almost a million of our youth drop out of school and enter the adult world with inadequate skills and with diminished chances of becoming productive citizens; countless others are denied the opportunities to develop to their fullest potential through effective vocational training, meaningful work experience, or higher education. For all of our children and youth the transition to adulthood is made difficult. We fail to provide avenues for learning adult roles, for acquiring skills, or some approved means by which youth's voice can influence a world in which they too must live.

We know that when these rights are granted, development will proceed favorably for most infants. Few children, however, encounter continuously those ideal circumstances that maximize their hereditary potential for health, competence, and humanity. At conception, at birth, and throughout development, there are vast variations and inequalities in the life chances of our young. Undoubtedly, many will continue to be psychologically damaged. If our more unfortunate are to become functioning and productive citizens, we believe they must be granted:

—*the right to receive care and treatment through facilities which are appropriate to their needs and which keep them as closely as possible within their normal social setting* yet, several millions of our children and youth—the emotionally disturbed, the mentally ill, the mentally retarded, the handicapped, and the delinquent—are not receiving such care. The reasons are innumerable. Many go untreated because the services are fragmented, or nonexistent, or because they discriminate by cost, class or color. Others are diagnosed and labeled without regard to their level of functioning. They are removed from their homes, schools, and communities and confined to hospital wards with psychotic adults or to depersonalized institutions which deliver little more than custodial care.

Going back as far as the first White House Conference on Children in 1909 we have repeatedly, and with considerable eloquence, announced our intentions to develop a strong, imaginative program to care for emotionally disturbed children. For example, the 1930 White House Conference on Child Health and Protection, composed of several thousand citizens and government officials, proclaimed that:

> The emotionally disturbed child has a right to grow up in a world which does not set him apart, which looks at him not with scorn or pity or ridicule—but which welcomes him exactly as it welcomes every child, which offers him identical privileges and identical responsibilities.

The 1930 White House Conference estimated that there were, at that time, at least two and one-half million children with well-marked behavioral difficulties, including the more serious mental and nervous disorders.

In the four decades since the issuance of that report, the care of the emotionally disturbed child in this country has not improved—it has worsened considerably. During the three years of its deliberations and fact-finding efforts the Commission has gathered together an impressive body of descriptive material on the plight of the emotionally disturbed child in America today.

Using the most conservative estimate from various school surveys, the National Institute of Mental Health estimates that 1,400,000 children under 18 needed psychiatric care in 1966.

Are they getting this treatment? Surveys of various psychiatric facilities, undertaken by the National Institute of Mental Health, show that nearly a million of those children needing psychiatric care in 1966 did not receive treatment. These estimates indicate that we are providing care to only one-third of our children who are in serious need of attention. An additional seven to ten percent or more are estimated, by school surveys, to need some help for emotional problems.

What happens to these emotionally sick children for whom there are no services in the community? Each year, increasing numbers of them are expelled from the community and confined in large state hospitals so understaffed that they have few, if any, professionals trained in child psychiatry and related disciplines. It is not unusual in this year 1969 to tour one of these massive warehouses for the mentally ill and come upon a child, aged nine or ten, confined on a ward with 80 to 90 sick adults. Our present data indicate that slightly over 27,000 children under 18 were under care in state and county mental institutions in 1966. On the basis of a trend which has been developing over the past few years, the National Institute of Mental Health estimates that by 1970 the number of children aged 10–14 hospitalized in these institutions will have doubled.

The National Institute of Mental Health also reports that thousands upon thousands of elderly patients now confined on the back wards of these state institutions were first admitted as children 30, 40, and even 50 years ago. A recent report from one state estimates that one in every four children admitted to its mental hospitals "can anticipate being permanently hospitalized for the next 50 years of their lives."

What happens if the disturbed child is fortunate enough to escape the state institution treadmill? There are a few private, residential treatment centers which care for about 8,000 children a year. Since the average cost to the parents of such hospitalization ranges from $30 to $50 a day, it is obvious that only those of our citizens who are in the higher income brackets can take advantage of such services. Even among those rarified income brackets the situation is far from satisfactory; for every child admitted to one of these private facilities, 10 or more are turned away because of lack of space. In 8 of our states, there are no such facilities, either public or private. In many of our states, there are no public units to care for children from low and middle income groups.

What happens to all our children who receive no help for emotional problems? Here the statistics become much less precise, since a vast majority of these children are literally lost. They are bounced around from training schools to reformatories to jails and whipped through all kinds of understaffed welfare agencies. No one is their keeper. No agency in the community is equipped to evaluate either the correctness of their placement or the outcome of such placement.

If they are sent to a training school, as recent testimony before a Senate Committee revealed, they generally receive poorer treatment than caged animals or adult convicts. Appearing in 1969 before a Senate Committee, Joseph R. Rowan, an expert on delinquency who is now director of the John Howard Association of Illinois, characterized these institutions for juveniles as "crime hatcheries where children are tutored in crime if they are not assaulted by other inmates or the guards first." Another witness, Arlen Specter, the District Attorney of Philadelphia, told the same committee that these so-called correctional institutions for juveniles take a 13 year old and in 12 years, turn out "a finely honed weapon against society."

Commenting on the failure of juvenile courts and juvenile correctional facilities to even begin to meet the manifest needs of emotionally disturbed and sociopathic children, Judge David Bazelon, a member of the Commission, noted in a recent talk that although this Nation is aware of the problem, it does not support funds to treat and care for these children *because it has really given up on them.*

We must ask ourselves whether we can continue to deny our children their inalienable rights. Can we continue to gamble with our Nation's future by allowing children to grow up in environments which we know are psychologically damaging—and compound this by lack of adequate care and treatment?

We have the knowledge and the riches to remedy many of the conditions which affect our young, yet we lack a genuine commitment to do so. We blind ourselves to the fact that we create most of the social problems of our young which we so deplore—infants who fail to thrive, seriously disturbed children in mental institutions, adolescent drug addiction, acts of violence and destruction by youth.

Our lack of commitment is a national tragedy. We know already that it is more fruitful to prevent damage to our young than to attempt to patch and heal the wounds. We know that much of the damage could be avoided in the first three years of life. We know that the basis for mental development and competence is largely established by the age of six. Yet we do not act on this knowledge. Studies indicate that most children, regardless of class or race, whether in the ghetto or in suburbia, do not receive the needed support and assistance from our society. But, it is the damaged, the vulnerable, and the poor who are given the least from our health, welfare, and educational services. Those who are the most helpless are the most neglected.

This Commission proposes a shift in strategy for human development in this Nation—one which will deploy our resources in the service of optimizing human development. We emphasize the critical need to concentrate our resources on the new generation and eliminate problems which later exact so high and tragic a price.

In the allocation of these resources, it is the consensus of most of the Commission's task force and committees that equal priority should be given to the following:

—Comprehensive services which will insure the maintenance of health and mental health of children and youth.
—A broad range of remedial mental health services for the seriously disturbed, juvenile delinquents, mentally retarded, and otherwise handicapped children and their families.
—The development of an advocacy system at every level of government to insure the effective implementation of these desired goals.

The services we propose should cover the entire range of childhood, from systematic maternal and infant care to the transition of the adolescent and college age youth into effective young adulthood.

It should be emphasized that fostering the development of human beings in this country is a means to an end—a means to stem the increasing numbers of people who have no meaningful role in society. Their services in health, education, welfare, and other human and community services are desperately needed and currently unused.

Commitment, genuine commitment, to our children and youth is, necessarily, the beginning. We must look honestly at the scope of the problem and begin *now* to follow our words by action. We must develop advocacy functions at all levels of government and society, functions which will insure that the needs of children and their families are being met. This commitment to advocacy means commitment to change. It means that we—as parents, educators, professionals and legislators—must participate and collaborate in change in national, state and local levels. We must reorder our priorities so that the developmental needs of children rank first in importance. The commitment requires finding effective ways to link our fiscal resources, services and manpower so that every infant will be guaranteed the continuous care and the opportunities required for his optimal development. The creation of an advocacy system means that we, at last, will act to insure the rights of our living and unborn young. For in our children lie our future and our hope for the fulfillment of our national goals. We must not—cannot afford to do less.

2. Child Psychiatry:
The Past Quarter Century

Leon Eisenberg

Historiography is a constant dialogue between past and present; it takes new form from the grounds of the shifting present. The historian 25 years hence will almost certainly view our recent past from perspectives quite different from our own, having at his command new viewpoints and more distance from the controversies in which we are still engaged. We can only hope he will be kind to those of us then still alive, and show due respect for our venerability if not for our perspicacity. I beg him to forgive me for limiting my survey mostly to this continent, but this is the only scene I know well enough to dare these comments.

Fortunately, our assessment of recent developments can take as its starting point the insightful and balanced comments of Professor Kanner, who, in a series of scholarly and delightfully literate publications,[33-35] has attended the birth and early childhood of child psychiatry. The paternity of this hybrid invites us to invoke the mechanism of superfecundation, involving as it did general psychiatry, the juvenile court movement, defectology, education, child development, psychoanalysis, pediatrics, and child guidance. Although textbooks concerned with the "mental diseases" and "insanity" of children had appeared before the turn of the century, they were primarily exercises in the imposition of adult nosology upon childhood disorders.[34] It was not until 1926 that Homburger[29] wrote the first treatise on the psychopathology of childhood that can be said to be informed by a concern for the child as a person, and it was not until 1935 that Kanner[36] published the first American textbook with the title *Child Psychiatry*. By the 1930's child guidance clinics were a burgeoning feature of the North American scene. Tramer's Zeitschrift für Kinderpsychiatrie had been founded, and Heuyer had organized an international congress in Paris under the title "Psychiatrie infantile."

The year that marks the opening of our survey (1943), appropriately

From the *American Journal of Orthopsychiatry,* 1969, **39,** 389–401. Copyright © 1969 by the American Orthopsychiatric Association, Inc. Reproduced by permission.

enough, was the year in which Professor Kanner[37] reported the previously undescribed syndrome that has come to be known as early infantile autism, the first instance of a psychotic disorder peculiar to childhood. To that point in time, the contributions of child psychiatry might be summarized in these terms: The desirability of multidisciplinary study of the child in his family had been well established. At an operational level this was reflected in the collaboration of the social worker, the psychologist, and the psychiatrist in the child guidance clinic and in the eligibility of all three groups for membership in the American Orthopsychiatric Association.[44 57 65] The first effective drugs, the amphetamines, had been introduced.[6] The thesis that adult disorders have antecedents in childhood experience had been broadly accepted; true, this idea had been introduced into psychiatry by Freud without the benefit of child study four decades earlier, but the accumulating clinical reports of child psychiatrists had given it—or at least appeared to have given it—empirical support.

The enthusiasm for prevention, again a doctrine enunciated at the turn of the century in the mental hygiene movement, now became the province of children's clinics. In much the same spirit that Victor Hugo had proclaimed that the opening of each new school meant the closing of a prison, the community was led to expect that each new child clinic made obsolete an adult mental hospital. However distant the day of its realization might seem, given the shortages of funding and manpower then as now, there was no lack of conviction that the control of mental illness could be attained by a proper network of child guidance clinics, training of school teachers, and education of parents. And this conviction was no mere matter of naive optimism on the part of our professional forebears; the nature of their daily clinical work with its high rates of symptomatic improvement in the children they cared for appeared to verify their beliefs.

Yet for all the honor due to child psychiatry for having pioneered a broader view of patient-family-community interaction than was then typical of adult psychiatry, our horizons were constricted by our focus on the clinical study of the individual patients and families who passed through our clinic doors. It is only in the last decade that we have begun to recognize that population studies are essential[62 63] and that clinic intake has unintended as well as deliberate bias built into it.[1] Once appropriate controls for social class were introduced, it became difficult to verify the widespread assumption that such variables as age and method of weaning, toilet training practices, sex education, or the parental attitudes measured by standard inventories distinguish clinic patients from other children.[48] Such factors do indeed vary significantly by social class but they fail to predict patienthood. In contrast to such factors, what did discriminate patients from controls in a study[48] of a sample of our clinic population was the experience of separation from parents by illness, death, or desertion and the occurrence of marital distress.

Many of the formulations which seemed to have explanatory value when applied in retrospect to patient populations that were skewed in unknown fashion by gate-keeping procedures disappeared into insignificance when appropriate sampling and control techniques were introduced.

Such errors, in my estimation, have stemmed in part from the isolation of the child guidance clinic from medicine, on the one hand, and from child development on the other. No physiologist would describe a normal heart in terms derived solely from the study of a failing one; had he done so, Starling would have concluded that ventricular output decreases rather than increases in relation to ventricular dilatation. Yet we have generalized from our clinical work with troubled families to theories of normal development. Freud's experience before the turn of the century should have warned us of the unreliability of our patients' reconstructions of their past; what he first thought to be historical events he later discovered to be fantasy. Yet he and we have persevered in our preoccupation with those fantasies in lieu of the more laborious task of accumulating detailed prospective accounts of the vicissitudes of development. It has been only in the last decade that systematic longitudinal studies by such careful workers as Professor Chess[70] and her collaborators have begun to supply the information necessary for a meaningful account of the interaction between temperamental characteristics, parental behaviors, and social experiences in generating personality traits.

It is therefore not surprising that the promissory note of prevention issued by the mental hygienists has not been able to be redeemed.[16] If theories of cause rested on such uncertain foundations, nonspecific interventions are not likely to have been highly productive. Indeed our decisions on the "suitability" of particular children for treatment seemed to have been based more on our class biases than on the patients' psychiatric needs.[68] [71]

The Furman et al.[67] study of voluntary psychiatric facilities, facilities supported by charitable as well as tax funds, identified preferential service to those health areas that were better off economically. The most recent survey,[49] carried out by the New York Council on Child Psychiatry under the sponsorship of the Joint Commission on the Mental Health of Children, decried the long waiting periods for screening, prolonged intake procedures, clinic hours inappropriate for working parents, and other factors which summed to produce high dropout rates and differential likelihoods for treatment such that the least ill and the least poor families (within clinic income ceilings) were those most likely to be treated psychotherapeutically.

On the other hand, the most significant long-term followup study[59] ever carried out in our specialty has documented the lamentable outcome of just those children least preferred by clinic intake policy, the antisocial, the aggressive, the disorganized. As Professor Robins and her co-workers have shown, the neurotic child, though still at higher risk for psychiatric illness in adulthood than classroom controls, has the best prognosis for favorable outcome even in the absence of care. Yet just such children are, or at least have been, preferentially sought by therapists. Mind you, this is no injunction to sprinkle psychotherapy on delinquents; there is little evidence that they benefit therefrom.[55] It is a call to concentrate our efforts on developing methods of care for those disorders that constitute the major threats to public health.[17]

To its credit, the past decade has seen the first systematic studies of the outcome of psychotherapy for children. In general, the findings have not been reassuring.[41][43] Although occasional studies, such as one my associates and I carried out,[18] do provide some evidence in favor of psychotherapy, most studies have been unable to provide systematic evidence of benefit when the treated are contrasted with waiting list or designated controls. This point requires clarification. Not to have found a difference is not equivalent to having demonstrated that there was *in fact* no difference. Measures of outcome employed in most studies are admittedly crude; significant differences in attitude and in values, which may stand a child and his parents in good stead for the future, may emerge from sensitive and skilled psychotherapy and not be reflected in symptom counts, given the evanescence of symptoms in children.[40] But the counterassertion that change *has* been produced requires documentation. It is yet to be forthcoming.

What is remarkable is how little effect these studies with their Scots verdict of "not proven" have had on professional practice. Surely, at the least, they should have led to major investment of energy and effort in studies to define the indications for, the best methods of, and the limitations to psychotherapy rather than what can only be compared to a religious conviction in the possession of an exclusive road to salvation. And for all the interest aroused by the newer forms of psychological treatment such as family therapy[3][4] and behavior therapy,[23] there has been just the same dearth of controlled studies and the same evangelical proselytizing by the newly converted. Let me make it clear if I can: I regard both of these innovations as substantial contributions. I plead only for the necessity of controlled evaluation of their efficacy. I urge only that we abandon the Doctrine of Panacea and instead begin with the more likely proposition that particular methods will best suit particular patients and that the obligation of the psychiatrist is to be competent with a variety of treatment methods from which he can choose the one best suited for the individual patient.

All too often, what has been the liberation of one generation becomes the bondage of the next. If we can fairly claim credit for the introduction of the team of psychologist, social worker, and psychiatrist, we are also guilty of having elevated it to what Kanner has termed "the holy trinity." Countless extra hours go into "interdisciplinary communication" in situations where one qualified professional could more effectively manage the problem without ending up talking to himself. More often, the "team" is used as a shibboleth when in fact there is not and cannot be a team simply by virtue of the relative distributions of time for the various disciplines at the clinic. There has been an ultimate blurring of roles as social workers have become junior psychiatrists—with no one doing the by now low prestige social work; as psychiatrists function exclusively as psychotherapists—with no one competent to do the neuropsychiatric evaluation; as psychologists can be distinguished from psychiatrists only by their lower earnings and lower caste. Need I argue that it is well past time for us to re-examine the training for each discipline in relation to its actual professional function[24] and to utilize whatever special skills each might have in relation to the real problems of real people? Do we offer something tangible and useful to those who seek our help or are we content to "cool them out"? With growing shortages of manpower and with the growing press of claimants for service, it would indeed be a mockery to waste our human resources on busy work. The crying need is for rigorous studies evaluating outcome as we introduce new clinics, new services, new programs for community mental health.[19]

A posteriori, it is easy to see the faults of an earlier era and to overlook the devoted efforts of the legion of dedicated workers who applied what they believed to be true in a humane effort to ameliorate the distress of children. For that, all credit to them. Most of us can do no better than reflect the social perceptions of our times. The past quarter century, marked by the defeat of fascism and the upturning of economic indices, was one of social optimism in which the poor disappeared from American consciousness if not from the slums of our cities. The publication of Michael Harrington's[26] *The Other America* in 1962 can be taken as a convenient marker for the cresting of a wave of public concern for the poor and the black which has given new impetus and more productive directions to research in child development.

I am convinced that research in cognitive and personality development as resultants of the interaction between experience and maturation has been the major productive thrust of the past decade. If we psychiatrists are to contribute to the welfare of children, these are the areas in which the most is to be learned and the most to be given.

Just as the moral treatment of the insane had flowered and died a century before we were to rediscover it as "milieu therapy" and "community mental health," the antecedents of contemporary concerns with the effects of exogenous factors on cognitive development trace back at least that far.[35] But with the explosive demographic changes in the postwar period—the migration of the poor into center city areas, the flight of the affluent into suburbs and the decline in the urban tax base—the public school crisis has provided a new imperative for a long-standing issue.

Whether one examines IQ scores, achievement test results, years of schooling, or almost any traditional index of academic success, one finds marked differences that co-vary with the social class of the child.[31] Given the millions of children who are performing at marginal levels on the standard measures of academic achievement,[12 64] it becomes an urgent matter to identify the source of this human wastage. In a necessarily brief scan of recent research, I propose to touch upon the following issues: test bias, prenatal and paranatal factors, postnatal nutrition, family style, the school and, finally, the effects of racism.

Logically, the first question to be raised is whether test score differences are "real" differences or merely artifacts of measurement. The answer depends upon what we suppose that the tests measure. If it is "innate ability," as the naive psychometrist may assert, then intelligence test score differences are simply irrelevant, since they register the interaction between biological potential and experience, with no way of distinguishing the one from the other.[20] The pragmatist may assert nonetheless: what matters is the functional result, whether it reflects environment, heredity, or both. Are the functional differences real? Again, the answer will be different for different measures. Pose the question this way: Are there real deficits in ability to solve standard arithmetic problems or to read standard English paragraphs? The answer is an unequivocal: "yes." And this answer is a significant one; for, whatever other skills an adult may have, if he cannot use and read standard English, he will be seriously handicapped in negotiating the middle-class terrain where the material rewards of society are to be obtained. But there remains another question of major importance: Is the child impaired in his ability to reason, or do the language and the symbols in which the problem has been coded account for his performance failure?

It is by now abundantly clear that there *are* major differences in syntax as well as in vocabulary between middle-class and lower-class languages[5] and between white and Negro dialects.[2 66 69] I would caution you against the widespread assumption that what is different is defective. Lower-caste language may be dysfunctional in a middle-class world but it may also convey every subtle nuance of meaning within the indigenous culture. However, the Negro child attending first grade may be facing the task of learning a new language as well as of learning to read, at one and the same time. If this analysis is correct, it may account in part for his performance breakdown; Mexican Indian children learn to read more readily if they are taught with primers transcribed in their own dialect rather than in the Spanish they are just beginning to master.[45]

Moreover, a former colleague of mine, Professor Sonia Osler,[50 51] has demonstrated that lower-class children are able to profit from training (in learning to solve a concept problem) quite as well as middle-class children with a mean IQ some 15 points higher. Indeed, she calls our attention to how much *less* often there is any report of deficit when tasks involving *new* learning are given to such children in contrast to tests reflecting cumulative accomplishment. In our own studies[21] on children in Project Head Start, we have demonstrated statistically significant gains in such measures of "IQ" as the Peabody Picture Vocabulary Test and the Goodenough-Harris after no more than a 10-week enrichment experience. I do *not* mean to maintain—and indeed I do *not* believe—that there are *not* significant impairments in the academic function of some of these children by the time of school-leaving age. But I would emphasize that (1) the differences are exaggerated by the linguistic code factor and (2) the ability to learn is preserved to an extent far greater than conventional test scores are able to register. Both of these propositions have important implications for compensatory education programs.[25]

The second series of studies salient to this review concerns the prenatal and paranatal factors that influence brain development. Professors Pasamanick and Knobloch,[39 52] in a masterful series of investigations, have identified a "continuum of reproductive casualty" that extends at one end from spontaneous abortion and stillbirth, through mental deficiency and epilepsy, to learning disabilities and behavior disorders at the other end.

The underlying brain injuries are related to complications of pregnancy and parturition (toxemia, bleeding, infection, prematurity), complications which occur at significantly higher risk among the poor, the black, the unmarried, the underaged, and the overaged mother. These complications appear to result from an interaction between inadequate diet, poor prenatal care, poor housing, and gross stress, each of which is associated with pregnancy outcome.[76]

Sequential followup studies[73][74] have provided unequivocal evidence that the low birth-weight infant shows a high rate of neuropsychiatric disorder which results in serious impairment of academic performance.

But the hazards that surround the perinatal period—unacceptable and needless as they are—should not be mistaken for the major source of academic failure. In a recent 10-year followup of a pregnancy cohort in Kauai, the authors concluded: "The overwhelming number of children with problems at age 10 had relatively little or no perinatal stress, but they had grown up in homes low in socioeconomic status, educational stimulation, and emotional support."[72]

The third related area of research centers on nutritional factors, both before and after birth. Although earlier studies of maternal diet during pregnancy had been inconclusive because birth-weight was used as the outcome measure, recent studies[9][10] have indicated that low protein diet during pregnancy can lead to permanent stunting of subsequent adult stature even in animals not noticeably different at birth. A diet deficient in protein during the nursing period can induce permanent stunting in whole body and organ growth even when a free diet is made available to the young after weaning. Although the brain is proportionately less influenced than is total body weight, it does show significant growth retardation and the affected animals display poor performance in problem-solving situations.[15]

To turn to human data, the developmental quotient of children with kwashiorkor is markedly retarded and may not recover even after dietary repletion.[13] In a study[14] of children whose stature was taken as an index of earlier nutritional impairment, the authors found significant developmental delay in intersensory integration. More recently, Winick,[75] employing DNA (desoxyribonucleic acid) content as a measure of cell number, has shown that there is a marked restriction in brain cell growth in malnourished infant animals. Careful DNA measurements on human infants adequately nourished but dead of poisoning or infection has indicated that brain cell number continues to increase until five to six months of age. When these control values were compared with those from five children who died of severe malnutrition in the first year of life, there was a marked reduction in the number of brain cells in these infants, two of whom demonstrated a cell number less than 40% of normal!

Thus, it would appear that severe protein deficiency may wreak its havoc on intellectual development by interfering with cell multiplication during these crucial early months of development. The question that remains to be answered is whether this is a threshold phenomenon, appearing only when protein malnutrition exceeds some set value or whether it is graded and may appear in moderately malnourished children. Professor Monckeburg[46] of Chile has recently reported an association between developmental level, physical growth retardation, and level of protein intake as measured by careful dietary histories.

Here we confront a problem of world-wide significance, applying not only to the savage starvation that obtains in the underdeveloped countries but as well to the malnourished youngsters who populate Appalachia, the black ghettos of our cities, the black belt of the South, the Indian and Eskimo reservation of North America, and the Mexican-American and Puerto Rican enclaves scattered through the United States.[30][47] All of the facts may not be in, but those we do have demand a massive commitment by the wealthy nations of the world to ensure that no child starves. To await the final refinements in nutritional research is to condemn another generation of children to intellectual crippling—in Biafra, in Guatemala, in India, in pockets of poverty in our cities. Even as we study, we must act. We, who as students of development are aware of the grim toll of malnutrition, must take the lead in persuading our governments of the urgency of prompt intervention.

The fourth area of study moves us from the biosocial to the psychosocial sphere. The urban slum child grows up in a home bereft of books and often of newspapers, restricted in geographic experience to the few blocks surrounding his dwelling, denied stimulating cultural vistas, and limited to learning a nonstandard language.[32][38] His parents, like himself, are likely to have been earlier victims of limited educational exposure and to have cognitive styles which differ significantly from those modal for the larger society.

Professor Hess,[27][28] now of Stanford University, has conducted a number of significant studies employing the technique of direct laboratory observation of mothers and their 4-year-old children during sessions in which the mother was asked to teach each of three simple previously mastered tasks to her child. Her strategies of control, her teaching styles, her language, and her affective behavior were carefully observed during this interaction. As expected, the middle-class children performed at higher levels on a variety of measures than did the lower-class children, all of them Negro in these studies. There were clear associations between maternal control strategies, teaching styles, language, and affective behavior and the child's test performance.

It should come to us as no revelation that the mother is the child's first teacher, but to say this is not to have identified the particular aspects of the mother-child relationship which are significant in the learning process and thereby to have indicated the critical points at which guided intervention can improve her skills. The work of Professor Hess has moved us a significant step in this direction.

Thus far, we have presented evidence that the child arrives at school already different in his mode of function from the middle-class child for whom teaching styles have been designed. What of the effect of the school itself? School administrators are wont to displace the responsibility for his subsequent failure on to the "defects" of the child, whether they assert those defects to be congenital or acquired. Although it is somewhat more fashionable today to lay the blame on the home, the vehemence with which the defect theory is asserted implies the inherent nature and the incorrigibility of the defect.

That the schools have not succeeded in helping the child who arrives at its doors different from the middle-class norm is clear enough from the school achievement studies and dropout rates described earlier. Not only do they not succeed in reducing the achievement gap, but the test data demonstrate an ever-increasing disparity.[12] Can it be that the overcrowded, understaffed, undersupplied, and discipline-oriented schools found in the urban slum may in fact actively contribute to a child's failure? I cannot here review an extensive literature which suggests that this may indeed be the case,[53] but will call attention to several representative studies.

In the Head Start research referred to earlier,[21] Dr. Keith Conners was able to demonstrate that the amount of improvement in a class of children could be correlated with measures of the teacher's cognitive, disciplinary, and affective styles. Unhappily, the characteristics associated with better performance were those incompatible with the rigid authoritarian attitude of urban school teachers suggested by a survey of teachers carried out at the same time. Anecdotal reports and clinical experience suggest that many school teachers expect little and are not surprised when they get little from black children. And yet the importance of expectation has been demonstrated to be a major influence on performance.[60]

In a California study, Professor Rosenthal[61] and his associates administered a pretest to first grade children, a number of whom were chosen at random to be identified to their school teachers as being likely to show great improvement during the school year. Not only did the teachers (in rating these children at the end of the year) describe them in more positive terms but the children themselves performed significantly better on achievement tests at the end of the year. And yet chance alone had dictated the selection of these "bloomers." The investigators did not, as ethical considerations dictated, single out other children as dull or likely to fall behind. But the data from this study, together with a wealth of supporting material from other studies on social expectation, make it clear that depression of scores would have been recorded if such a companion study of likely dullards had been attempted.

I suggest to you that such a "study" has been being carried out for the past 50 years in public education because of our failure to imbue teachers with a concept of cognitive development that emphasizes its dependence upon the positive reinforcement of appropriate experience in the context of a warm and supporting human relationship. I suggest to you that it is not the children who fail but the schools that have failed, and that it is we who have failed because of our lack of involvement in the critical area of teacher education.

The final—and in many ways the most important—factor in this saga of human waste is racism: the attitudes and beliefs that deny full humanity to those who differ from us in color or culture. It is little comfort for Americans to recognize that this is a phenomenon found in Britain as well as the United States, in Nigeria as well as in South Africa, in India as well as in Poland, in Israel as well as in Egypt. The biosocial and psychosocial factors thus far discussed are intertwined with racism. True, they occur even in its absence; witness the deprivation experienced by the poor regardless of ethnicity. But the intolerable burdens are multiplied by the housing ghettos, the employment barriers, the lower pay scales, and the barrage of psychological insult directed against those who are visibly different.[11] [56]

Given the greater biological hazards *and* the cultural differences that militate against attaining economic success, the further assault of a dominant culture that systematically degrades the characteristics that establish one's identity makes the task of growing up whole a particularly difficult one for the black child.[8] If one is to attain a sense of potency—a conviction of one's manliness or womanliness—one must have a belief in the effectiveness of his own efforts as a determinant of personal attainment. But how can a conviction of personal competence be attained when skin color if one is black, automation if one is unskilled, illness if one is denied medical care, false imprisonment if one cannot obtain legal assistance—all issues beyond personal control—destroy the job, the savings, the dreams of the hardest working and the most diligent?[22]

There is one antidote that may serve as a soul-saving measure while the major struggle for human dignity is being fought. And that antidote, not without its own toxicity, is pride in race. We have begun to observe the growing strength in the United States of a movement that asserts that black is beautiful and that African culture is better than Western. United by common beliefs, black communities have begun to assert the rights of local control in policing, business interests, schooling, and urban planning. I count all of this a distinct *psychological* gain for the black and for the white community; whether it will succeed *politically* is still an open question.

When we turn to the public school crisis, we find the movement for local autonomy confronted by the vested interests in job and tenure of the educational establishment, from the most underpaid teacher to the most prestigious school-board member. Mechanisms to enable both local control and job security to survive remain to be invented, but a significant shift in power is inevitable. In essence, the black community confronts us with these incontrovertible facts: integration has not moved forward in meaningful fashion in the 15 years since the Supreme Court decision; black children are not learning effectively in the schools run *for* them by the white establishment; the longer they wait for "goodwill" and "gradualism," the more their children will fall by the academic wayside. Could black-run schools do worse? I do not believe so. Successes have been attained by "street academies" established by militant volunteers. There is, as I see it, good reason to support black power. It accepts the segregated housing patterns and school distributions as unavoidable phenomena of the near future. At least some of the spokesmen for black control anticipate a time when reunion and reintegration will be possible once the blacks have obtained political power as attested by the history of each of the immigrant groups to these shores. Will this prove to be true? It is the more likely to be true the greater the commitment of professionals to its success. It will provide us with a unique opportunity to study the interaction between self-concept and personal development if we make ourselves available to the new schools as contributors to their growth and investigators of the progress of their pupils. For they, no less than we, will want to learn where they succeed and where they fail and what will accelerate their development. Mind you, this will require that we be willing to learn even as we teach, that we abandon the arrogance of our own pretensions as standard bearers, that we become active participants and not merely "neutral" observers.

To close on a historical note, I would recall to you a paper written 35 years ago by Joseph Brenneman,[7] a distinguished pediatrician of his time, who gave his paper the ominous title "The Menace of Psychiatry." He decried the armchair speculations, the absence of empirical data, and the confusing psychological theories that served only to upset parents and alienate pediatricians. In response, James Plant of the Essex County Juvenile Clinic wrote "The Promise of Psychiatry." His concluding paragraph included these statements:

> We are, as a people, going through great changes in the matter of human relationships. Whether you like it or not, the families which are your clientele are finding themselves face to face with new and profound social problems. These matters affect the conduct and health of the patients and serve to make every family part of our clientele, because every family is having to adjust itself to these changes. You cannot escape these problems and their implications to the child's health by deprecating them, nor can you solve or understand them by setting up a beautiful little experimental station where they do not exist.... The promise of psychiatry is the promise that if the pediatrician will address himself to these problems he will face a vista of rare challenge.... Personally, I am sorry if he is only afraid of that challenge.[54]

And now let me jump forward three decades and echo the words of Walter Orr Roberts, president of the American Association for the Advancement of Science:

> Never before has the opportunity been so great. We have the knowledge and the means to achieve a living environment of unprecedented quality. And we can do this not only for one nation but for all who travel with us on this planet. I have no illusions that it will be easy to achieve what we want from our civilization and our moment in history. It will clearly be a long and hazardous job, for scientist and citizen alike, to reach our goal for the human condition. But, as Thornton Wilder said, "every good and excellent thing stands moment by moment at the razor edge of danger, and must be fought for." Can we not wage the right kind of fight for the goal of the century twenty enlightenment?[58]

References

1. Bahn, A., C. Chandler, and L. Eisenberg. 1961. Diagnostic and demographic characteristics of patients seen in outpatient psychiatric clinics for an entire state. Amer. J. Psychiat. 117:769–777.
2. Baratz, J. 1968. Linguistic and cultural factors in teaching reading to ghetto children. Center for Applied Linguistics, Washington. Mimeo.
3. Bell, J. 1961. Family Group Therapy. Pub. Hlth. Mono. No. 64.
4. Bell, N., and E. Vogel (eds). 1960. The Family. Free Press, Glencoe, Ill.
5. Bernstein, B. 1961. Social class and linguistic development. *In* Economy, Education and Society, A. Halsey, ed. Free Press, Glencoe, Ill.: 288–314.
6. Bradley, C. 1937. Behavior of children receiving amphetamine. Amer. J. Psychiat. 94: 577–585.
7. Brenneman, J. 1931. The menace of psychiatry. Amer. J. Dis. Child, 42:376–402.
8. Brown, C. 1965. Man-Child in the Promised Land. Macmillan, New York.
9. Chow, B., Q. Blackwell, and R. Sherwin. 1968. Nutrition and development. Borden Rev. Nutritional Res. 29: 25–39.
10. Chow, B., et al. 1968. Maternal nutrition and metabolism of the offspring: studies in rats and man. Amer. J. Publ. Hlth. 58: 668–677.
11. Clark, K.: Dark Ghetto: Dilemmas of Social Power. 1965. Harper and Row, New York.
12. Coleman, J. 1966. Equality of Educational Opportunity. U.S. Dept. of Health, Education and Welfare, Washington.
13. Cravioto, J., and B. Robles. 1965. Evolution of adaptive and motor behavior during rehabilitation from Kwashiorkor. Amer. J. Orthopsychiat. 35: 449.
14. Cravioto, J., E. Delicarde, and H. Birch. 1966. Nutrition, growth, and neurointegrative development. Pediat. 38: 319–372.
15. Dubos, R., D. Savage, and R. Schaedler. 1966. Biological Freudianism: lasting effects of early environmental influences. Pediat. 38: 789–800.
16. Eisenberg, L. 1962. Preventive psychiatry. Ann. Rev. Med. 13: 343–360.
17. Eisenberg, L., and E. Gruenberg. 1961. The current status of secondary prevention in child psychiatry. Amer. J. Orthopsychiat. 31: 355–367.
18. Eisenberg, L., C. Conners, and L. Sharpe. 1965. A controlled study of the differential application of outpatient psychiatric treatment for children. Jap. J. Child Psychiat. 6: 125–132.
19. Eisenberg, L. 1968. The need for evaluation. Amer. J. Psychiat. 124: 1700–1701.
20. Eisenberg, L. 1967. Clinical considerations in the psychiatric evaluation of intelligence. *In* The Psychopathology of Mental Development, J. Zubin and G. Jervis, eds. Grune & Stratton, New York.
21. Eisenberg, L., and C. Conners. 1966. Final report OEO Contract 510. Mimeo.
22. Eisenberg, L. 1968. Racism, the family and society: a crisis in values. Ment. Hyg.
23. Eysenck, H. 1960. Behavior Therapy and The Neuroses. Pergamon Press, London.
24. Freedman, A. 1966. The great training robbery??? Amer. J. Orthopsychiat. 36: 590.
25. Gordon, E. 1965. A review of programs of compensatory education. Amer. J. Orthopsychiat. 35: 640–651.
26. Harrington, M. 1962. The Other America: Poverty in the United States. Macmillan, New York.
27. Hess, R., and R. Bear, (eds). 1968. Early Education. Aldine, Chicago.
28. Hess, R. 1968. Maternal behavior and the development of reading behavior in urban Negro children. Center for Applied Linguistics, Washington. Mimeo.
29. Homburger, A. 1926. Vorlesungen Uber Die Psychopathologie des Kindesalters. Springer, Berlin.
30. Hunger and Malnutrition in America. 1967. Hearings before the Subcommittee on Employment, Manpower, and Poverty of the Committee on Labor and Public Welfare. U.S. Senate, 90th Congress, July 11 and 12, 1967. U.S. Govt. Printing Office, Washington.
31. Hunt, J. 1961. Intelligence and Experience. Ronald Press, New York.

32. John, V. 1963. The intellectual development of slum children. Amer. J. Orthopsychiat. 33: 813–822.
33. Kanner, L. 1957. Child Psychiatry. Charles C. Thomas, Springfield, Ill. 3rd Edit.: 1–32.
34. Kanner, L. 1959. The thirty-third Maudsley lecture: trends in child psychiatry. J. Ment. Sci. 105: 581–593.
35. Kanner, L. 1964. A History of the Care and Treatment of the Mentally Retarded. Charles C. Thomas, Springfield, Ill.
36. Kanner, L. 1935. Child Psychiatry, First Edit. Charles C. Thomas, Springfield, Ill.
37. Kanner, L. 1943. Autistic disturbances of affective contact. Nerv. Child. 2: 217–250.
38. Keller, S. 1963. The social world of the urban slum child: some early findings. Amer. J. Orthopsychiat. 33: 823–831.
39. Knobloch, H., and B. Pasamanick. 1966. Prospective studies on the epidemiology of reproductive casualty: Methods, findings, and some implication. Merrill-Palmer Quart. Behav. and Devel. 12: 27–43.
40. Lapouse, R., and M. Monk. 1958. An epidemiological study of behavior characteristics of children. Amer. J. Publ. Hlth. 48: 1134–1144.
41. Levitt, E. 1957. The results of psychotherapy with children. J. Consult. Psychol. 21: 189–196.
42. Levitt, E. 1958. A comparative judgemental study of "defection" from treatment at a child guidance clinic. J. Clin. Psychol. 14: 329–432.
43. Levitt, E. 1959. A followup evaluation of cases treated at a community child guidance clinic. Amer. J. Orthopsychiat. 29: 337–349.
44. Levy, D. 1968. Beginnings of the child guidance movement. Amer. J. Orthopsychiat. 38: 799–804.
45. Modiano, N. 1968. National or mother language in beginning reading: A comparative study. Center for Applied Linguistics, Washington. Mimeo.
46. Monckeburg, F. 1968. Presentation to the second Western Hemisphere Nutrition Congress, San Juan.
47. North, H. 1968. Research issues in health and nutrition in early childhood. OEO Project Head Start, Washington. Mimeo.
48. Oleinick, M., A. Bahn, L. Eisenberg, and A. Lilienfield. 1966. Early socialization experiences and intrafamilial environment. Arch. Gen. Psychiat. 15: 344–353.
49. O'Neal, P., and L. Robins. 1958. The relation of childhood behavior problems to adult psychiatric status. Amer. J. Psychiat. 114: 961–969.
50. Osler, S., and E. Scholnick. 1968. Effects of stimulus differentiation and inferential experience on concept attainment in disadvantaged children. J. Exp. Child. Psychol.
51. Osler, S. Transfer of training effects in disadvantaged and middle-class children. In preparation.
52. Pasamanick, B., and H. Knobloch. 1966. Retrospective studies on the epidemiology of reproductive casualty: old and new. Merrill-Palmer Quart. Behav. and Dev. 12: 7–26.
53. Passow, A. (ed.). 1963. Education in Depressed Areas. Columbia Univ. Press, New York.
54. Plant, J. 1932. The promise of psychiatry. Amer. J. Dis. Child, 44: 1308–1320.
55. Powers, E., and H. Witmer. 1951. An Experiment in the Prevention of Delinquency. Columbia Univ. Press, New York.
56. Report of the National Advisory Commission on Civil Disorders. 1968. Bantam Books, New York.
57. Richmond, J. 1968. Future projections for orthopsychiatry. Amer. J. Orthopsychiat. 38: 809–813.
58. Roberts, W. 1968. Letter from the president. AAAS Bull., Sept. 1968.
59. Robins, L. 1966. Deviant Children Grown Up. William and Wilkins, Baltimore.
60. Rosenthal, R., and L. Jacobson. 1968. Pygmalion in the Classroom. Holt, Rinehart and Winston, New York.
61. Rosenthal, R. 1966. Experimenter Effects in Behavioral Research. Appleton-Century-Crofts, New York.

62. Rutter, M., and P. Graham. 1966. Psychiatric disorder in ten- and eleven-year-old children. Proc. Roy. Soc. Med. 59: 382–387.
63. Rutter, M. 1966. Children of Sick Parents. Oxford Univ. Press, London.
64. St. John, N. 1968. Minority group performance under various conditions of school ethnic and economic integration. IRCD Bull. 4(1).
65. Shakow, D. 1968. The development of orthopsychiatry. Amer. J. Orthopsychiat. 38: 804–809.
66. Shuy, R. 1968. Some consideration in developing beginning reading materials for ghetto children. Center for Applied Linguistics, Washington. Mimeo.
67. Silverman, J. 1968. As reported in Frontiers of Hospital Psychiatry 5(14).
68. Solnit, A. 1966. Who deserves child psychiatry? J. Amer. Acad. Child Psychiat. 5: 1–16. L. Eisenberg. Discussion. Ibid. 17–23.
69. Stewart, W. 1968. Continuity and change in American Negro dialects. Center for Applied Linguistics, Washington. Mimeo.
70. Thomas, A., S. Chess, and H. Birch. 1968. Temperament and Behavior Disorders in Children. New York Univ. Press. New York.
71. Tuckman, J., and M. Lavell. 1959. Attrition in psychiatric clinics for children. Publ. Hlth. Rep. 74: 309–315.
72. Werner, E., et al. 1968. Reproductive and environmental casualties: A report on the ten-year followup of the children of the Kauai pregnancy study. Pediat. 42: 112–127.
73. Wiener, G., et al. 1965. Correlates of low birth weight: psychological status at six to seven years of age. J. Pediat. 35: 434–444.
74. Wiener, G., et al. 1968. Correlates of low birth weight: psychological status at eight to ten years of age. Pediat. Res. 2: 110–118.
75. Winick, M. 1968. Nutrition and cell growth. Nutr. Res. 26: 195–197.
76. Wortis, H., and A. Freedman. 1968. The contribution of social environment to the development of premature children. Amer. J. Orthopsychiat. 35: 57–68.

3. Models, Myths, and Manpower

George W. Albee

Let me begin by citing some of the more prevalent myths that affect our whole approach to mental disorder and that ultimately, if we continue to believe them, will be disastrous for the "mental health movement."

The first, and most pervasive, myth is that people who exhibit disturbed and disturbing behavior are *sick*. From this fundamental conceptual error everything else that follows is a castle built on sand. I have discussed at length elsewhere[1] this basic defect in our conceptual model, so I will not belabor the point here. Let me simply say that this argument did not originate with me, and that it cannot be dismissed as a reflection of an interprofes-

From *Mental Hygiene*, 1968, **52**, 168–180. Copyright 1968 by the National Association for Mental Health. Reproduced by permission.

sional dispute. The most thoughtful psychiatrists today are saying the same thing.

There are many signs that the overextension of the sickness concept is beginning to bother medical people. In an editorial in *Mental Hygiene*[2] there was considerable soul-searching about the appropriateness of calling every deviate "sick." The editorial states:

> We who labor in the field of mental hygiene have much to do. Can we take on all the troubles of the world and offer our special help and protection to all who deviate from the standard? One sees two dangers in this generosity: first, the increasing dilution of our efforts to the point where we try to do so much for so many that we do so little for everybody, and, second, the danger of creating a model of conformity, so that we place little labels on all who fail to conform. And that label will read—you know what—"sick, sick, sick."

The editorial also asks whether the whole field of deviation belongs to psychiatry or only clinically recognizable forms of "sickness." "Is an unhappily married couple sick? . . . . Is it sickness that drives a person to alcohol or narcotics? Or sickness that drives an addict to crime to get the money to buy the solacing balm that he so sorely needs? Is truancy at school or work a kind of sickness?"

Obviously, the answer to these questions is, "No."

Periodically the National Institute of Mental Health (NIMH) issues a statement to the effect that "mental illness" is the third most serious health problem facing the nation (after heart disease and cancer), and often the NIMH shares the further intelligence that alcoholism is our fourth largest health problem.

These statements are used to impress Congress, and the American people, with the need for more research funds to find the mysterious cause of these "diseases" and for more training funds for medical and paramedical personnel. Psychiatrist Don D. Jackson,[3] thoroughly disenchanted with this approach, says, "We must not allow the public to think of mental disorders as they do heart disease or cancer, or some day they will turn on us with the righteous anger of those who have been misled."

Jackson also puzzles over the fact that

> Each year data are collected that provide strong evidence for the fact that mental disorders, including schizophrenia, arise out of personal relationships. Each year we seem to rediscover this fact, splicing out the rest of the year with dreams of glory about the *biochemical* cause of schizophrenia, and new happy pills.

Robert Coles,[4] an articulate, literate psychiatrist at Harvard who has done brilliant work both with students and with the poor, argues that we already know much, if not most, of what there is to know about psychodynamics and the causes of mental disorder. He says: "As for what can legitimately be called psychiatric disorders, I am not at all convinced that anything 'new' will be discovered to 'cure' them. I am not even sure that we ought to call them 'disorders' or 'diseases.' In this case, the language we use becomes misleading."

Psychiatrist Coles goes on to say:

> One can expect a variety of metabolic disorders and their psychiatric manifesta-
> tions to disappear as scientists catch up with errant genes and flawed glands.
> But what pills will ever dissolve the anxiety and fear that go with life itself? What
> will psychiatry ever know that it does not know now about the damage done
> by thoughtless, cruel parents to vulnerable children? What further "frontiers"
> do we really have to conquer, when it comes to such subjects as despair, brutality,
> envy?

The second of the persistent myths suggests that the manpower picture
is improving in the professional fields concerned with the care of the mentally
disordered. This myth suggests that there will soon be enough mental health
care for everyone.

According to the manpower projections of the NIMH, our nation is to
see an annual increment of more than a thousand psychiatrists beginning
this year, and this increment is to increase to something like 1,300 new
psychiatrists a year by 1972. With only 7,500 new physicians graduating from
our medical schools each year, and with the competition of all the other
medical specialties for residents, who are in short supply, I simply cannot
see how these projections are accurate.

During the first half of the present decade, the annual growth of the American Psychiatric Association membership was only slightly more than five
hundred persons, despite a very hard-sell campaign to increase the number
of psychiatrists in the country. In short, I believe that there is considerable
evidence to suggest that our nation is falling *behind* each year in the production of the number of psychiatrists required to maintain our present ratio
of psychiatrists to population. Everyone agrees that we are shorter and
shorter of physicians. It is hard to understand how we can be gaining ground
in psychiatry when the prerequisite to psychiatric residency training is medical training.

The official figures of the NIMH claim a remarkable increase in the number
of psychiatrists and other mental health professionals during the current
decade. It is very hard to understand how this increase came about when
the number of physicians trained in this country is at least 3,500 a year
below the number required for us to stay even, but NIMH publishes figures
that prove its point. I can supply detailed facts and figures that indicate
exactly the opposite conclusion. I believe we are not even holding our own
in producing professionals. Further, even if we were to double our production, there could be no significant increase in services available to the poor,
where the real need is, because our professionals will not work in tax-
supported agencies serving the poor!

Nor would there be any improvement in care outside the suburban-
university axis, where all the care is now delivered—none, for example, in
rural areas, where care is practically non-existent.

Perhaps it is irreverent of me to ask where this large number of new
psychiatrists is finding employment. Clearly it is not in the state hospitals.

A recent survey revealed that in well over one-third of all the state hospitals in this country there was only one to four psychiatrists. This means that in well over a third of all state hospitals very little, if any, psychiatric attention is available to the inmates.

I also find it difficult to know how we will staff the 2,000 comprehensive community mental health centers scheduled to be built by 1980. At the present time there are nearly two thousand psychiatric clinics scattered throughout the United States. Another recent survey reveals that *two-thirds* of these clinics do not have a *single* full-time psychiatrist on their staffs. If we cannot staff community clinics with even one solitary full-time psychiatrist, how are we going to staff 2,000 comprehensive centers? Yet the NIMH has estimated that at least seventeen professional people will be required to staff each center.

In talking about staffing the new centers, Dr. Stanley Yolles[5] says: "As a general pattern, it appears that the median for psychiatrists is 2; for psychologists, 2.8; for social workers, 4.3; and for nurses, 7.8. The greater number of nurses is, of course, a reflection of 24-hour staffing needs in the inpatient services."

Yolles sounds the persistent theme that is being played by the National Institute of Mental Health:

> The growth of manpower training in the four core professions is heartening, even though the 1960 baseline was so low that the increases have not as yet been sufficient to close the gap between supply and need. All indications point to a continued manpower shortage if the existing rate of training of professional personnel does not increase. Even so, the 1965 statistics represent an increase of 44% over the 1960 total for psychiatrists, psychologists, social workers and nurses. This growth rate is quite spectacular when compared to a 19% increase over the same five-year period in the five major health professions of medicine, dentistry, nursing, environmental health and health research.

Statistics can be made to perform all sorts of tricks if properly, or improperly, used. To add together psychiatrists, nurses, social workers, and others, and then to calculate the per cent increase in this heterogeneous bag, tells us very little about where we are going in mental health man-power.

More than half of all the psychiatrists in the country are located in the five states New York, California, Pennsylvania, Massachusetts, and Illinois. The rural states have relatively few; and, although these states represent 35 per cent of the population, they claim only 13 per cent of the psychiatrists. What good is it to try to double our professional number if everyone flocks to the favored states and to a private practice in suburbia?

Seeing a double standard of health care is not the result of a jaundiced view. As responsible an observer as Dr. William H. Stewart,[6] Surgeon General of the United States Public Health Service, says, "The armed forces suffer, as does the Nation as a whole, from . . . a two-class system of health care—excellence for some of our people and mediocrity or nothing for the rest."

Professor Henry Weihofen,[7] of the University of New Mexico School of

Law, scores the double standard of care even in our *public* clinics, which, though claiming to be non-discriminatory, manage to give preferential treatment to the middle class over the lower class. He writes:

> Because psychiatrists understandably prefer "good" patients—those who are sensitive and sophisticated with social and intellectual standards similar to their own—the poor who become patients frequently get inferior treatment, even in the public clinics that purport not to make distinctions between paying and non-paying patients. A recent survey revealed that even a public clinic excluding those able to pay for private psychiatric care still distinguished its patients by social class. Not only were patients from upper social classes accepted for treatment more often, but their treatment was more apt to be given by a senior or more experienced member of the staff.

Professor Weihofen believes that it is the poor who really need treatment, and they need it close to their homes. (Originally this was the purpose of the comprehensive centers, but this notion has dropped out of the picture lately.) He suggests that "perhaps the answer . . . is a neighborhood service center staffed by non-professionals, perhaps people from the low-income neighborhoods themselves . . ." And he adds:

> These suggestions do not, of course, bring a solution to what is inescapably the essential problem—psychiatrists' lack of interest in dealing with the lower socioeconomic classes. That solution would seem to lie in immediate and intensive self-examination about the purpose of psychiatry. Is not the ultimate aim to alleviate misery and suffering in men of all classes?

We are largely neglecting the poor, the children, the aged, the disadvantaged; yet these groups have the most pervasive problems—especially children and adolescents.

Although there are nearly two thousand outpatient psychiatric clinics in the United States, the majority of these are in large urban areas. A recent report identified only 56 clinics in rural areas, and only 50 of these served children. This means that only 3 per cent of all our clinics are in those rural areas in which one-third of all people under 18 years of age live. There are six of these rural clinics located in the 17 southern states, where the rural population of people under 18 years is approximately seven and a half million.

I agree with Erik Erikson's indictment that the most deadly of all possible sins is "the mutilation of a child's spirit." Our society is guilty of doing terrible things to children. For the past three years I have been a consultant to a juvenile court. No hand has the skill to write, nor any tongue the words to tell, of the mindless cruelty, the stifling hopelessness, the infinite emptiness, and the callous indifference suffered by innocent children in this fair land.

Leonard Ganser,[8] Director of Mental Hygiene for Wisconsin, provides some startling figures on the number of persons receiving public assistance who are also suffering from mental disorders. He reports that under Title 4 of the Social Security Act (Aid to Families with Dependent Children) are

223,472 cases in which father, mother, or child is suffering from a mental condition. Practically none of these are being treated. Approximately 6,300 persons under Title 10 (Aid for the Blind) are suffering also from mental conditions. And 137,448 permanently and totally disabled persons (Title 14) are receiving federal assistance. Combining these three groups gives a total of 367,243 persons receiving public assistance and therefore "medically indigent" and eligible for outpatient care under Title 19 of Medicare.

But the problem does not even stop here. According to Ganser, studies in several states have shown that, for every medically indigent person receiving public assistance, there is another one in the community who should be, but isn't. In other words, the ratio is one to one, which means that there are well over 700,000 poor persons with a mental disorder for whom no one is concerned.

Poor people have always had a higher rate of emotional disturbance because of the stresses they must face in their daily lives. They have a greater need for intervention or for good institutional care because it is especially difficult to take care of a disturbed person in overcrowded and inadequate housing. And feeding an unemployed, unproductive relative is an excessive financial burden for many families.

Although it is true that half of all first admissions for mental disorder are to general hospitals, an unbelievable 95 per cent of disturbed people hospitalized on any given day are in "prolonged care hospitals," a polite term for human warehouses.

Meanwhile, we are told that we are catching up, and that unspecified new "group approaches" are going to solve our problems.

Every press release and public statement about developments in psychiatric methods emphasizes the importance of "new techniques" that are bringing new hope to the "troubled and diseased minds" of mental patients. Uniformly, among the methods cited are group therapy and related techniques, such as family therapy. Unhappily, the facts do not fit the publicity. A recent survey done by Margaret Conwell,[9] of the U.S. Public Health Service, found that 80 per cent of all "mental" patients treated are seen in psychiatrists' offices. Young people under 25 and older persons over 65 are not frequently seen. A psychiatrist's patient is most likely to be white, upper-middle-class, female, and neurotic (confirming Ryan's[10] Boston survey results). Fewer than 4 per cent of the psychiatric patients were in group or family therapy. The very large majority were being seen in individual psychotherapy.

Practically everyone now agrees that individual psychotherapy is *not* the answer to the nation's needs for intervention with disturbed citizens. The American Psychiatric Association published a "white paper" on manpower in March 1966,[11] with the approval of its Council. This paper says:

> It is inherent in bringing psychiatric services to all citizens who need them that prolonged individual psychotherapy is quite impracticable on a wide scale. Short intensive treatment techniques, utilizing pharmacotherapy, supportive counseling, group and family therapy, in general hospitals, private hospitals, by private practitioners, and in outpatient settings are the order of the new day.

This, though an honest statement of psychiatric chauvinism, hardly seems a conceptual breakthrough. Psychiatry is always at a loss when it tries to dream up some alternative to the traditional one-to-one method. It always refers vaguely to group techniques and family therapy, then trails off into generalizations such as "and other innovative practices."

We hear a great deal about the "psychiatric revolution" and about emerging new patterns of patient care. Yolles,[5] in a discussion of 173 community mental health centers already functioning, makes the bold new approach sound more like the timid old approach. He says, "New outpatient services will be established by 45 per cent of the current centers, and an additional 40 per cent plan to improve and expand existing therapeutic approaches used in outpatient techniques—including individual and group psychotherapy, family therapy and chemotherapy." What is new about these?

Another widely shared illusion has it that our nation is about to undertake to train a large number of semiprofessional, or middle-level, mental health workers who will soon move into the mental hospitals and mental health centers to be the numerous ancillary people needed to do middle-level-skill jobs.

There are at least two significant reasons why this will not happen. The first of these is that all first-class mental health training facilities are already swamped with applicants for advanced training in the core disciplines; and, because status accrues to those programs that train the highest-level professional people, first-class centers will resist any training demands that cut into their commitments to the core disciplines. Secondly, it will be very difficult to recruit lower-order semiprofessionals into careers in hospital settings. The status hierarchy, or pecking order, in the hospital is well defined, and bachelor's-level workers are far down the list. A school teacher is accorded high status when employed in a school, but a school teacher employed in a hospital may not even rate a key to the staff lavatory.

Another myth has it that, although there may never be enough psychiatrists to go around, psychiatry is extending its influence far beyond its actual number by treating the "gatekeepers of the society." This myth argues that psychiatric time is being spent with leaders and opinion-molders who, as a consequence of deepened and broadened self-knowledge, will spread positive influence by being more effective leaders and teachers. This ripple effect, it is alleged, makes psychiatric time go a long way beyond the consulting room.

The truth of the matter is that the most common psychiatric patient is an upper-middle-class, white, non-Catholic female between the ages of 30 and 40. She is college educated, and she is often in one of the professions. She is usually nervous because she is not married, or nervous because she is. She is hardly a gatekeeper, in the usual sense.

Still another common misconception involves the belief that the new comprehensive community mental health centers are going to be available to all citizens regardless of economic level, race, creed, or age, and irrespective of their social origin. Walter Barton,[12] in his introduction to the volume *The Community Mental Health Center*, says, "This program should provide treatment for all persons of all ages, and for all types of psychiatric illness. It should be broad enough in concept to meet the requirements of the individual patient at the various stages of his illness." Dr. Barton makes it clear that he is not talking about the privileged few, but about everyone. He says that this "program . . . provides total mental health services to meet the total needs of the community."

The reality is very different. When the regulations finally were written, they were very carefully structured to permit general hospitals with psychiatric wards to qualify for construction funds for centers if the hospital agreed to allocate as few as 10 per cent of the beds to indigent people. I want to be certain that this is clear to you. Some 70 per cent of the mental health center construction plans approved so far are for centers to be located in general hospitals. These hospitals are required to use no more than 10 per cent of the new beds, built with federal matching funds, for the poor. This means that the hospital may use 90 per cent of the new beds for middle-class mental patients who have hospitalization insurance. These people can be admitted, of course, only by one of the private psychiatrists who control these beds by virtue of being on the staff of the hospital. Obviously, the people admitted to these beds also must have funds to pay for their private medical care.

These considerations will limit sharply the number of poor people served as inpatients. The counter argument advanced in response to irreverent observations such as these is that the comprehensive centers consist of more than just beds, and that the indigent poor may participate in all the other programs represented in the comprehensive center concept. But general hospitals are not renowned for their free clinical programs for the mentally disordered poor. Little such help will be available.

This leads us to the *next* misconception—that the comprehensive centers will be beehives of activity, with all sorts of programs for all sorts of people. We are subjected to an idealized view that there will be ongoing programs for children, for alcoholics, for the aged, for discharged state hospital patients, for multiproblem families, for teenagers, for delinquents, and so on.

Reality is, again, quite different. In order to qualify for construction funds under the law, it is necessary only to have inpatient and outpatient services, partial hospitalization including day care, emergency hospitalization, and consultation services to community agencies. Reading these requirements carefully makes it clear that a center can be funded in any general hospital that owns a psychiatric ward with practically no change in the ongoing routine save the creation of some sort of day-care center. All of the other important services are "desirable components," but are not required for funding.

When the Joint Information Service of the APA and NAMH three years ago polled state mental health directors, executive directors of state Mental Health Associations, presidents of local Psychiatric Association branches, and anyone else who might know, they found only 234 facilities in the whole country that offered inpatient and outpatient service and at least *one* of the other three essential elements. They finally chose 11 centers that best represented the comprehensive mental health center concept.[12] It is instructive to read the results of their study of these outstanding 11 centers.

They found individual psychotherapy was the most usual method of treatment. They found services for children practically non-existent. They found that practically all of the centers avoid the problems of alcoholism, mental retardation, the disorders of old age, and other chronic difficulties. Few did anything in vocational rehabilitation. Only one of the 11 "outstanding" centers had a separate division concerned specifically with community consultation. Even these *best* centers had serious staffing problems; they found it almost impossible to recruit enough professional personnel on a full-time basis. Most of the centers were not engaged in research, even on the effectiveness of their own programs.

Now these comprehensive centers are supposedly going to replace, or make obsolete, many of the worst components of the state hospital system!

There is a growing double standard of care for mental disorder in our society, and the inequity is growing year by year. Poor people are the ones who suffer most. A bed in a general-hospital psychiatric unit costs, on the average, $50 per day. In general, staffing is good and care is intensive in the general hospital. Psychiatric fees are, of course, over and above the cost of the room. But, because middle-class and upper-class people today are almost universally covered by hospitalization insurance, the mentally disordered person from these favored groups goes to the general hospital. He stays a short time and gets intensive treatment and then goes home with a supply of drugs.

The poor, on the other hand, who do not have hospitalization insurance, must be sent to the public, state hospital. A recent statement by the American Psychological Association describes state mental hospitals as "lower class horrors." In most states the horrors are far more horrible than you can imagine. But the poor will not be treated in the centers in general hospitals, and the state hospitals will get worse.

Dr. David Vail,[13] who is Medical Services Director for the State of Minnesota, has been a sharp critic of the new centers. He summarizes his position:

> A basic problem is that the Comprehensive Centers drive developed out of the admitted failure of state mental hospitals and state mental health programs generally to solve the problems before them. But can one best bring about change in an institution by setting up another institutional system?

Indeed, concern about the appropriateness of the comprehensive community mental health centers model has been expressed by some of the most responsible and thoughtful leaders in American psychiatry. Dr. Lawrence S. Kubie says:[14]

> I see red because the public is being deceived into thinking the millennium has arrived ... The public has been oversold on what it can be provided with in services.
> If the planners can't deliver what is promised, the people will feel sold down

the river. The mental health movement will suffer a setback and there will be a hopeless reversion to the custody of mental institutions, the very thing we seek to avoid.

There is nothing in community psychiatry that hasn't been a part of all psychiatric service for years. There is nothing new here but a catch phrase and government money. I have no objection to government money but I do have an objection to selling the market short.

In the *Community Mental Health Journal*,[15] there was a report of a survey of psychiatrists in New York State on whether they would be willing to spend time working in a comprehensive mental health center. The findings were quite clear. Psychiatrists employed in state hospitals were quite eager to consider full-time positions in mental health centers. Psychiatrists in private practice were unwilling to consider full-time positions, but were willing to give "a few hours a week."

The centers are going to deplete further the small professional staffs in the state hospitals to the extent that they hire any permanent psychiatric personnel. More likely, the centers will provide one more source of occasional consultation for the busy private practitioner.

When all is said and done, the whole problem boils down to certain basic essentials. If we build comprehensive community mental health centers where psychiatrists will work—in the general hospitals—these centers will not treat the poor. And if we build the centers for the poor, in tax-supported neighborhood centers, psychiatrists will not work in them. We can have centers serving the middle class *with* psychiatric care or we can have centers serving the lower class *without* psychiatrists. Centers serving the poor must be tax supported because the poor cannot pay for care themselves and do not have hospitalization insurance.

The comprehensive centers will fail for the same reasons that the state hospitals are a failure. Because American medicine believes that medical care must be paid for by the user, with as little outside interference or mediation between doctor and patient as possible, the system shuts out the poor; but it is the poor who have the most urgent need.

This double standard of care for mental disorders is nothing new. More than a hundred years ago, in the State of Massachusetts, more than half of the "native insane" were cared for in private retreats, whereas more than 90 per cent of the "foreign insane" were sent to poorly supported public institutions for "treatment." *Foreign Insane Pauperism* became a common diagnosis right after the beginning of the waves of European immigration. Kennard[16] ascribes the change in approach and effectiveness as follows:

> Accompanying this shift in attitude, an increase in size of the institution, and the abandoning of the practices of the era of moral treatment was a greater emphasis on organic factors and etiology. The Worcester State Hospital which had recovery rates of 50% in the 1830's showed only 5% in 1880. It was in this era that the patterns of segregation, control and custody, became dominant in the mental hospital.

Today, a hundred years later, Ryan's[10] Boston mental health care survey found that persons being admitted to the *public* mental hospitals were people who were poor, older, and isolated from any meaningful social group. Residentially they came from those sections of the city "blighted by poverty, family disorganization, slums and racial segregation . . ."

Let me discuss for a moment some of our current illusions about state mental hospitals.

One of these is the persistent myth that most of the inmates are psychotic. If we look at the cold, statistical facts, accumulated by the Office of Biometry of the NIMH,[17] we find some remarkable details that contradict prevalent notions about the condition of people entering public mental hospitals.

First of all, some 50 per cent of all persons admitted to our state hospitals for the first time are not psychotic at all. They are classified variously as having "personality disturbances" (which is often a polite way of describing the alcoholic), or psychoneurosis, or transient situational personality disturbances, or even as being "without mental disorder." (This mysterious latter group, which numbered something over two thousand persons last year, apparently is hospitalized despite the fact that those so admitted have nothing seriously wrong mentally!)

It was a surprise to me to learn that only 19 per cent of persons first admitted to our public hospitals across the country are diagnosed as schizophrenics. Indeed, only about one-quarter of *all* first admissions, including the schizophrenic group, are called functionally psychotic. In short, only one person in four admitted can be defined as functionally psychotic. Another quarter of those admitted for the first time suffer from chronic brain syndromes, most of them elderly people who certainly do not belong in a state hospital. I repeat: Half the first admissions are not even psychotic!

To pull these data together, let me summarize by saying that perhaps no more than one person in ten admitted to a state hospital for the first time belongs in a protective environment. Elderly senile people, alcoholics, and others lumped together as persons with personality disorders or psychoneurosis, who together constitute nearly three-quarters of all first admissions to mental hospitals, simply don't belong there! The remaining quarter is really the smaller pool from which might be drawn the limited number of persons society must lock up. But what percentage of functionally psychotic people are truly dangerous? If you will agree that not more than half are dangerous, we are down close to 10 per cent of all present first admissions. And, if you agree that many of *these* people would not be dangerous if properly controlled by intensive care programs, we arrive at a point at which we have practically eliminated the need for the state mental hospital for first admissions altogether.

Still another illusion that has wide currency suggests that treatment in the state mental hospitals is getting better. Indeed, this illusion has been around for a long time. More than a hundred years ago Dorothea Dix went around the country assuring the state legislatures that, if only they would build state mental hospitals, most of the insane could be cured if brought to these hospitals during the early stages of their insanity. Later, historians of this period marked this as the beginning of the "cult of curability."

Between 1841 and 1881 Miss Dix traveled up and down the land cajoling and arguing the state legislatures into building insane asylums. She is given credit for the establishment of at least 32 such institutions in this country, and many more in Canada and in Scotland.

It was not long before it became clear that there was no magic cure available inside the walls of the asylum. As early as 1856 a report of the Commission on Lunacy in Massachusetts[18] pointed out that the insane were *not* being cured as rapidly, nor in as great numbers, as the earlier enthusiastic reports had promised. The Commission said: "The public found that it had been deceived, and, naturally enough, conceived a distrust of enterprises that required the aid of support over and above the unadulterated truth. It was seen that many patients did not recover, and that the incurables continued and accumulated."

A great deal has been made, in recent years, of the reversal and downturning that have occurred in the curve representing the total number of people in public mental hospitals. Many state commissioners have made dramatic speeches hailing the medical triumphs that at long last have halted the seemingly inexorable upward movement of the curve; most state hospital systems have fewer residents today than they had five years ago.

Two factors are primarily responsible for this state of affairs, and neither involves a medical triumph.

The first is the fact that there has been a phenomenal expansion in hospitalization insurance in recent years and that most of this insurance, typified by Blue Cross, has provided 30 to 45 days of paid hospitalization for "mental illness." This has meant that many people from the lower middle class upward are taken to a general hospital psychiatric unit, rather than to jail or to the state hospital. The number of first admissions of persons with mental conditions to general hospitals now is approximately the same as to state hospitals.

The second factor responsible for the decrease in public hospital residents is the massive use of chemicals that dull the behavior of persons with psychosis, making them less frightening, less troublesome to care for, and therefore less of a threat to their families. As a consequence, many psychotics are living at home; and, although they often are still psychotic, they are not occupying beds for an uninterrupted lifetime in the state hospital, as was once the case.

However, the readmission rate is high. If the patients forget to take their chemicals, their disturbing behavior emerges and their families hustle them back to the hospital, so that many hospitals speak of "the revolving door," with people coming and going, rather than coming and staying.

Both of these factors have provided a temporary pause in the demand for beds, but the time is approaching when population growth and increased demands for care under present models will require beds that our institutions are not preparing and that will not be available.

According to the *New England Journal of Medicine,*[19] "If mental hospitals are to avoid reaccumulating long-term inpatients the need to provide alternatives to inpatient care is of urgent concern. Unless alternatives are provided promptly and found to be effective such a reaccumulation seems inevitable."

There was a time in the Western world when poverty was a crime. To be a pauper, to be hopelessly in debt, was grounds for imprisonment. Today we read with horror about the thousands of unfortunates who were thrown into debtors' prisons, or transported to the New World as indentured servants, because they were guilty of the crime of poverty. A hundred years from now, men may look back on the harsh and inhuman treatment of the mentally disordered today in the bleak prisons we call state mental hospitals with the same kind of disbelief and horror.

Human beings simply do not have to spend their lives in these places. But they are going to if we persist in believing that they have illnesses that require medical treatment and long-term hospitalization.

For example, a research project of considerable importance has been conducted and reported from the Olympic Mental Center in the State of Washington. There, Hanford and colleagues[20][21] have been able to demonstrate that an unselected full range of people between the ages of 14 and 60 admitted to a state mental hospital could be returned to the community in a very short period of time. The median length of institutionalization for their unselected group was 21 days. Over 75 per cent returned to the community within two and a half months. Altogether, 95 per cent of nearly four hundred patients returned to the community under this program. Despite the brief time in the institution, the readmission rate did not increase; and a follow-up indicated that subsequent time in the institution was significantly reduced.

There is a kind of owl-faced platitude, usually delivered with great pompousness, that says that the social and behavioral sciences lag behind the physical and biological sciences. If only—it is alleged—we could make faster progress in the behavioral sciences, if only we could learn as much about the human being as we know about the atom, then our problems would disappear. Frankly, this is nonsense. We *do* know a great deal in the behavioral sciences, but many of the things we know are threatening to the Establishment and threatening to the status quo. For example, we know very well that the nature of the social world of the infant and the child in the family is of critical importance in determining subsequent rates of emotional disorder. In our culture, the stable family is the best bulwark against emotional disorder; and efforts toward prevention will have to be directed to those social institutions that, directly or indirectly, affect family stability. In the case of hopelessly disrupted families, we must find ways of providing the best possible substitutes for the children affected.

What I'm saying is that we have already made the research breakthroughs. Research has already demonstrated that psychopathology increases as the integrity of the family is damaged or destroyed and that, conversely the amount of psychopathology is low in groups in which the stability and strength of the family are high. Children from strong, well-integrated families have very low lifelong rates of mental disorder, and children from broken or emotionally disrupted families have high subsequent rates. Now this is the heart of my argument; so let me dwell for a few minutes on the *impor-*

tance of the model, the conceptual model, we use to explain causation, because this determines the kind of institutions we develop; and they, in turn, determine the kind of manpower that is required. So long as the disease model prevails as the primary explanation for mental disorders, we are simply going to have too few medical and paramedical professionals attempting to *treat sick* people in hospitals and clinics with minimal effectiveness and appropriateness. When this model is replaced with a better one, we can think about training new kinds of professionals—closer, I think, to school teachers than to either psychologists or psychiatrists—to work with these disturbed people. I see new kinds of institutions—more like schools, residential schools, or residential rehabilitation centers, than like hospitals.

The kind of model we accept determines the kind of institutions we establish, which, in turn, determines the kind of personnel we need. I would predict, unless my crystal ball is hopelessly clouded, that eventually the direct interventionists will be bachelor's-level people working in institutions resembling training schools for children and adults.

To suggest, as I have been doing, that people now in state mental hospitals would be better off in a new kind of institution devoted to rehabilitation, relearning, and re-education is not a new idea at all. Exactly one hundred years ago Pliny Earle,[22] writing in the *American Journal of Insanity*, suggested that the psychopathic hospital should become more like a college. Dr. Earle wrote:

> The hospital, no less than the college, should have its established curriculum; and this should comprehend a course of exercises—hygienic, laborious, disciplinary, amusing, creative, instructive, and devotional. The patients should go from exercise to exercise as students from lecture to lecture. They would then be subjected, during a large part of the day, to restraining, diverting, and hence curative influences, instead of being left to lounge, apathetically, or to wander to and fro in their rooms or halls, subject to the wayward impulses of their disorder. Subdued thus for a while, the patient, as a general rule, would exert his self-control permanently and cease his abnormal demonstrations.
>
> One obstacle to the establishment of such curriculums is public opinion. Drugs and medicines may be forced upon a patient until, so far as recipiency is concerned, he becomes a perfect apothecary's shop, and all is right; but any attempt to force him to the genial, wholesome, and curative exercise of manual labor is an outrage on humanity!

I am convinced that, once society accepts the evidence that most neurotic and functionally psychotic behaviors represent learned patterns of disturbed behavior, the institutions that will be developed to deal with these will be *educational* in nature. It is already widely demonstrated that behavioral modification techniques can prevent or interrupt the desocialization that occurs on the back wards of state hospitals. By using college graduates with some special training in re-educational techniques it would be possible for society to develop new institutional forms requiring manpower that could be rather easily recruited and trained. Although it is difficult to describe institutions not yet conceived, it is possible that they will be combinations of present day-care centers but recast as small, tax-supported, state adult schools with heavy emphasis on occupational therapy, re-education, and rehabilitation. Bandura[23] has a similar vision. He says:

> The day may not be far off when psychological disorders will be treated not in hospitals or mental hygiene clinics but in comprehensive "learning centers", when clients will be considered not patients suffering from hidden psychic pathologies but responsible people who participate actively in developing their own potentialities.

Unless we develop a viable alternative to the illness model as an explanation of mental disorder, and unless we change our care delivery systems, we must face the next several decades with the realistic understanding that the mental health manpower picture is going to worsen because we cannot train enough professionals to meet the manpower needs of the institutions this model demands.

References

1. Albee, G. W.: The Relation of Conceptual Models to Manpower Needs. In: Cowen, E. L., Gardner, E. A., and Zax, M. (eds.): Emergent Approaches to Mental Health Problems. New York, Appleton-Century-Crofts, 1967, pp. 63–73.
2. Davidson, H. A.: *Mental Hygiene*, 51:5 (January), 1967.
3. Jackson, D. D.: Stanford Medical Bulletin, 20:202, 1962.
4. Coles, R.: The Progressive, 31(5):32, 1967.
5. Yolles, S.: Speech to the American Psychiatric Association, May 11, 1967 (mimeographed).
6. Stewart, W. H.: Speech to the Annual Meeting of the Association of Military Surgeons of the U. S., Washington, D.C., November 15, 1965 (mimeographed).
7. Weihofen, H.: Psychiatric News, 2(10):2, 1967.
8. Ganser, L.: Testimony before House Ways and Means Committee, March 13, 1966. Reprinted by the National Association of State Mental Health Program Directors (mimeographed).
9. Conwell, M.: News release from Department of Health, Education, and Welfare on speech to American Psychiatric Association, May 8, 1967 (mimeographed).
10. Ryan, W.: Distress in the City: A Summary Report of the Boston Mental Health Survey (1960–1962). Boston, The Massachusetts Association for Mental Health, The Massachusetts Department of Mental Health, and United Community Services of Metropolitan Boston, 1967.
11. American Psychiatric Association: White Paper Prepared by the Commission on Manpower. Washington, D.C., American Psychiatric Association, 1966.
12. Glasscote, R., *et al.*: The Community Mental Health Center. An Analysis of Existing Models. Washington, D.C., The Joint Information Service of the American Psychiatric Association and the National Association for Mental Health, 1964.
13. Vail, D.: Editorial in Mental Health Newsletter, State of Minnesota, 6:3 (March), 1966.
14. Kubie, L. S.: Quoted in feature story in Baltimore News American, Sunday, March 26, 1967.
15. Brown, A. C.: Community Mental Health Journal, 1:256, 1965.
16. Kennard, E.: Major Patterns of the Mental Hospital—U.S.A. In: Opler, M. (ed.): Culture and Mental Health, New York, Macmillan, 1959.

17. National Institute of Mental Health, Office of Biometry: Public Health Service Publication No. 1452, Part 2. Washington, D.C., U. S. Government Printing Office, 1966.
18. Commission on Lunacy of the State of Massachusetts: Report to Legislature. Reprinted in North American Review, 82:91, 1856.
19. Pugh, T. F.: New England Journal of Medicine, 271:672 (September), 1964.
20. Hanford, D. B.: Bulletin of the Division of Mental Health, Department of Institutions, State of Washington, 11:1, 1967.
21. Hummel, R. T., and Lubach, J. E.: Bulletin of the Division of Mental Health, Department of Institutions, State of Washington, 10:82, 1966.
22. Earle, P.: American Journal of Insanity, October, 1867.
23. Bandura, A.: Scientific American, 216(3):78, 1967.

Chapter Two

Role of the Family in Development of Psychopathology

Almost all theories of personality assign great importance to the influence of family relationships on development of personality. Probably the most significant of these theories is the psychoanalytic theory formulated by Sigmund Freud. According to this theory, the most influential experiences in one's entire life-span are those encountered in the family circle in the first few years of childhood (Freud, 1933). The orthodox Freudian view of psychosexual stages of development, and Erikson's (1963) modifications of this theory, suggest that experiences encountered in relation to infantile feeding, toilet training, and sexuality during the preschool years play a paramount role in determining the kind of personality traits and psychopathological tendencies the individual will show in later life.

Stages of Psychosexual Development

These crucial phases in the first six years of life, each involving some basic problem or crisis to be resolved between parents and child, are known as the oral stage, the anal stage, and the phallic stage of psychosexual development. For example, the phallic or early genital stage is that in which the male child is believed to experience the Oedipus complex and the female child the Electra complex. Essentially, these complexes refer to the fact that the child between the ages of 4 to 6 years is supposed to be sexually attracted to the opposite-sex parent and feel hostility and resentment toward the same-sex parent. In the normal family circle, these conflicts are usually resolved without undue trauma, and from these intra-family encounters the growing child learns how to cope with authority figures. In the view of orthodox Freudians, unsatisfactorily resolved Oedipal and Electra complexes are destined to lead to psychological maladjustment that will be evidenced in many areas of interpersonal relationships in adulthood.

According to these psychoanalytical conceptions, by the time the child reaches school age, much of his basic personality structure has been established for life. Psychoanalytic theory maintains that on entering school the child also enters what is known as the latency stage of psychosexual development. In the original Freudian theory, this particular stage was not considered to have important formative influences. However, Erikson has placed considerable emphasis on the acquisition of the personality characteristics of industry and competence through mastery of problems first encountered during this so-called latency stage.

The final psychosexual period in orthodox Freudian theory is the genital stage, which is usually reached in the early teens and coincides with the attainment of physical sexual maturity. The young adolescent acquires secondary sexual characteristics and is faced with the resolution of adult-type genital conflicts. Erikson sees adolescence as the time when the individual must acquire a sense of identity as opposed to role diffusion. This sense of identity carries with it a mastery of the problems of childhood and a readiness to face the challenges of the adult world.

While orthodox psychoanalytic theory does not concern itself with psychosexual development beyond this point in the life span, in Erikson's modified theory, personality formation continues long past the genital stage and does not cease until death. At any rate, both Freud and Erikson, who are certainly two of the most influential theorists concerned with child development, make it abundantly clear that throughout early and middle childhood, relations between parents and child are of crucial importance in determining the psychological well-being of the child.

More specifically, according to Erikson's theory, in each developmental phase there is a psychosocial crisis to be resolved, and satisfactory outcome of the dilemma is largely determined by parent-child relations. Erikson locates the foundation for all later development in the oral phase. It is in this initial phase of development that the child acquires either a sense of basic trust or a sense of mistrust. Such personality attributes as optimism and confidence are believed to derive from a warm, loving, gratifying relationship between mother and child during this stage. From successful experiences in the second developmental stage, which coincides with Freud's anal stage, according to Erikson the child acquires a sense of autonomy as opposed to feelings of shame and doubt. The third preschool phase in Erikson's model, which coincides with Freud's phallic stage, is that in which the normal child acquires a sense of initiative and overcomes any sense of guilt. As mentioned above, the school-age child is faced with problems that will result in acquiring either a sense of industry or a sense of inferiority that will color much of what he attempts or accomplishes in later life.

Sullivan's Interpersonal Theory

Another personality theorist who stresses the early mother-child relationship is Sullivan (1953). His viewpoint, which is known as the interpersonal theory of psychiatry, maintains that from the very first day of life the child is part of an interpersonal situation; throughout life, whatever is distinctly human is largely determined by social interactions. According to this theory, anxiety is a product of interpersonal relations and is transmitted originally from mother to infant. It is believed that the child is able to empathize with the mother and perceive her feelings even without verbal communication or understanding. From the mother's behavior toward him, the child develops a concept of the "good-me" or the "bad-me" and learns how to perform in order to avoid feelings of anxiety that result from threats to his security. This is believed to be the foundation on which the child acquires the self-concept that is so important in guiding his interpersonal behavior in later life. In other words, interactions between mother and infant lead to feelings of security or anxiety that result in a rudimentary self-perception of being good (and therefore safe from danger) or being bad (and therefore likely to be rejected). Much of this social learning occurs long before the child is able to comprehend intellectually the nature of the events taking place in the world around him. However, the person's view of himself and his ways of interacting with other people at later stages in his life-span will be largely determined by how threatened or secure he felt during these earliest years in his psychosocial development. It would certainly seem from this theoretical position that being buffeted around between institutions, neighbors' or relatives' homes, or foster homes at an early age would undermine any feelings of security and self-worth that might have been established on the basis of a stable and gratifying relationship between mother and child.

Harlow's Studies of Infant Monkeys

While most personality theorists have derived their formulations from observations of human children, Harlow's (1965) contribution is based on his well-known studies of infant monkeys. His program of experimental investigation has demonstrated most convincingly that infant monkeys raised in social isolation, and thus deprived of a normal relationship with a mother-figure during the first months of life, show abnormal postures, bizarre behaviors, and inadequate peer relationships when later placed with other monkeys. It is extremely difficult to overcome the emotional and behavioral deficits in these experimentally produced "neurotic" monkeys, especially if the social isolation and absence of environmental stimulation is instituted at an early age and for a considerable length of time. Moreover, Harlow's longer-range observations have revealed that monkeys who were deprived of a normal mothering relationship in infancy later made very inadequate parents and were extremely rejecting and hostile toward their own offspring.

Effects of Institutionalization

From this brief review of childhood conflicts and the personality traits that result from them long before the child reaches adolescence, it should be obvious that interpersonal relations within the family must be of crucial importance. But what of those unfortunate children whose parents are absent during their formative years? These are the unwanted children, the neglected, abused, emotionally or physically handicapped youngsters who are placed in institutional settings for varying lengths of time. When not institutionalized, they are raised in foster homes and other types of agency-supported settings designed to substitute for the normal family living that through no fault of their own has been denied to them.

Older studies, several of which are now regarded as classics, have suggested that institutionalization at an early age is certain to have negative consequences. Goldfarb (1943a, 1943b, 1945) published several papers reporting that children who were institutionalized early in life fared very poorly when later compared with those who had been reared in normal family settings. These children showed deficits both in intellectual functioning and in personality adjustment.

Spitz (1945, 1946) published several influential but highly controversial reports of what he termed "hospitalism." According to Spitz, studies showed that children suffer greatly when they are deprived of a normal mothering relationship during the first year of life. They showed phenomena termed "anaclitic depression" and "marasmus," which are signs of severe grief reaction and physical illness evidenced by infants who are removed from their mothers for various reasons. If the children were cared for by their own mothers even in institutional settings (for example, in prison), they fared very well. However, if they were placed in impersonal, understaffed orphanages and were cared for by overworked caretakers, they showed the previously mentioned unhealthy and unhappy characteristics. Thus these studies and most other reports of institutionalization at an early age show undesirable, detrimental, and lasting negative effects on the child.

A long-range follow-up study by Skeels (1966) showed differential effects of contrasting types of institutional experiences in childhood. This is a very unusual and valuable investigation, both from the viewpoint of methodology and findings obtained. The study began in the early 1930s and covered a span of 30 years. It involved 25 infants who were wards of the state and were placed in an orphanage in Iowa. Intelligence testing showed them all to be mentally retarded. Due to crowded conditions at the orphanage, 13 of these children were transferred as "house guests" to an institution for the retarded. The children were all under 3 years of age at the time of this transfer. They were placed under the care and companionship of retarded women who showered these youngsters with attention and affection. The remaining 12 children stayed in the orphanage where they received very little stimulation, attention, or love. Over a period of two years, the children in the group transferred to the institution for retarded women showed an average gain of 29 IQ points, whereas the group that remained in the orphanage showed an average loss of 26 IQ points. This is truly a remarkable difference between two groups who only two years before had performed at a very similar retarded level on intelligence tests.

An initial follow-up study conducted three years after termination of the original study found that 11 of the 13 children in the transferred group had been placed in adoptive homes and had maintained their earlier gains in intelligence. The two who were still living in the institution with the retarded women had declined in rate of mental growth. At the time of this follow-up study, all children who had remained in the orphanage were still mentally retarded to a marked degree. In the few children in this group who showed gains in intellectual functioning there had been improved environmental experiences subsequent to the original study.

A unique feature of this investigation is that a longer-range follow-up study, after a lapse of 21 years, located and obtained information on every one of the original group of children. It was found that the two groups had maintained their divergent patterns of competency into adulthood. All 13 children in the transferred group were self-supporting and none was institutionalized. Their educational and occupational achievements compared favorably with the general population. Most of them had married and had children who were perfectly normal from the viewpoint of IQ and school achievement. According to Skeels (1966), "Their adult status was equivalent to what might have been expected of children living with natural parents in homes of comparable sociocultural levels."

Adult follow-up findings from the 12 children who had spent their entire early childhood in the unstimulating environment of the orphanage were much different. One died in adolescence following continued institutionalization and four were still residents in state institutions. While the adopted children had completed a median of the twelfth grade, those in the comparison group had completed a median of less than the third grade. As indicated above, four members of the latter group (36 percent) were still institutionalized and unemployed. Those who were employed, with only one exception, were engaged in menial work with very limited incomes. Only two members of this group had married, with one marriage producing a mentally retarded child and the other resulting in a family of normal children.

Skeels points to the vast amounts of money spent on those patients who remained wards of the state, and postulates that " ... if the children in the contrast group had been placed in suitable adoptive homes or given some other appropriate equivalent in early infancy, most or all of them would have achieved within the normal range of development, as did the experimental subjects [p. 56, 1966]." Taking a strong stand against mere custodial care, Skeels concludes that " ... sufficient knowledge is available to design programs of intervention to counteract the devastating effects of poverty, sociocultural deprivation, and maternal deprivation [p. 56, 1966]"

The Issues

In the first paper in this chapter, Henry B. Biller and I present an integrative review and discussion of literature bearing on the role of parent-child interactions in the development of personality and childhood psychopathology. A large portion of this comprehensive paper is devoted to the importance of the father in child development. The intention here is not to de-emphasize the mother's role, but to call attention to the neglected issue of the effects of father-child relations on personality formation in sons and daughters (Biller, 1971).

While the father has been relatively ignored in much previous writing on child development, there is rather voluminous literature on effects of different kinds of mothering. Excellent reviews of effects of infant care (by Caldwell), separation from parents (by Yarrow), and consequences of parental discipline (by Becker) can be found in Hoffman and Hoffman's (1964) *Review of Child Development Research.*

The next paper in this chapter, by Martin L. Heinstein, is designed to dispel certain myths concerning breast-feeding. Among the many unresolved issues pertaining to mother-child interactions, the matter of breast-feeding seems to have been particularly subject to stereotyped thinking. It is commonly assumed that breast-feeding is a sign of a good mother and that children are certain to benefit psychologically from this early feeding experience. Heinstein, however, shows that this issue is much more complex than has been commonly thought. This paper is included both because of its theoretical and practical significance and to counterbalance the father emphasis in the opening paper.

In the third paper, Richard Q. Bell provides a scholarly review and discussion of another traditionally neglected issue in child psychology—the effects of children on parents. Theorists and investigators have tended to favor a one-way perspective, looking for the effects of parents on personality development of their offspring. Bell, however, stresses that family interactions are multi-directional, with parents' emotional adjustment being influenced by their children's personality and behavior.

Thus, from these three papers, the reader should become aware of: (1) the importance of the father in child development, (2) unsubstantiated myths regarding breast-feeding, and (3) the direction of effects in parent-child relations.

References

Biller, H. B. *Father, child, and sex role.* Lexington, Mass.: Heath, 1971.

Erikson, E. H. *Childhood and society.* (2nd ed.) New York: Norton, 1963.

Freud, S. *New introductory lectures on psychoanalysis.* New York: Norton, 1933.

Goldfarb, W. The effects of early institutional care on adolescent personality. *Journal of Experimental Education,* 1943, **12,** 107–129. (a)

Goldfarb, W. Infant rearing and problem behavior. *American Journal of Orthopsychiatry,* 1943, **13,** 249–266. (b)

Goldfarb, W. Psychological privation in infancy and subsequent adjustment. *American Journal of Orthopsychiatry,* 1945, **15,** 247–255.

Harlow, H., & Harlow, M. K. Learning to love. *American Scientist,* 1965, **54,** 244–272.

Hoffman, M. L., & Hoffman, L. W. (Eds.) *Review of child development research.* Vol. 1. New York: Russell Sage Foundation, 1964.

Skeels, H. M. Adult status of children with contrasting early life experiences: A follow-up study. *Monographs of the Society for Research in Child Development,* 1966, **31** (No. 3, Serial No. 105).

Spitz, R. A. Hospitalism: An inquiry into the genesis of psychiatric conditions in early childhood. *The Psychoanalytic Study of the Child.* Vol. I. New York: International Universities Press, 1945.

Spitz, R. A. Anaclitic depression. *The Psychoanalytic Study of the Child.* Vol. II. New York: International Universities Press, 1946.

Sullivan, H. S. *The interpersonal theory of psychiatry.* New York: Norton, 1953.

4. Parent-Child Relations, Personality Development, and Psychopathology

Henry B. Biller
Anthony Davids

A wealth of data indicates that parents play an important role in the psychological development of their children. Unfortunately, much of the research and theory does not take into account the complexity of family dynamics. In particular, the mother's influence has often been focused on to the exclusion of father-child and father-mother interactions. In addition, there has been a lack of consideration of the differential effects of parent-child relations as a function of sex of parent and sex of child.

We take the position that much of the parents' influence is based on the type of models they represent to their children. In our research and clinical experience, we have found that children's imitation of their parents has very important consequences in their personality development. Our goal is to review relevant research, with particular emphasis on the importance of paternal behavior and father-mother interaction. This article by no means represents an exhaustive coverage of the literature. Our main goal is to acquaint the reader with some important findings and issues. The material in this article draws extensively from parts of previous reviews (Biller, 1970, 1971b; Biller & Weiss, 1970).

The Father-Son Relationship

This section contains an examination of how the quality of the father-son relationship and father-absence may be associated with certain developmental deficits and difficulties. It is speculated that many psychological handicaps can be viewed as being in varying degrees related to sex-role development problems of paternally deprived boys (Biller, 1971a).

Cognitive Functioning

Several investigators have found that father-absent children often suffer from intellectual deficits. Deutsch's (1960) studies are particularly interesting and indicate that the father-absent black child compared to the father-present black child scores significantly lower on intelligence and academic achievement tests. Father-absence often seems to be a significant factor in the complex and debilitating process of cultural deprivation. It is possible to infer from some of the evidence that among lower-class blacks, father-absence is particularly inhibiting for both the interpersonal and cognitive development of the male child (for example, see Bronfenbrenner, 1967; Pettigrew, 1964).

Kimball (1952) examined familial antecedents of variations in scholastic performance of highly intelligent adolescent boys enrolled in a residential preparatory school. She compared the underachieving boys with a group of boys randomly selected from the total school population. In terms of sentence completion test responses, significantly more of the boys in the underachieving group appeared to have negative relationships with their fathers. Davids (1972) has reported similar findings from group psychotherapy conducted with bright adolescent underachievers.

An interesting but rather unsystematic clinical investigation studied elementary school boys who had at least average intelligence, but scored one to two years below expectation on standard achievement tests (Grunebaum, Hurwitz, Prentice, & Sperry, 1962). The fathers of the underachieving boys were reported to feel generally inadequate and to consider themselves failures; they did not seem to offer their sons adequate models of male competence. Most of the fathers viewed their wives as being superior to them and their wives generally shared this perception. There was evidence that the mothers were involved in undermining both their husbands' and sons' feelings of adequacy.

Blanchard and Biller (1971) attempted to assess the effects of different levels of father-availability on the academic functioning of third-grade boys. They explored both the impact of father-absence and the degree of father-son interaction in the father-present home. The boys in the study were of average intelligence and were from working-class and lower-middle-class backgrounds. Subjects were matched (age, IQ, socioeconomic status, presence or absence of male siblings) and categorized as early father-absent (beginning before age three), later father-absent (beginning after age five), low father-present (less than six hours per week), and high father-present (more than two hours per day). Class grades and academic achievement test scores were examined, and it was found that the academic performance of the high father-present group was very superior to the other three groups. The early father-absent boys were clearly underachievers, the late father-absent and low-father-present boys usually functioned slightly below grade level, and the high father-present group performed above grade level.

Boys from high father-present families appear more likely to actualize their intellectual potential than do boys from families in which the father is absent or relatively unavailable. Highly available fathers seem to afford their sons models of perseverance and achievement motivation. The father can provide his child an example of a male functioning successfully outside of the home atmosphere. Frequent opportunity to observe and imitate his father seems to facilitate the development of the child's overall instrumental competence. Having a highly competent father would not seem to facilitate a child's intellectual development if the father is not consistently accessible to the boy or if the father-child relationship is negative in quality (that is, if the father is generally critical and frustrating with his child).

Carlsmith (1964) found that upper-middle-class high school boys who were father-absent in their early childhood (up to and before the age of five) were more likely than boys who were father-present to have a feminine patterning of aptitude test scores. In contrast to the usual male pattern of math score higher than verbal score, father-absent boys were more likely than father-present boys to have a verbal score higher than their math score. The likelihood of feminine patterning appeared to be positively related to the length of father-absence and negatively related to the child's age at the onset of father-absence. Citing evidence from other studies, Carlsmith reasoned that such a score pattern was a reflection of a feminine-global conceptual style.

Although Carlsmith (1964) did not specifically analyze her data to see how the father-absent and father-present males' verbal and mathematical aptitudes compared in absolute terms, it appears that the father-absent group tended to be equal or superior in verbal aptitude to the father-present group, though inferior in mathematical aptitude. Since academic achievement in most fields is so heavily dependent on verbal ability, father-absent middle-class children may not be greatly handicapped. Hilgard, Neuman and Fisk's (1960) findings are suggestive. In an interview study in a university town, they found that some men who had lost their fathers during childhood tended to be highly successful in academic pursuits despite, or possibly because of, a conspicuous over-dependence on their mothers. The middle-class maternally overprotected boys in Levy's (1943) study also did superior work in school, particularly in subjects requiring verbal facility, but their performance in mathematics was not at such a high level, which seems consistent with Carlsmith's (1964) findings.

In homes in which the father is absent or relatively unavailable, the mother seems to assume the primary role in terms of dispensing reinforcements and emphasizing certain values. In fact, one could predict that a father-absent boy who strongly identified with an intellectually oriented mother would be at an advantage in certain facets of school adjustment since he might find the transition from home to the typically feminine-oriented classroom quite comfortable; such father-absent boys might be expected to do particularly well in tasks where verbal skills and conformity are rewarded. (The influence of the mother-child relationship is discussed in more detail in a later section of this paper).

If a relationship does hold between father-absence and certain types of cognitive functioning, it must be remembered that father-absence *per se* is only one of many variables responsible for such a relationship. The values of the mother and the peer group are extremely important. Among children in the lower class, father-absence usually intensifies lack of exposure to certain cognitive experiences. In addition, many boys in their masculine overcompensation perceive intellectual tasks and school in general as "feminine." The school situation, which presents women as authority figures with strong demands for obedience and conformity, is particularly antithetical to such boys' conscious values and desperate attempts to feel masculine. Many of them develop an almost phobic reaction concerning intellectual matters (Biller, 1971a).

Impulsive and Antisocial Behavior

Mischel (1961) reported data relating father-absence and impulse control. He studied preferences for delayed or immediate gratification in 8- and 9-year-old West Indian children. The criterion of father-absence was simply whether the father was living at home. Father-absent children showed a stronger preference for immediate gratification than did father-present children. For instance, they significantly more often chose a small piece of candy for immediate consumption rather than waiting a week for a large candy bar.

Meerloo (1956) postulated that a lack of accurate time perception is common among father-absent children. According to him, " . . . the father symbolizes punctuality and adherence to time schedules . . . [and] he represents social order and social functioning." It is interesting to note that antisocial acts are often impulsive as well as aggressive. Davids (1972) has shown that institutionalized emotionally disturbed boys tend to be present-oriented, impulsive, and unable to delay gratification. Many of those child psychiatric patients diagnosed as "passive-aggressive personality" come from family backgrounds in which the father-son relation has been either absent or characterized by hostility and rejection. The father seems to serve as a representative of social order, and his absence or inadequacy often leads to deficiencies in the child's conscience development (Hoffman, 1971).

Miller (1958) concluded that lower-class boys from female-based homes, in their constant effort to prove their masculinity, are more often involved in antisocial (at least by middle-class standards) acts than are father-present boys. Delinquency can have many different etiologies. What may be postulated is that some cases of delinquency are a result of masculine overcompensation, particularly among father-absent boys. Bacon, Child, and Barry (1963), in a cross-cultural study, found that degree of father-absence as defined by family structure was related to the existence of theft and personal crime in particular societies. Those societies with a predominantly monogamous nuclear family structure tended to be rated low in the amount of theft and personal crime; societies with a polygamous mother-child family structure tended to be rated high in both theft and personal crime. Bacon, Child, and Barry suggested that such antisocial behavior was a reaction against a female-based household and an attempted assertion of masculinity. Overcompensating preadolescent and adolescent boys are important role models in lower-class neighborhoods.

Glueck and Glueck (1950) found that over two-fifths of the adolescent delinquent boys they studied were father-absent as compared with less than one-fourth of a matched non-delinquent group. Siegman (1966) collected medical students' responses to a questionnaire and found that those who had been without a father for at least one year during their first four years of life, compared to those who had been continuously father-present, admitted to a greater degree of antisocial behavior in childhood. Anderson (1968) found that a history of paternal absence was much more frequent among boys committed to a training school. He discovered that among the non-delinquents who had experienced father-absence, there was a much higher rate of father-substitution (such as a stepfather or father-surrogate) between the ages of 4 and 7 than was found for the delinquent group. There are also a large number of psychiatric referrals with the presenting complaint of aggressive acting-out behavior made by mothers of preadolescent and adolescent father-absent boys (MacDonald, 1938; Wylie & Delgado, 1959). Clinical study of such boys often reveals severe sex-role conflicts.

Father-present juvenile delinquents appear to have very poor relationships with fathers. Bach and Bremer (1947) discovered that preadolescent delinquent boys produced significantly fewer father fantasies on projective tests than did a non-delinquent control group. The delinquents portrayed fathers as lacking in affection and empathy. Similarly, Andry (1962) found that delinquents characterized their fathers as glum, uncommunicative, and as employing unreasonable punishment and little praise. Andry's findings are consistent with those of Bandura and Walters (1958), who reported that the relationship between delinquent sons and fathers is marked by rejection, hostility, and antagonism.

On the other hand, some investigators report that boys who have positive relationships with their fathers are likely to engage in constructive and prosocial gang behavior (Crane, 1951; Thrasher, 1927). It is also noteworthy that boys who commit delinquent acts by themselves seem to have more negative relationships with their fathers than do boys who commit delinquent acts with other gang members. Such findings suggest that deficits in fathering may interfere with the formation of the boy's peer relationships.

Interpersonal Relations

A number of studies have revealed that father-absent boys have more difficulty in forming satisfying peer relationships than do father-present boys (for example, Mitchell & Wilson, 1967; Stolz, 1954; Tiller, 1958). Father-absent boys may be less popular with their peers than father-present boys because they more often lack a secure masculine sex-role orientation (Biller, 1968b, 1969b; Biller & Bahm, 1971).

Payne and Mussen (1956) reported that adolescent boys who were similar to their fathers in terms of responses to the California Personality Inventory were rated as significantly more friendly by their teachers than boys who had responses markedly different from their fathers. Evidence from the Mussen, Young, Godding, and Morante (1963) study also indicated that positive father-son relationships were associated with successful peer relationships and self-confidence among adolescent males. Hoffman (1961) reported similar results and discovered that elementary-school-age boys from mother-dominant homes had much more difficulty in their peer relationships than did boys from father-dominant homes. Several investigators have found that masculine development is impeded in mother-dominant homes (for example, see Biller, 1969a; Hetherington, 1965; Moulton, Burnstein, Liberty, & Altucher, 1966). It appears that for boys, the presence of a masculine father, a positive father-son relationship, generally sex-appropriate behavior, and popularity with peers are strongly related.

There is much evidence that a warm relationship with an active, competent father is very important in a boys' sex-role development (Biller, 1971a). For example, Biller (1969a) found a strong association between kindergarten-age boys' masculinity, particularly in relation to self-concept and perceived paternal involvement (paternal nurturance, decision-making, and so on). Furthermore, paternal influence in father-mother interactions was positively related to the boys' perceptions of the degree of their fathers' active participation in their families.

Other analyses of the data in Biller's study revealed the complex influences of family interactions on boys' sex-role development. Several of the boys who were not very masculine had fathers who were very influential in terms of father-mother interaction and generally seemed masculine but also appeared to be controlling and restrictive of their son's behavior. For instance, this type of dominant father seemed to punish his son for disagreeing with him. The boy's masculine development appears most facilitated when his father is active and involved in the family and also allows and encourages the boy to be assertive and independent. Moreover, in families where the mother and father competed for the decision-making function, boys were often very restricted. It may be that when the wife does not allow her husband to be dominant, he is apt to attempt to dominate his son in a restrictive and controlling manner.

Some investigators have suggested that father-absent males are more prone than are father-present males to become homosexual. Both West (1959) and O'Connor (1964) reported that homosexual males more often than neurotic males had histories of long periods of father-absence during childhood. West (1967) presents an excellent review of available data pertaining to the antecedents of male homosexuality: males who as children are father-absent or have ineffectual fathers and are involved in an intense, close-binding relationship with their mothers seem particularly likely to develop a homosexual pattern of behavior. A close-binding sexualized mother-son relationship seems more common in father-absent homes than in father-present homes and may, along with other related factors, lessen the probability of the boy entering into meaningful heterosexual relationships (Davids, Joelson, & McArthur, 1956). There is also evidence that a significant proportion of homosexuals, as children, were discouraged by their mothers from participating in masculine activities and were reinforced for feminine behavior (for example, see Bieber, 1962; Gundlach, 1969).

Males who have been father-absent often appear to have difficulty in forming lasting heterosexual relationships. Winch (1949, 1950), in a questionnaire study, found that father-absence among males was negatively related to degree of courtship behavior (defined as closeness to marriage). Among college males, a very high level of emotional attachment to mothers was also found to be negatively related to degree of courtship behavior. Hilgard, Neuman, and Fisk (1960) described the continued mother-dependency among males whose fathers died when they were children, if their mothers did not remarry: only one of the ten men who fit this category reportedly showed a fair degree of independence in a marital relationship. Pettigrew's (1964) study with working-class blacks also suggests that father-absent males have difficulty jn their heterosexual relationships. He found that father-absent males compared to father-present males were more likely to be single or divorced.

Much of the difficulty that some manifestly masculine father-absent lower-class males experience in forming meaningful heterosexual relationships may also be associated with a compulsive rejection of anything they perceive as related to femininity (Miller, 1958). Many lower-class males seem intent on constantly proving that they are not homosexual and/or effeminate. In their efforts to prove themselves masculine, they frequently engage in a "Don Juan" pattern of behavior, making one conquest after another and never forming a stable emotional relationship with a female.

Personal Adjustment

Frequent opportunities for observing a competent adult male in a variety of situations seem important in the development of the boy's maturity and responsibility. An investigation by Bronfenbrenner (1961) indicated that the amount of time adolescent boys spent with their fathers was positively related to the amount of leadership and responsibility they displayed in school. On the basis of their findings, Mussen et al. (1963) concluded that instrumental achievement striving was more frequent among adolescent boys with adequate (affectionate) father-son relationships than among those with inadequate father-son relationships.

Reuter and Biller (1973) studied the relationship between various combinations of perceived paternal nurturance-availability and college males' personality adjustment. A family background questionnaire was designed to assess perceptions of father-child relationships and the amount of time fathers spent at home. The personal adjustment scale of Gough and Heilbrun's Adjective Check List and the socialization scale of the California Psychological Inventory were used to measure personality adjustment. High paternal nurturance combined with at least moderate paternal availability and high paternal availability combined with at least moderate paternal nurturance were related to high scores on the personality adjustment measures. A male who has adequate opportunities to observe a nurturant father can imitate his behavior and develop positive personality characteristics. The father who is both relatively nurturant and relatively available may, himself, have a more adequate personality adjustment than other types of fathers.

In contrast, high paternal availability combined with low paternal nurturance and high paternal nurturance combined with low paternal availability were associated with relatively low scores on the personality adjustment measures. Males who reported that their fathers were home much of the time but gave them little attention perceived themselves as undependable and insecure. It may be that the relatively unnurturant father is an inadequate model and that his consistent presence is a detriment to the boy's personality functioning. In other words, the boy with an unnurturant father may be better off if his father is not very available. In such a case the boy may be less influenced in a negative manner. This speculation is consistent with evidence that suggests father-absent boys may show better personality adjustments than boys with passive, ineffectual fathers (Biller, 1971a).

Males who were high in paternal nurturance but low in paternal availability also seemed to be handicapped in their psychological functioning. The boy with a highly nurturant but seldom home father may feel frustrated that his father is not home more often and/or may find it difficult to imitate such an elusive figure.

The results of some studies suggest that males who have been father-absent during childhood generally have lower achievement motivation and experience less career success than do males who have been father-present during childhood (for example, see McClelland, 1961; Veroff, Atkinson, Feld, & Gurin, 1960). The father-absent boy often seems to have much difficulty in learning how to delay gratification of his needs and control his impulses. One might therefore predict that father-absent boys would find it very frustrating to persist in arduous situations and in meeting certain long-term responsibilities. Suedfield (1967) found that among Peace Corps volunteers, those who were father-absent during childhood were much more likely not to complete their scheduled overseas tours than were those who had not been father-absent. Reasons for premature termination were associated with problems of adjustment and included some psychiatrically based decisions.

Psychoanalytic theorists such as Freud and Fenichel viewed anxiety as a primary outcome of father-absence. Their emphasis was on anxiety springing from the unresolved Oedipal situation (Fenichel, 1945), but the frequent economic and social insecurity of the father-absent family also cannot be ignored. Koch (1961) found that father-absent nursery school children (eight boys and three girls) were more anxious as measured on a projective test of anxiety than a matched group from intact families; the father-absent children more often selected unhappy faces for the central child depicted in various situations than did the matched group.

Father-absence does not necessarily lead to maladjustment, although the probability of maladjustment appears higher for father-absent than for father-present individuals. Studies indicating a higher-than-average frequency of interpersonal and cognitive difficulties among father-absent individuals have already been reviewed. It is not surprising that many studies have suggested that father-absent children often act very immature and show a high rate of behavior problems relating to school adjustment, both academic and interpersonal (for example, Garbower, 1959; Gregory, 1965a; Holman, 1953). Methodological limitations make for problems in interpreting most such studies. In particular, many of the studies do not analyze data in terms of sex of child and do not use control groups of non-problem children.

Some studies suggest that individuals who have been father-absent are likely to exhibit, to a pathological degree, feelings of loss and depressed behavior. Beck, Sehti, and Tuthill (1963) found that paternal absence before the age of four is particularly likely to lead to depression. It may be that loss of father due to death is more strongly related to chronically depressed behavior than is loss of father due to other factors. However, the available studies concerning father-absence and depressed behavior, though of heuristic value, have not been carefully controlled. For instance, many of the subjects suffering from paternal loss in these studies have frequently also had a history of institutionalization.

There is a growing literature suggesting that father-present males having inadequate fathering, compared to those with adequate fathering, are much more likely to develop severe behavior disturbances and/or schizophrenia (see Farina, 1960; Kayton & Biller, 1971; Lidz, Parker, & Cornelison, 1956). Lack of paternal involvement and often correlated maternal domination of the family seem particularly common in the development of psychopathology. Adequate personality development seems facilitated in families in which the father clearly represents a positive masculine role, the mother a positive feminine role.

There is also accumulating evidence indicating that severely disturbed and/or schizophrenic behavior is associated with abnormalities in sex-role development (Biller & Poey, 1969; Gardner, 1967; Kayton & Biller, 1972; McClelland & Watt, 1968). A look at the files of child guidance centers suggests that both paternal deprivation and inadequate sex-role development are much more common among disturbed children than among children in the general population, but methodologically sound studies must be conducted. Rates of childhood father-absence among adult patients classified as neurotic (Madow & Hardy, 1947; Norton, 1952) and as schizophrenic (Oltman, McGarry, & Friedman, 1952; Wahl, 1956) are higher than among the general population.

Gregory (1965b) critically reviewed many of the relevant studies and emphasized some of the methodological pitfalls in comparisons involving the relative incidence of mental illness among father-present and father-absent individuals; lack of consideration of the possible effects of socioeconomic status is a major shortcoming of most of the studies. Cobliner (1963) presented some provocative findings suggesting that father-absence is more likely to be related to serious psychological disturbance in lower-class rather than middle-class individuals. Middle-class families, particularly with respect to the mother-child relationship, may have more psychological as well as economic resources with which to cope with father-absence.

The Mother-Son Relationship

This section contains a description and discussion of data relating to the mother's influence, particularly with respect to the paternally deprived boy.

Matriarchal Homes

A striking example of maternal domination occurs in matriarchal families, which are very common in lower-socioeconomic neighborhoods (Miller, 1958). Matriarchal families seem to be particularly prevalent among lower-class blacks (see Dai, 1953; Pettigrew, 1964). Certainly there are black families of lower-socioeconomic status in which the father is an integral member, but there seem to be a great many in which the father is absent or a relatively peripheral member.

Dai's (1953) observation that girls are usually preferred to boys by lower-class black women is supported by Rohrer and Edmonson's (1960) findings. In the latter study, black women were asked about their adoption preferences and they overwhelmingly said that they would prefer to adopt girls rather than boys. The lopsided preference for girls by black women seems in marked contrast to the finding that middle-class white women prefer to have a first-born male child (Dinitz, Dynes, & Clarke, 1954).

Maternal attitudes relating to males, particularly to the father, are also important in the personality development of children in intact homes. Grunebaum et al. (1962), in a clinical study of academically underachieving boys, contended that a contributing factor to the boys' difficulties was the mothers' perceptions that their husbands were inadequate and incompetent. Comparing high school boys' self-descriptions with the boys' perceptions of their fathers, Helper (1955) found son-father similarity significantly related to the mother's approval of the father as a model for the child. Sears (1953) reported that kindergarten-age boys who took the feminine role in doll play had mothers who, among other things, were highly critical of their husbands.

How the mother perceives the father and how she communicates about him to her son can be of much significance in her son's personality development (Bach, 1946; Biller, 1971a). It seems particularly important that the absent father's masculinity be described in positive terms. For instance, his general competence in dealing with his environment and his strength and physical prowess would connote his masculinity in our society. On the other hand, specific depreciation of the father's masculinity, such as occurs in the lower-class black matriarchal family, might lead the young boy to avoid acting masculine at least until he came into contact with his male peer culture. Kardiner and Ovesey (1951), discussing the lower-class black matriarchal family, stated that "The greatest damage to the group as a whole is done by the injury in the boy's mental life to his parental ideal. He never hears the father's role lauded, only condemned [p. 347]."

The mother's attitude regarding masculinity and men, including her reactions to her son's masculine behavior, forms a significant part of the mother-son relationship. Her perception of the boy's father frequently seems to generalize to her son. However, it could be predicted that the degree to which a mother perceives her son as similar to his father is related to the boy's behavioral and physical characteristics as well as to particular maternal attitudes. For example, if her son very much resembles his father facially and physically, it seems more likely that the mother would expect the boy's behavior to approximate his father's than if there was little father-son resemblance. As Bell (1968) points out, the stimulus value of the child and his impact on parental behavior has not received sufficient research attention.

Maternal Overprotection

In families where maternal overprotection exists, the father generally seems to play a very submissive and ineffectual role (Levy, 1943). Where the father is absent, the probability of a pattern of maternal overprotection seems to be increased. Most fathers are very critical of having their children overprotected and most fathers also serve as models for independent behavior. The child's developmental stage at the onset of father-absence is an important variable. The infant or pre-school-age, father-absent boy seems likely to be overprotected by his mother, whereas if father-absence begins when the boy is older, he might be expected to take over many of the responsibilities his father had previously assumed.

Comparing the family histories of 20 first-grade children rated as overdependent by their teachers with 20 matched children, Stendler (1954) found that overdependency was common in families in which the father was absent or ineffectual. Of the 20 overdependent children, 13 lacked the consistent presence of the father in the home during the first three years of life as compared to only six in the control group. In addition, the six relatively father-absent children in the control group had generally been without their fathers for a much shorter time than the overdependent children. Stendler pictured the role of the father as one that discouraged the mother's overprotecting tendencies and actively encouraged independent activity.

The analysis of Stolz et al. (1954) of retrospective maternal reports suggested that mothers whose husbands were away in military service tended to restrict their infants' locomotor activities to a greater extent than did mothers whose husbands were present. Tiller (1958) reported similar results with mothers of 8- and 9-year-old Norwegian children whose fathers were seldom-home sailors. With respect to both sons and daughters, these mothers were more overprotective, as judged by maternal interview data and by the children's responses to a structured doll play test, than were the mother of matched father-present children. Biller (1969b) also found that mothers of father-absent boys were less encouraging of masculine behavior than were mothers of father-present boys. In the father-absent families, many of the mothers' informal responses suggested that they were very fearful of their children being physically injured.

Some studies suggest that maternal overprotection is relatively infrequent among lower-class families (Heckscher, 1967; McCord, McCord, & Thurber, 1962; Rohrer & Edmonson, 1960); that is, socioeconomic status seems related to the frequency of maternal overprotection. A lower-class mother may have less opportunity to overprotect a father-absent son because she is more often engaged in a full-time job than is a middle-class mother (Heckscher, 1967). Second, compared to middle-class families, there seems less of a social stigma attached to father-absence among lower-class families, especially among lower-class black families (King, 1945). A mother without a husband who has young children is a more common phenomenon in the lower class. The middle-class mother may be more predisposed to feel guilty because her child, particularly her son, is being deprived of a father. She may be more likely to try to make this up to the boy by overprotecting and overindulging him.

On the other hand, there is evidence to suggest that maternal rejection and neglect are quite common among husbandless lower-class mothers (Heckscher, 1967; Kardiner & Ovesey, 1951; McCord, McCord, & Thurber, 1962). Lower-class mothers without husbands seem particularly concerned with their own needs and their day-to-day existence and often withdraw from their children. There is some evidence that boys are more often rejected than girls (see Beller, 1967; Dai, 1953; Pettigrew, 1964).

In any case, either overprotection or rejection would seem to reduce the probability of the boy's feeling a sense of worth in terms of his maleness. However, it does seem that maternal indifference or rejection would make a boy more prone to be indiscriminately influenced by the gang milieu. The maternally overprotected father-absent boy may be quite timid and retiring in peer interactions, whereas it seems more probable that the maternally rejected father-absent boy will act out aggressively and choose masculine activities and attitudes in order to gain the respect of his peers. Nevertheless, both overprotected and rejected father-absent boys seem likely to be low in underlying masculinity of their self-concepts.

The frequent negative attitude of lower-class mothers toward their sons and males, in general, seems to contribute to the meaningfulness of the gang milieu for boys. The boy who feels neglected or rejected can have his needs for attention, recognition, and affection satisfied by becoming a member of a gang. Masculinity of an aggressive acting-out nature (in relation to typically middle-class standards) is valued by the gang, and behaviors perceived as feminine are fearfully avoided. Such an atmosphere may help bolster the boy's self-image if he has the ability to perform in an aggressive-competitive manner, but it often leads to rigid and narrow interpersonal and cognitive functioning. For example, because women are usually authority figures in the school situation, many boys resent participation in intellectual pursuits, perceiving such activities as feminine.

The general economic and social difficulties of the husbandless mother cannot be overlooked (Glasser & Navarre, 1965; Kriesberg, 1967). Kriesberg (1967) clearly summarized the frequent plight of the mother whose husband is absent: "His absence is likely to mean that his former wife is poor, lives in poor neighborhoods, and lacks social, emotional, and physical assistance in childrearing. Furthermore, how husbandless mothers accommodate themselves to these circumstances can have important consequences for their children [p. 288]." The degree to which the fatherless family has available social and economic resources influences the child's interpersonal and educational opportunities. The lower-class child seems even more disadvantaged by fatherlessness than does the middle-class child.

Paternal deprivation often leads to an increase in the intensity of the emotional relationship between mother and child, especially during infancy and early childhood. Stephens (1962) presented cross-cultural evidence indicating that long post-partum taboos prohibiting sexual activity tend to make mothers closer to their children and less husband-centered. In such societies mothers apparently are more attentive and succorant as well as more indulgent of dependency in their young children than mothers in societies in which post-partum taboos are of short duration. There is also some interesting anthropological data suggesting that males often experience sex-role conflicts in societies in which children, during their first few years of life, have a relatively exclusive relationship with their mothers (Bacon, Child, & Barry, 1963; Burton & Whiting, 1961; Stephens, 1962).

Levy (1943) reported that excessive physical contact is a frequent concomitant of maternal overprotection (and paternal underinvolvement). Of 19 cases of maternal overprotection involving boys, he found that six of the boys slept with their mothers long past infancy, three of them during adolescence. In almost one-half of the clinical cases involving father-absent preadolescent and adolescent boys in Wylie and Delgado's (1959) study, mother and son slept together in the same bed or bedroom. In reviewing relevant psychoanalytic case studies, Neubauer (1960) described how difficult sex-role development is for the young father-absent boy who has a highly sexualized relationship with his mother. Such an intense relationship affords the boy little opportunity to interact with masculine role models.

Stoller (1968) described several boys who felt that they were really females. These transsexual boys had extremely close physical relationships with their mothers. Mutual body contact during infancy was especially intense and there was much evidence that the mothers reinforced many forms of feminine behavior in their sons. It is of particular interest that in none of these cases was the father masculine or actively involved in the family. Stoller's book is replete with references to his and other therapists' case studies suggesting that disturbed sex-role and sexual development in males is associated with an overly intense, relatively exclusive mother-son relationship.

Such family structure variables as birth order and age and sex of siblings can interact with maternal behavior to influence the father-absent child's personality development. If a father-absent boy is an only child or the only boy in all-female family, the probability of maternal overprotection seems increased. On the other hand, if the boy, during his early years, has frequent opportunity to interact with older male siblings, peers, or adults who encourage the development of his autonomy and assertiveness, the chances of a close-binding mother-son relationship seemed lessened.

Positive Mothering

Some researchers have suggested that the mother-son relationship can have either a positive or a negative effect on the paternally deprived child's personality development. Such a conclusion was reached by McCord, McCord, & Thurber (1962) when they analyzed social workers' observations of 10- to 15-year-old lower-class boys. They found that the presence of a rejecting and/or disturbed mother was related to various behavior problems (sexual anxiety, regressive behavior, and criminal acts) in father-absent boys, but father-absent boys who had seemingly well-adjusted mothers were much less likely to have such problems.

Pederson (1966), studying military families, reported evidence suggesting that psychologically healthy mothers may be able to counteract the effects of father-absence. Mothers of a group of emotionally disturbed 11- to 15-year old boys were themselves found to be significantly more disturbed (in terms of the Minnesota Multiphasic Personality Inventory) than mothers of a comparable group of non-disturbed children. Both the emotionally disturbed and non-disturbed children had experienced relatively long periods of father-absence, but it was only in the disturbed group that degree of father-absence was related to level of emotional disturbance (measured by the Rogers Scale of Adjustment).

Hilgard, Neuman, and Fisk (1960), in an investigation of adults who as children had fathers who died, stressed the importance of the mother's ego strength. The mother's ability to use her own and outside resources and assume some of the dual functions of mother and father with little conflict appeared strongly related to her child's adjustment as an adult. Hilgard et al. emphasized that such women had been relatively feminine while their husbands were alive but that they were secure enough in their basic sex-role identifications to perform some of the traditional functions of the father after he had died. These researchers also felt that the mother's ego strength rather than her warmth or tenderness was the essential variable in her child's adjustment. Excessive maternal warmth and affection may be related to maternal overprotection, particularly among father-absent children.

A mother who is generally dominant and competent in interpersonal and environmental interaction can provide her child with an effective model. However, parental dominance seems to facilitate a child's personality development only if the dominant parent allows the child sufficient freedom and responsibility to imitate effective parental behaviors that he has observed (Biller, 1969a). A serious problem that the young boy from a typical matriarchal family faces is that his mother often does not allow or encourage him to display competent behaviors. The mother frequently seems to interfere with the boy's attempts at mastery and to reward his dependency upon her.

It seems reasonable to suppose that a mother could facilitate her father-absent boy's sex-role development by having a positive attitude toward the absent father and males in general and by consistently encouraging masculine behavior in her son. Biller (1969b) found that for father-absent kindergarten-age boys, degree of maternal encouragement of masculine behavior, as measured by a multiple-choice questionnaire, was significantly related to masculinity as assessed by a game preference measure and a multidimensional rating scale filled out by teachers. In father-absent families, mothers who accepted and reinforced aggressive and assertive behavior appeared to have much more masculine sons than mothers who discouraged such behavior.

Sears, Rau, and Alpert (1965) found that parents who permitted and accepted aggressive and assertive behavior in their pre-school-age sons had highly masculine sons. In contrast, boys low in masculinity were found to have parents who were anxious, non-permissive, and severely punishing of aggression. These findings are consistent with earlier investigations (for example, Baldwin, Kalhorn, & Breese, 1949) reviewed by Becker (1964), which reported that restrictive and autocratic parents tend to have passive, conforming, and dependent children whereas permissive and democratic parents tend to have active, assertive, and independent children.

Since the father-son relationship appears more critical than the mother-son relationship when the father is present (Biller & Borstelmann, 1967), it could be predicted that maternal encouragement and expectations concerning sex-appropriate and sex-inappropriate behavior are less important when the father is present than when he is absent. For instance, a masculine and salient father would seem able to outweigh the effects of a mildly overprotective mother. However, it is hypothesized that maternal behavior is the most critical variable in facilitating or inhibiting the young father-absent boy's masculine development. It is assumed that the mother can, by reinforcing specific responses and expecting masculine behavior, increase the boy's perception of the incentive value of the masculine role. This, in turn, would seem to promote a positive view of males as salient and powerful, thus motivating the boy to imitate their behavior.

An overview of previous research (Biller, 1971a) suggests that father-absence generally has more of an effect on the boy's sex-role orientation (his underlying perception and evaluation of his maleness and/or femaleness) than it does on his sex-role preference (his choice of particular sex-typed activities and attitudes) or his sex-role adoption (how masculine and/or feminine his behavior is in social or environmental interaction). Sex-role preference and sex-role adoption seem easier to influence, at least after a child reaches school age, than does sex-role orientation, and it may be that maternal behavior during the pre-school years has more impact on the boy's sex-role preference and sex-role adoption than it does on his sex-role orientation. However, it could be speculated that if a father-absent boy learns a masculine preference and adoption on the basis of both consistent maternal and peer-group reinforcement, then he is likely to view himself and his masculinity positively and to develop a masculine sex-role orientation at least by his middle school years.

There is some evidence that father-absence before the age of 5 has more effect on the boy's sex-role development than does father-absence after the age of 5 (Biller, 1971a), and it may be that the mother-child relationship is particularly important when the boy becomes father-absent early in life. Biller and Bahm (1971) discovered that degree of perceived maternal encouragement for aggressive and assertive behavior was highly related to the masculinity of junior high school boys who had become father-absent before the age of 5. Among the early father-absent boys, perception of clear-cut maternal encouragement for appropriate sex-typed behaviors, as assessed by a Q-sort technique, was associated with high masculinity of self-concept, as measured by an adjective check list.

It is hoped that future research will lead to delineation of the kinds of maternal behaviors and dimensions of the mother-child relationship that are relevant to the father-absent boy's personality development. In the next section, some research concerning the effects of father-absence on the girl's personality development is reviewed; it would seem that investigators studying the impact of father-absence should systematically examine possible differential effects of the mother-child relationship as a function of sex of child. Findings from such research may be useful for programs designed to maximize the interpersonal and intellectual potential of father-absent children and to help mothers in father-absent families to become more effective parents.

The Father-Daughter Relationship

As can be seen from literature cited in previous sections, the father's impact on personality development has been increasingly recognized by contemporary theorists and researchers. However, the focus has been on the father-son relationship with relatively little acknowledgement of the importance of the father-daughter relationship. In this section, we attempt to review ideas and findings relevant to understanding what influence adequate and inadequate fathering may have on personality development of females.

Feminine Development

Femininity in social interaction seems to involve expressiveness of warmth and affection, sensitivity to the needs of others, and skill in understanding and communicating feelings. Feminine interests and preferences tend to center around domestic, social, and caretaking activities (Biller, 1971a). A fundamental part of the girl's sex-role development seems to be the positive acceptance of herself as a female. The father's particular relationship with his daughter seems very important in her sex-role development. He may foster the establishment of a positive feminine identity by valuing her and encouraging the development of her potentialities (Biller, 1971a).

Feminine behavior in the girl seems to be related to how the father defines his role as a male to his daughter and how he differentiates his masculine role from the feminine role. Mussen and Rutherford (1963) suggest that "the father's possession of a high degree of masculinity of interests and attitudes and his active encouragement of the girl's participation in appropriate sex-typed activities tend to foster the girl's development of appropriate sex-role preference [p. 603]." Thus, whereas the mother behaves in a relatively feminine manner to both her male and female children, if the father differentiates between masculine and feminine roles, his daughter may be more able to establish and maintain a secure sense of femininity. Mussen and Rutherford also found that fathers of highly feminine first-grade girls encouraged their daughters more in sex-appropriate activities than did fathers of unfeminine girls. Sears et al. (1965) reported a significant correlation between girls' femininity and their fathers' expectations of their participation in feminine activities.

Participation by the father in a secure and consistent relationship—emotionally warm, stable, and democratic—with his daughter seems to provide a highly significant ingredient for her feminine development. It appears that the more a father participates in constructive interplay with his daughter, the more adequate will be her sex-role and personality development.

The results of Fish and Biller's (1973) investigation are consistent with the supposition that the father plays an important role in the girl's personality development. College girls' perceptions of their relationships with their fathers during childhood were assessed by means of an extensive family background questionnaire. Subjects who perceived their fathers as having been very nurturant scored high on the Adjective Check List personal adjustment scale, as did those who perceived their fathers as having been very positively involved with them. In contrast, subjects who perceived their fathers as having been highly rejecting scored extremely low on the personal adjustment measure.

Hoffman (1961) found that girls from mother-dominant homes had difficulty relating to the opposite sex and were disliked by boys. She suggested that both sexes, but girls to a lesser extent, "will have self-confidence and feel accepted by others, show a positive assertiveness in the peer group, have skills, like others, be well-liked, and exert influence if the father is the dominant parent, if he has a positive emotional involvement with his children, and if he disciplines them [pp. 104–105]."

Hetherington (1965) did not find a significant difference between the sex-role preferences of girls from father-dominant versus mother-dominant families. A later study (Hetherington & Frankie, 1967) further supports the hypothesis that parental dominance is a less crucial factor in the development of girls than it has been found to be with boys. Hetherington (1965) suggested that a mother could be more dominant than her husband, yet not be dominant in other relationships (that is, relationships with other women) and that such a mother might have other feminine traits with which her daughter could identify.

Biller (1969c) suggested that for kindergarten-age girls, it does not seem crucial that the mother be perceived as more dominant than the father, but that the daughter's feminine development is facilitated if the mother is seen as a generally salient controller of resources. In his study, girls perceived their fathers as more competent and decision-making, their mothers as more limit-setting, and both parents as similar in nurturance. He found a subgroup of girls whose femininity scores were low and who perceived their mothers as relatively high in decision-making and limit-setting but quite low in nurturance and competence. One might speculate that the optimal level of father-dominance would be moderate rather than extreme, since in such a home the mother would be seen as a "salient controller of resources" yet in a general context of paternal involvement. Biller and Zung's (1972) study suggests that very high maternal control and dominance hampers the girl's as well as the boy's development. They found that high maternal control and intrusiveness were associated with high anxiety and sex-role conflict among elementary school girls.

Family Milieu

The personality development of children appears to be highly dependent on the family milieu. The absence of the father from the home may dramatically upset the dynamics of family life. In addition to economic considerations related to the loss of the father in the family, the mother-child relationship may be adversely affected by the absence of the husband's emotional support. Data supporting the view that father-absence influences the girl's personality development has come from research by Lynn and Sawrey (1959), who examined the effects of father-absence on Norwegian boys and girls in the second grade. The specific effect of father-absence on the girls in this study consisted of greater-than-average dependency on their mothers.

Based on their findings in projective doll-play sessions, Sears, Pintler, and Sears (1946) report that "there is no indication that the girls are more frustrated when the father is present; on the contrary, his absence is associated with greater aggression, especially self-aggression [p. 240]." These writers speculate that such aggressive behavior may be a function of the father-absent girl's conflict with her mother. Heckel (1963) reported frequent school maladjustment, excessive sexual interest, and social acting-out behavior in fatherless preadolescent girls. Such behavior may be a manifestation of intense frustration stemming from unsuccessful attempts to find an adult male figure with whom they can form a meaningful relationship. Father-absent girls often seem to manifest a variety of symptoms which to some degree reflect maladjustment. It appears that these developmental problems are related to the complex interaction of father-absence, maternal behavior, and pre-separation family adjustment.

The father influences his daughter's personality development in terms of his relationship with his wife, who acts as a primary model for his daughter. If the father meets his wife's needs she may, in turn, be able to interact more adequately with her children. Bartemeier (1953) considers the wife's emotional health, self-regard, and capacity for appropriately nurturing her children to be influenced by her husband's attitudes and behavior. Bartemeier emphasized that the father's own history is a significant factor in determining his behavior as a husband and father. Inadequate fathering may be a reflection of underlying conflicts in the husband that upset his complementary relationship with his wife.

According to Becker, Peterson, Luria, Shoemaker, and Hellmer (1962), conduct problems are generally found in children whose parents are not only arbitrary but overly emotional as well. In some of the cases they studied, the mother was tense and thwarting while the father showed inadequate concern with the family. He was found to be a poor enforcer of discipline, particularly of rules established by his wife. Maladjusted and domineering fathers, on the other hand, contributed to shyness and emotional overactivity in their children. This inadequacy of fathering was evident in the husband's lack of a harmonious relationship with his wife, his arbitrary power assertions, and his lack of warmth in dealing with his family.

Sopchak (1952) and Lazowick (1955) presented findings supporting the proposition that inadequate fathering is related to emotional disorders in females. Sopchak (1952) studied the effects of poor identification with the father on college women. He summarized his results as follows: "Women with tendencies toward abnormality as measured by the MMPI show a lack of identification with their fathers. . . . Masculine women identify with their fathers less than feminine women . . . and identification with the father is more important in producing normal adjustment than is identification with the mother [p. 164–165]." Lazowick (1955) has also studied the influence of inadequate identification with the father and concluded that a high degree of manifest anxiety in undergraduate women is related to the absence of an adequate father-daughter relationship.

A healthy father-identification for the girl seems to consist of understanding and empathizing with the father. It can also include the sharing of certain of the father's values and attitudes as long as these do not interfere with the daughter's development of a feminine self-concept and an expressive mode of social interaction. When the father plays an active and competent masculine role in the family, his daughter is more likely to imitate his non-sex-typed positive attributes and be more adaptable and less narrow in her behavior repertoire than when he is unmasculine or aloof. The probability of the girl spurning her femininity seems high in such a situation (that is, with a competent father who encourages her valuation of her femininity) *only* if her mother is cold and rejecting or somehow unable to express acceptance, warmth, and nurturance toward her.

Inappropriate or inadequate fathering is often related to the development of homosexuality in females. For instance, Bené (1965) reported that female homosexuals felt their fathers were weak and incompetent and Kaye (1967) found that fathers of female homosexuals (as compared to control group fathers) tended to be puritanical, exploitative, and feared by the daughters as well as possessive and infantilizing. Kaye also presented evidence that suggests female homosexuality is associated with rejection of femininity early in life. Clinical data suggest that fathers who do not accept their daughter's femininity (because they wanted sons and/or are threatened by feminine behavior) can have a very destructive effect on their daughter's personality development (see Seward, 1946; West, 1967).

Lidz and Lidz (1949) conclude that inadequate fathering is a significant antecedent in the development of schizophrenia; such maladjustment is considered to be associated with a lack of stable paternal involvement in childhood. Research by Hamilton and Wahl (1948) revealed that among a population of hospitalized schizophrenic women, almost 75 percent of them experienced some inadequacy of fathering.

Lidz et al. (1956) attempted to specify the nature of insufficient fathering for schizophrenic females. Fathers in severe conflict with their wives—who contradict their wives' decisions and degrade their wives in front of their daughters—were most notably inadequate in their family relationships. Such men were considered to maintain rigid and unrealistic expectations regarding their wives' conformity to their arbitrary authority. As a result of disappointment in these expectations, such fathers "would like to mold their daughters to fit their needs [p. 128]." In conclusion, these researchers state: "In our experience, it is the daughter who sides with the father and seeks his love who becomes psychotic. She cannot follow the mother in her development and the father's demands are too inconsistent, unrealistic, and hostile. In some instances, acceptance of the father's tenets would require pathological distortion of reality [p. 128]."

It thus appears that certain maladjustive tendencies are fostered by distorted expectations, power assertions, or the complete passivity of the father. The effects of paternal inadequacy may leave the child generally limited in social experience. Concomitant with limited social experience may be the child's inability to develop fully her interpersonal potential and a narrowing of perspective regarding her own adequacy as a person.

Literature cited in this section has suggested many ways the father's behavior can facilitate or inhibit the girl's personality development. Parental childrearing practices, discipline, social attitudes, and personality appear to be important factors, but there is a tremendous need for more systematic research.

Overview and Implications

In this section, in addition to describing some relatively unexplored research avenues, we will discuss certain practical applications of existing knowledge relating to the parents' role in personality development.

Research Considerations

A major goal of this article is to stimulate further research examining the impact of parent-child relationships on the adequacy of personality development. A great many studies have been reviewed and various interpretations and speculations have been made. However, most of the statements put forth should be viewed as hypotheses deserving more systematic research rather than as established facts.

Most of the studies of parent-child relationships and personality development have methodological deficiencies or limited generality. In most investigations, the father's behavior is not directly assessed; instead, maternal or child reports of paternal behavior are used. In many studies, the sources of evidence about parental behavior and the child's behavior are not independent, leading to problems of interpretation. More studies assessing the amount of consistency among observer ratings of familial interactions and children's and parents' perceptions of parent-child relationships should be done.

Most studies of parent-child relationships and the child's development have been of a correlational nature. Often the child's perception of parents (see Davids & Hainsworth, 1967) or some report of the parents' behavior is related to a measure of the child's personality development. For instance, when significant correlations are found between the degree to which a boy perceives his father as nurturant and the boy's masculinity, it is usually assumed that paternal nurturance has been an antecedent of masculine development. But it could be reasoned that fathers become nurturant and accepting towards their sons when their sons are masculine and rejecting when their sons are unmasculine. Longitudinal research would be particularly helpful in determining the extent to which certain paternal behaviors are antecedents of particular dimensions of children's behavior.

Studies of father-absent children have revealed some clues as to the influence of parent-child relationships. In addition to the obvious theoretical and practical relevance of studying the effects of father-absence, a possible methodological justification is that father-absence is a "naturalistic" manipulation; it can be argued that father-absence must be an antecedent rather than a consequence of certain behaviors in children. However, many researchers have treated father-absence in an overly simplistic fashion. In many studies, there has been no specification of such variables as length and age of onset of father-absence, and the sex of the child. Few researchers have matched father-absent and father-present children; potentially important variables such as IQ, SES, sociocultural background, birth order, sibling distribution, and availability of father surrogates have rarely been taken into account, either in subject matching or in data analysis.

Individual differences among father-absent and paternally deprived children should be carefully explored. For instance, many paternally deprived children have very adequate interpersonal adjustments. For example, case study analysis of some of the 5-year-old father-absent boys in Biller's (1968a, 1969b) studies suggests that boys who are relatively mesomorphic are likely to be less retarded in their masculine development than are boys with unmasculine physiques. A child's physique has a certain stimulus value in terms of the expectations and reinforcements it elicits from others and it may, along with correlated genetic and physiological factors, predispose the boy toward success or failure in particular types of activities. Individual differences in children's constitutional-temperamental and cognitive predispositions and the impact of the child on the parent (as well as vice versa) must be taken into account if we are to gain a more thorough understanding of child development (Davids, 1968).

Some data suggest that surrogate parental models can facilitate personality development. Systematic studies, possibly exposing groups of paternally deprived children in varying degrees to father-surrogates and mother-surrogates, need to be done. For example, we have little controlled data concerning the effects of different amounts of father-availability in the intact home on the child's personality development or the degree of possible benefit or remediation gained by the presence of a step-parent at various age levels. When the father is present, it appears that the quality of the father-child relationship is more important than the amount of time the father is available (Biller, 1968a, 1971a). However, much further investigation of variations of both quantitative and qualitative paternal availability in the father-present home should be conducted.

The timing of fathering and father-absence appears quite important. Longitudinal studies would be valuable in revealing factors in the pre-paternal absence and father-child and father-mother relationships that may be very important to the child's personality development as well as to immediate familial adjustment following father-absence. The husband-wife relationship before the birth of the child (Davids, 1968), the expectant father's attitudes toward children, and the parents' adjustment during pregnancy (Davids & DeVault, 1962) should also be examined in terms of their possible linkage with post-partum father-child interaction. In particular, father-child interaction during the child's first few years of life should be studied in great detail.

Inadequate fathering or father-absence predisposes children toward certain developmental deficits. However, there are many paternally deprived children who are generally well adjusted, and such children should be more carefully studied. The quality of the mother-child relationship, particularly, is important in the personality development of the paternally deprived child. Studies comparing paternally deprived individuals having different types of adjustments in terms of their relationships with their mothers would be quite revealing. There is a paucity of investigations attempting to relate individual differences in mothering in father-absent homes and the child's personality development. Variations in sociocultural background, particularly those reflected in terms of prevalent patterns of mothering, may lead to marked differences between father-present and father-absent children in some societies and subgroups but not in others.

Girls' as well as boys' personality development may be adversely affected by paternal inadequacy and paternal absence. Some data suggest that the extent and direction of sex differences varies with respect to which dimensions of personality development are considered. There is great need for much more systematic research if one is to come to any firm judgment regarding the differential impact of variations in fathering as a function of sex of child.

These suggestions are just some of the possible directions for future research. Despite limitations and deficiencies in investigations relating to the effects of fathering on personality development, many generalizations were put forth because of the apparent consistency of available data. On the basis of the related generalizations that paternal deprivation often leads to problems in personality development and that adequate fathering can positively influence many facets of personality development, certain practical implications follow.

Practical Applications

Applications of existing knowledge should not be divorced from research endeavors. Whenever feasible, treatment and preventive projects should be integrated with research programs and vice versa (Davids, 1972).

Although controlled research is lacking, there are many illuminating descriptions of how psychotherapists have attempted to help emotionally disturbed children who are father-absent or suffer from inadequate fathering (see Forrest, 1967; Meerloo, 1956; Neubauer, 1960). Unfortunately, the emphasis on the mother-child relationship in most child psychotherapy has often obscured the father's role.

It seems that therapists would strengthen their impact on the father-absent or paternally disadvantaged child by also working with the child's actual or potential father surrogate. This could be accomplished by consultation, but engaging the father surrogate and child in joint sessions (or in groups with other children and father surrogates) might be even more beneficial. The use of modeling and related behavior techniques such as those described by Bandura (1969) seems a particularly worthwhile course to explore in individual, family, and group therapy with paternally deprived children. In many cases, the probability of successful treatment could be greatly increased if knowledge concerning the process of positive fathering were integrated into the psychotherapy process, especially in family therapy (Biller, 1971a).

The availability of father surrogates is important for father-present children with inadequate fathers, as well as for father-absent children. Glueck and Glueck (1950) reported that delinquent boys who form a close relationship with a father surrogate often resolve their antisocial tendencies. Similarly, Trenaman (1952) found that young men who had been chronically delinquent while serving in the British army were able to be helped by relationships with father surrogates. Some father-absent children have very effective father surrogates in their own families or find an adequate role model among older peers or teachers. A paternally deprived child may be particularly responsive to a male therapist because of his motivation for male companionship. Rexford (1964), in describing the treatment of young antisocial children, notes that therapists are more likely to be successful with father-absent boys than with boys who have strongly identified with an emotionally disturbed, criminal, or generally inadequate father. Older well-adjusted boys might prove to be very salient and influential models for younger paternally-deprived boys.

Various organizations (Big Brother, YMCA, Boy Scouts, athletic teams, churches, settlement houses) provide many children with father surrogates. With further professional consultation and cooperation and additional community support (especially more father surrogates), such organizations could be of even greater benefit to more children. A very important implication from available research is that even in the second and third years of life, the child's personality development can be greatly influenced by the degree and type of involvement of a father or father surrogate; group settings such as Head Start can be used as vehicles to provide father surrogates for those children (both boys and girls) who could profit from them.

It would seem that nursery schools, kindergartens, and elementary schools could have a greater positive influence on children if more male teachers were available (Biller, 1971a). Male teachers might be able to facilitate certain types of cognitive functioning in paternally deprived children as well as contributing to their interpersonal development. Institutionalized children, including those who are orphaned or emotionally disturbed, could benefit from a larger proportion of interaction with competent males (Davids, 1972). For example, Nash's (1965) data suggest that having institutionalized children live in a situation in which they are cared for and supervised by a husband-wife team is beneficial for their sex-role development.

Education and the mass media can play a significant role in making prospective fathers and father surrogates more aware of the significance of the father in child development and, along with other programs, might lessen the number of families that become father-absent. Reinforcement, in terms of financial and other support for fathers remaining with their families (in contrast to the current rewarding of father-absence by many welfare departments), might do much to keep some families intact and reconstitute other families.

Perhaps preventive programs can be developed especially for families that seem to have a high risk of becoming father-absent; individuals from certain sociocultural backgrounds and with particular personality patterns seem highly vulnerable to divorce or separation (Loeb & Price, 1966; Pettigrew, 1964). Systematic techniques to determine the potential consequences of father-absence for a family where separation or divorce is being contemplated should be developed. There are many families in which both the parents and the children would be able to function better subsequent to divorce. It also seems that when the divorce process is taking place, more consideration should be given to whether in certain cases all or some of the children might benefit more from remaining with their fathers than with their mothers.

The mother in the paternally deprived family must not be neglected; her reaction to husband-absence may greatly influence the extent to which father-absence or lack of father availability affects her children. She is often in need of psychological as well as social and economic support (Glasser & Navarre, 1965; Kriesberg, 1967). Educational and therapeutic groups such as Parents without Partners (Freudenthal, 1959; Schlesinger, 1966) appear to be very helpful. Biller and Smith (1972) described a welfare mothers' group in which one of the central goals was to help husbandless mothers deal constructively with their social and familial problems. Wylie and Delgado (1959) discussed their therapeutic techniques with father-absent sons and their mothers. Many useful suggestions for mental health professionals working with the father-absent family are available (see Despert, 1957; Kriesberg, 1967; Lerner, 1954).

An important function of community mental health efforts, both in terms of prevention and treatment, could be to supply father surrogates to groups of paternally deprived children; far-reaching community, state, and government programs are needed. The great number of children, particularly those in generally disadvantaged circumstances, who do not have consistent and meaningful contact with an adult male creates a serious situation that must be corrected if these children's growing social and educational opportunities are to be realized (Moynihan, 1965).

We have emphasized the influence of both the father's role and paternal deprivation on personality development. The possible impact of variations in fathering on different aspects of sex-role, cognitive functioning, interpersonal relationships, and psychopathology has been explored. Throughout, we have stressed that the effects of fathering or lack of fathering cannot be considered apart from other factors. Developmental periods, sex of child, constitutional variables, sociocultural milieu, sibling constellation, availability of surrogate models, and individual differences are some of the factors that must be considered. We hope that the speculative formulations and directions for future research described here will stimulate further scientific inquiry and understanding of the parents' role in development of personality and psychopathology.

REFERENCES

Anderson, R. E. Where's Dad? Paternal deprivation and delinquency. *Archives of General Psychiatry,* 1968, **18,** 641–649.

Andry, R. G. Paternal and maternal roles in delinquency. In *Deprivation of maternal care.* Public Health Paper No. 14. Geneva: World Health Organization, 1962.

Bach, G. R. Father-fantasies and father typing in father-separated children. *Child Development,* 1946, **17,** 63–80.

Bach, G. R., & Bremer, G. Projective father fantasies of pre-adolescent delinquent children. *Journal of Psychology,* 1947, **24,** 3–17.

Bacon, M. K., Child, I. L., & Barry, H., III. A cross-cultural study of correlates of crime. *Journal of Abnormal and Social Psychology,* 1963, **66,** 291–300.

Baldwin, A. L., Kalhorn, J., & Breese, F. A. The appraisal of parent behavior. *Psychological Monographs,* 1949, **63,** No. 1 (Whole No. 299).

Bandura, A. *Principles of behavior modification.* New York: Holt, Rinehart and Winston, 1969.

Bandura, A., & Walters, R. H. Dependency conflicts in aggressive delinquents. *Journal of Social Issues,* 1958, **14,** 52–65.

Bartemeier, L. The contribution of the father to the mental health of the family. *American Journal of Psychiatry,* 1953, **110,** 277–280.

Beck, A. T., Sehti, B. B., & Tuthill, R. W. Childhood bereavement and adult depression. *Archives of General Psychiatry,* 1963, **9,** 295–302.

Becker, W. C. Consequences of different kinds of parental discipline. In M. L. Hoffman & L. W. Hoffman (Eds.), *Review of child development research: I.* New York: Russell Sage Foundation, 1964.

Becker, W. C., Peterson, D. R., Luria, Z., Shoemaker, D. S., & Hellmer, L. A. Relations of factors derived from parent interview ratings to behavior problems of five-year-olds. *Child Development,* 1962, **33,** 509–535.

Bell, R. Q. A reinterpretation of the direction of effects in studies of socialization. *Psychological Review,* 1968, **75,** 81–95.

Beller, E. K. Maternal behaviors in lower-class Negro mothers. Paper presented at the meeting of the Eastern Psychological Association, Boston, April 1967.

Bené, E. On the genesis of female homosexuality. *British Journal of Psychiatry,* 1965, **3,** 815–821.

Bieber, I. *Homosexuality: A psychoanalytic study.* New York: Basic Books, 1962.

Biller, H. B. A multi-aspect investigation of masculine development in kindergarten-age boys. *Genetic Psychology Monographs,* 1968, **76,** 89–139. (a)

Biller, H. B. A note on father-absence and masculine development in young lower-class Negro and white boys. *Child Development,* 1968, **39,** 1003–1006. (b)

Biller, H. B. Father dominance and sex role development in kindergarten-age boys. *Developmental Psychology,* 1969, **1,** 87–94. (a)

Biller, H. B. Father-absence, maternal encouragement and sex-role development in kindergarten-age boys. *Child Development,* 1969, **40,** 539–546. (b)

Biller, H. B. Maternal salience and feminine development in young girls. *Proceedings of the 77th Annual Convention of the American Psychological Association,* 1969, **4,** 259–260. (c)

Biller, H. B. Father-absence and the personality development of the male child. *Developmental Psychology,* 1970, **2,** 181–201.

Biller, H. B. *Father, Child, and Sex-Role.* Lexington, Mass.: D. C. Heath, 1971. (a)

Biller, H. B. The mother-child relationship and the father-absent boy's personality development. *Merrill-Palmer Quarterly,* 1971, **16,** 227–241. (b)

Biller, H. B., & Bahm, R. M. Father-absence, perceived maternal behavior, and masculinity of self-concept among junior high school boys. *Developmental Psychology,* 1971, **4,** 178–181.

Biller, H. B., & Borstelmann, L. J. Masculine development: An integrative review. *Merrill-Palmer Quarterly,* 1967, **13,** 253–294.

Biller, H. B., & Poey, K. An exploratory comparison of sex-role related behavior in schizophrenics and non-schizophrenics. *Developmental Psychology,* 1969, **1,** 269.

Biller, H. B., & Smith, A. E. An AFDC mothers group: An exploratory effort in community mental health. *Family Coordinator,* 1972, **21,** 287–290.

Biller, H. B., & Weiss, S. The father-daughter relationship and the personality development of the female. *Journal of Genetic Psychology,* 1970, **114,** 79–93.

Biller, H. B., & Zung, B. Perceived maternal control, anxiety, and opposite sex-role preference among elementary school girls. *Journal of Psychology,* 1972, **81,** 85–88.

Blanchard, R. W., & Biller, H. B. Father availability and academic performance among third-grade boys. *Developmental Psychology,* 1971, **4,** 301–305.

Bronfenbrenner, U. Some familial antecedents of responsibility and leadership in adolescents. In L. Petrullo & B. M. Bass (Eds.), *Leadership and interpersonal behavior.* New York: Holt, Rinehart and Winston, 1961.

Bronfenbrenner, U. The psychological costs of quality and equality in education. *Child Development,* 1967, **38,** 909–925.

Burton, R. V., & Whiting, J. W. M. The absent father and cross-sex identity. *Merrill-Palmer Quarterly,* 1961, **7,** 85–95.

Carlsmith, L. Effect of early father-absence on scholastic aptitude. *Harvard Educational Review,* 1964, **34,** 3–21.

Cobliner, W. G. Social factors in mental disorders: A contribution to the etiology of mental illness. *Genetic Psychology Monographs,* 1963, **67,** 151–215.

Crane, A. R. A note on pre-adolescent gangs. *Australian Journal of Psychology,* 1951, **3,** 43–46.

Dai, B. Some problems of personality development among Negro children. In C. Kluckhohn, H. A. Murray, & D. M. Schneider (Eds.), *Personality in nature, society, and culture.* New York: Knopf, 1953.

Davids, A. A research design for studying maternal emotionality before childbirth and after social interaction with the child. *Merrill-Palmer Quarterly,* 1968, **14,** 345–354.

Davids, A. *Abnormal children and youth: Therapy and research.* New York: Wiley-Interscience, 1972.

Davids, A., & DeVault, S. Maternal anxiety during pregnancy and childbirth abnormalities. *Psychosomatic Medicine,* 1962, **24,** 464–470.

Davids, A., & Hainsworth, P. D. Maternal attitudes about family life and child-rearing as avowed by mothers and perceived by their underachieving sons. *Journal of Consulting Psychology,* 1967, **31,** 29–37.

Davids, A., Joelson, M., & McArthur, C. Rorschach and TAT indices of homosexuality in overt homosexuals, neurotics, and normal males. *Journal of Abnormal and Social Psychology,* 1956, **53,** 161–172.

Despert, L. J. The fatherless family. *Child Study,* 1957, **34,** 22–28.

Deutsch, M. Minority group and class status as related to social and personality factors in scholastic achievement. *Monograph of the Society for Applied Anthropology,* 1960, **2,** 1–32.

Dinitz, S., Dynes, R. R., & Clarke, A. C. Preferences for male or female children: Traditional or affectional. *Marriage and Family Living,* 1954, **16,** 128–130.

Farina, A. Patterns of role dominance and conflict in parents of schizophrenic patients. *Journal of Abnormal and Social Psychology,* 1960, **61,** 31–38.

Fenichel, O. *The psychoanalytic theory of neurosis.* New York: Norton, 1945.

Fish, K. D., & Biller, H. B. Perceived childhood paternal relationships and college females' personal adjustment. *Adolescence,* 1973, in press.

Forrest, T. The paternal roots of male character development. *The Psychoanalytic Review,* 1967, **54,** 81–99.

Freudenthal, K. Problems of the one-parent family. *Social Work,* 1959, **4,** 44–48.

Garbower, G. *Behavior problems of children in Navy officers' families: As related to social conditions of Navy family life.* Washington, D.C.: Catholic University Press, 1959.

Gardner, G. G. The relationship between childhood neurotic symptomatology and later schizophrenia in males and females. *Journal of Nervous and Mental Disease,* 1967, **144,** 97–100.

Glasser, P., & Navarre, E. Structural problems of the one-parent family. *Journal of Social Issues,* 1965, **21,** 98–109.

Glueck, S., & Glueck, E. *Unravelling juvenile delinquency.* New York: Commonwealth Fund, 1950.

Gregory, I. Anterospective data following childhood loss of a parent: I. Delinquency and high school drop-out. *Archives of General Psychiatry,* 1965, **13,** 99–109. (a)

Gregory, I. Anterospective data following childhood loss of a parent: II. Pathology, performance, and potential among college students. *Archives of General Psychiatry,* 1965, **13,** 110–120. (b)

Grunebaum, M. G., Hurwitz, I., Prentice, N. M., & Sperry, B. M. Fathers of sons with primary neurotic learning inhibition. *American Journal of Orthopsychiatry,* 1962, **32,** 462–473.

Gundlach, R. H. Childhood parental relationships and the establishment of gender roles of homosexuals. *Journal of Consulting and Clinical Psychology,* 1969, **33,** 136–139.

Hamilton, D. M., & Wahl, J. G. The hospital treatment of dementia praecox. *American Journal of Psychiatry,* 1948, **105,** 346–352.

Heckel, R. V. The effects of fatherlessness on the pre-adolescent female. *Mental Hygiene,* 1963, **47,** 69–73.

Heckscher, R. T. Household structure and achievement orientation in lower-class Barbadian families. *Journal of Marriage and the Family,* 1967, **29,** 521–526.

Helper, M. M. Learning theory and the self-concept. *Journal of Abnormal and Social Psychology,* 1955, **51,** 184–194.

Hetherington, E. M. A developmental study of the effects of sex of the dominant parent on sex-role preference, identification, and imitation in children. *Journal of Personality and Social Psychology,* 1965, **2,** 188–194.

Hetherington, E. M., & Frankie, G. Effects of parental dominance, warmth, and conflict on imitation in children. *Journal of Personality and Social Psychology,* 1967, **6,** 119–125.

Hilgard, J. R., Neuman, M. F., & Fisk, F. Strength of adult ego following bereavement. *American Journal of Orthopsychiatry,* 1960, **30,** 788–798.

Hoffman, L. W. The father's role in the family and the child's peer-group adjustment. *Merrill-Palmer Quarterly,* 1961, **7,** 97–105.

Hoffman, M. L. Father-absence and conscience development. *Developmental Psychology,* 1971, **4,** 400–406.

Holman, P. Some factors in the etiology of maladjustment in children. *Journal of Mental Science,* 1953, **99,** 654–688.

Kardiner, A., & Ovesey, L. *The mark of oppression.* New York: Norton, 1951.

Kaye, H. E. Homosexuality in women. *Archives of General Psychiatry,* 1967, **17,** 626–634.

Kayton, R., & Biller, H. B. Perception of parental sex-role behavior and psychopathology in adult males. *Journal of Consulting and Clinical Psychology,* 1971, **36,** 235–237.

Kayton, R., & Biller, H. B. Sex role development and psychopathology in adult males. *Journal of Consulting and Clinical Psychology,* 1972, **38,** 208–210.

Kimball, B. The sentence completion technique in a study of scholastic underachievement. *Journal of Consulting Psychology,* 1952, **16,** 353–358.

King, C. E. The Negro maternal family: A product of an economic and cultural system. *Social Forces,* 1945, **24,** 100–104.

Koch, M. B. Anxiety in preschool children from broken homes. *Merrill-Palmer Quarterly,* 1961, **1,** 225–231.

Kriesberg, L. Rearing children for educational achievement in fatherless families. *Journal of Marriage and the Family,* 1967, **29,** 288–301.

Lazowick, L. M. On the nature of identification. *Journal of Abnormal and Social Psychology,* 1955, **51,** 175–183.

Lerner, S. H. Effect of desertion on family life. *Social Casework,* 1954, **35,** 3–8.

Levy, D. M. *Maternal overprotection.* New York: Columbia University Press, 1943.

Lidz, R. W., & Lidz, T. The family environment of schizophrenic patients. *American Journal of Psychiatry,* 1949, **106,** 332.

Lidz, T., Parker, N., & Cornelison, R. R. The role of the father in the family environment of the schizophrenic patient. *American Journal of Psychiatry,* 1956, **13,** 126–132.

Loeb, J., & Price, J. R. Mother and child personality characteristics related to parental marital status in child guidance cases. *Journal of Consulting Psychology,* 1966, **30,** 112–117.

Lynn, D. B., & Sawrey, W. L. The effects of father-absence on Norwegian boys and girls. *Journal of Abnormal and Social Psychology,* 1959, **59,** 258–262.

MacDonald, M. W. Criminal behavior in passive, effeminate boys. *American Journal of Orthopsychiatry,* 1938, **8,** 70–78.

Madow, L., & Hardy, S. W. Incidence and analysis of the broken family in the background of neurosis. *American Journal of Orthopsychiatry,* 1947, **17,** 521–528.

McClelland, D. C. *The achieving society.* New Jersey: Van Nostrand, 1961.

McClelland, D. C., & Watt, N. F. Sex role alienation in schizophrenia. *Journal of Abnormal Psychology,* 1968, **73,** 226–239.

McCord, J., McCord, W., & Thurber, E. Some effects of paternal absence on male children. *Journal of Abnormal and Social Psychology,* 1962, **64,** 361–369.

Meerloo, J. A. M. The father cuts the cord: The role of the father as initial transference figure. *American Journal of Psychotherapy,* 1956, **10,** 471–480.

Miller, W. B. Lower-class culture as a generating milieu of gang delinquency. *Journal of Social Issues,* 1958, **14,** 5–19.

Mischel, W. Father-absence and delay of gratification. *Journal of Abnormal and Social Psychology,* 1961, **62,** 116–124.

Mitchell, D., & Wilson, W. Relationship of father-absence to masculinity and popularity of delinquent boys. *Psychological Reports,* 1967, **20,** 1173–1174.

Moulton, P. W., Burnstein, E., Liberty, D., & Altucher, N. The patterning of parental affection and dominance as a determinant of guilt and sex-typing. *Journal of Personality and Social Psychology,* 1966, **4,** 363–365.

Moynihan, D. P. *The Negro family: The case for national action.* Washington, D.C.: United States Department of Labor, 1965.

Mussen, P. H., & Rutherford, E. Parent-child relationships and parental personality in relation to young children's sex-role preferences. *Child Development,* 1963, **34,** 589–607.

Mussen, P. H., Young, H. B., Godding, R., & Morante, L. The influence of father-son relationships on adolescent personality and attitudes. *Journal of Child Psychology and Psychiatry,* 1963, **4,** 3–16.

Nash, J. The father in contemporary culture and current psychological literature. *Child Development,* 1965, **36,** 261–297.

Neubauer, P. B. The one-parent child and his Oedipal development. *Psychoanalytic Studies of the Child,* 1960, **15,** 286–309.

Norton, A. Incidence of neurosis related to maternal age and birth order. *British Journal of Social Medicine,* 1952, **6,** 253–258.

O'Connor, P. J. Aetiological factors in homosexuality as seen in R. A. F. psychiatric practice. *British Journal of Psychiatry,* 1964, **110,** 381–391.

Oltman, J. E., McGarry, J. J., & Friedman, S. Parental deprivation and the "broken home" in dementia praecox and other mental disorders. *American Journal of Psychiatry,* 1952, **108,** 685–694.

Payne, D. E., & Mussen, P. H. Parent-child relations and father-identification among adolescent boys. *Journal of Abnormal and Social Psychology,* 1956, **52,** 358–362.

Pederson, F. A. Relationships between father-absence and emotional disturbance in male military dependents. *Merrill-Palmer Quarterly,* 1966, **12,** 321–331.

Pettigrew, T. F. *A profile of the Negro American.* Princeton: Van Nostrand, 1964.

Reuter, M., and Biller, H. Perceived paternal nurturance—Availability and personality adjustment among college males. *Journal of Consulting and Clinical Psychology,* 1973, in press.

Rexford, E. N. Antisocial young children and their families. In M. R. Haworth (Ed.), *Child psychotherapy,* New York: Basic Books, 1964.

Rohrer, J. H., & Edmonson, M. S. *The eighth generation.* New York: Harper, 1960.

Schlesinger, B. The one-parent family: An overview. *Family Life Coordinator,* 1966, **15,** 133–137.

Sears, P. S. Child-rearing factors related to playing of sex-typed roles. *American Psychologist,* 1953, **8,** 431 (Abstract).

Sears, R. R., Pintler, M. H., & Sears, P. S. Effect of father-separation on pre-school children's doll-play aggression. *Child Development,* 1946, **17,** 219–243.

Sears, R. R., Rau, L., & Alpert, R. *Identification and child rearing.* Stanford: Stanford University Press, 1965.

Seward, G. H. *Sex and the social order.* New York: McGraw-Hill, 1946.

Siegman, A. W. Father-absence during childhood and antisocial behavior. *Journal of Abnormal Psychology,* 1966, **71,** 71–74.

Sopchak, A. L. Parental "identification" and tendency toward disorder as measured by the MMPI. *Journal of Abnormal and Social Psychology,* 1952, **47,** 159–165.

Stendler, C. B. Possible causes of overdependency in young children. *Child Development,* 1954, **25,** 125–146.

Stephens, W. N. *The Oedipus complex: Cross-cultural evidence.* Glencoe, Ill.: Free Press, 1962.

Stoller, R. J. *Sex and gender.* New York: Science House, 1968.

Stolz, L. M. *Father relations of war-born children.* Stanford: Stanford University Press, 1954.

Suedfield, P. Paternal absence and overseas success of Peace Corps volunteers. *Journal of Consulting Psychology,* 1967, **31,** 424–425.

Thrasher, F. M. *The gang.* Chicago: University of Chicago Press, 1927.

Tiller, P. O. Father-absence and personality development of children in sailor families. *Nordisk Psyckologi's Monograph Series,* 1958, **9,** 1–48.

Trenaman, F. *Out of step.* London: Methuen, 1952.

Veroff, J., Atkinson, J., Feld, S., & Gurin, G. The use of thematic apperception to assess motivation in a nationwide interview study. *Psychological Monographs,* 1960, **74,** (Whole No. 499).

Wahl, C. W. Some antecedent factors in the family histories of 568 male schizophrenics of the U.S. Navy. *American Journal of Psychiatry,* 1956, **113,** 201–210.

West, D. J. Parental relationships in male homosexuality. *International Journal of Social Psychiatry,* 1959, **5,** 85–97.

West, D. J. *Homosexuality.* Chicago: Aldine, 1967.

Winch, R. F. The relation between loss of a parent and progress in courtship. *Journal of Social Psychology,* 1949, **29,** 51–56.

Winch, R. F. Some data bearing on the Oedipus hypothesis. *Journal of Abnormal and Social Psychology,* 1950, **45,** 481–489.

Wylie, H. L., & Delgado, R. A. A pattern of mother-son relationship involving the absence of the father. *American Journal of Orthopsychiatry,* 1959, **29,** 644–649.

5. Influence of Breast Feeding on Children's Behavior

Martin L. Heinstein

Breast feeding has at times been singled out as the royal road to successful mothering and mental health for the child. Freud, through his concept of orality, made the nursing experience of the infant a central issue in the study of personality. His clinical findings and speculations about oral gratification and deprivation have received a great deal of attention in the literature about child development.

Nevertheless, the effects of various nursing regimes on a child's physical and emotional development are still essentially unknown. Equally obscure are the influences which induce a mother to feed her child from the breast.

Reprinted with permission from *Children,* 1963, **10**, 93–97, Children's Bureau, Office of Child Development, U.S. Department of Health, Education, and Welfare.

Few facts have been established despite speculation dating back to Hippocrates and a considerable amount of recent research.

A decline in the proportion of mothers in this country who breast feed has been apparent over the past several decades, although significant geographic differences have been noted in the frequency of the practice.[1-3] Research carried on in the 1930's and 1940's showed mothers from lower socioeconomic groups undertaking breast feeding more frequently and weaning their children later than mothers with higher socioeconomic status. Some recent studies indicate that these differences may now no longer exist or may even have been reversed.[4] [5]

Much of the research about the influence of breast feeding on child development has suffered from some obvious defects. None of the studies have attempted to evaluate the personality of the mother doing the feeding as well as the type of feeding being done. Nor have the studies taken into account the possibility that a tense, breast-feeding mother may present a more disturbing environment for an infant than a relatively relaxed, bottle-feeding mother. Furthermore, few, if any, studies have looked for possible differences in reactions on the part of male and female children, or to possible variability of response with the age of the child. Behavior disturbances apparent at the time of weaning may not be present at subsequent stages of development.

Studies have usually relied too heavily on retrospective data. Reports from mothers several years later on how they fed their babies and their children's later reactions are likely to be unreliable. Moreover, investigators have usually studied only special groups, such as middle-class families or children being treated at a clinic. Few studies have used samples representative enough of the general population to permit broad deductions.

The study to be reported upon here made use of longitudinal data collected on a representative sample of children—a sub-sample of every third child born in Berkeley, Calif., from January 1, 1928, to June 30, 1929. The data covered a period from the birth of the child to 18 years of age. Behavior problems of the children during the preschool period, middle childhood, and adolescence were looked at in relation to whether or not the children were breast fed, the length of their nursing experience (whether from breast or bottle, or both), and the family atmosphere during the nursing period.

The term *nursing* will be used in this article, as it was in the study, to refer to the period of breast and bottle feeding, or both. *Length of nursing* was determined by fixing the time at which the child was weaned to the cup.

The 47 boys and 47 girls in the sample had been studied intensively for physical, mental, and personality development by the Institute of Human Development at the University of California, Berkeley. Data were also available on the general characteristics of the parents, the mother's relations to the child, and the socioeconomic status of the family. Testing and intensive, open-ended interviews had been conducted periodically over the 18-year period. The sample and program of data collection have been described in previous publications.[6]

Study Variables

The main variables considered in this study were: (1) breast feeding without supplementary nursing; (2) length of nursing; (3) the warmth of the mother toward the child; (4) the nervous stability of the mother; (5) the marital adjustment of the parents; (6) and the behavior problems of the child. The warmth of the mother was determined by a combined average rating of the mother's closeness to the child, general friendliness, and expressiveness of affection toward her child.

The behavior of the child was evaluated both from reports of the mother, starting when the child was 21 months old, and interviews with the child starting when he was 6 years old. Ratings on behavior problems such as temper tantrums, thumb-sucking, fears, and enuresis were used for the preschool period and middle childhood. The results of projective testing by the Thematic Apperception and Rorschach tests were the basis for behavior assessment in late childhood and adolescence. Ratings of the personalities of the parents, their relations to each other and to their children were based on the reports of the intensive interviews.

While no other studies to date have looked into the joint influence of the mother's personality and the nursing process on the child's behavior, a number have focused on the characteristics of mothers who did and of those who did not breast feed. Some of these studies have been based in part on the supposition that the mother's personality and her feelings toward the child are related to her decision to breast feed or not. For example, Levy at one time maintained that weaning was an index of maternal rejection.[7]

On the other hand, two studies[8] [9] reported 16 years apart found no evidence that breast feeding was related to whether the mother wanted the child or to the degree of warmth of the mother toward the child. One of them, however, indicated "that breast feeding probably does have some special implications for quite a good many mothers, and that those who have a strong sense of modesty or anxiety about sex, in general, may avoid breast feeding."[9] Another study found that the "biologic type" of mother prefers to breast feed and to avoid a rigid schedule, while the "modern urban type" tends to bottle feed on a rigid schedule.[10]

In the present study, none of the variables used to define the mother-child relations or the general family atmosphere was found to be significantly related to breast feeding. For example, factors such as the warmth of the mother toward the child or the marital adjustment of the parents were not associated with breast feeding or with the duration of breast feeding. Thus the data can hardly be interpreted as representing evidence that breast feeding is a reliable measure of maternal acceptance of the child.

The socioeconomic status of the family, however, was associated with the duration of breast feeding. For both boys and girls, the lower the socioeconomic status of the family, the older the age of the child at weaning from the breast.

The relationship of lower socioeconomic status with longer duration of breast feeding is consistent with the results of other studies using breast-feeding data from about the same period (1928–29). As already mentioned, more recent investigations tend to indicate no differences in this respect between social classes while some studies report longer or more breast feeding by middle-class mothers. Possibly the recent rise in the proportion of mothers from lower socioeconomic groups who are working outside the home has decreased the opportunity for breast feeding among them. At the same time, the emphasis in pediatric and child development publications on the psychological benefits of breast feeding for the child has probably been influential in fostering positive attitudes toward breast feeding among middle-class mothers. The relatively greater decline of breast feeding among mothers of the lower socioeconomic levels may also mean, at least in part, that these mothers have reached standards of child care followed by middle-class mothers several decades ago.

Health and Behavior Problems

The study gave no evidence of breast feeding being positively related to favorable growth or general health of the child. On the contrary, length of breast feeding for both boys and girls correlated negatively with the rate at which the children reached various heights—one index of maturation. Four of six overall health ratings also correlated negatively with breast feeding. The health ratings were based on periodic physical examinations and frequency of illness. The study was not designed, however, to answer specific questions about the relation of breast feeding to health.

The study also failed to reveal significant differences in incidence of problem behavior between breast-fed or bottle-fed children—whether boys or girls. The findings of previous studies are noticeably inconsistent in this respect. In four studies, children who had been breast fed for 4 to 10 months were better adjusted than children who had been breast fed shorter or longer periods. Three studies reported that the later the weaning from the breast the fewer the behavior problems. Two other studies, in direct contrast to the first four mentioned, indicated that the best adjustment was among subjects breast fed for very short periods or not at all, or for a long period (11 or 12 months). Four other investigations found no significant differences in behavior according to the length of breast feeding.[11]

Parental Factors and Nursing

Psychologists who are influenced by learning theory and psychiatrists who place more emphasis on interpersonal transactions than on libidinal drives have regarded the personal-social environment of the child as fundamentally more important than a particular nursing regime. They have maintained that positive, early relationships of the child with the parents, particularly the mother, are likely to carry over to other later interpersonal relations.

The results of this study revealed that in general the daughters of the more stable or of the warm mothers had fewer behavior problems. For boys, only the warmth of the mother was associated in any degree with positive behavior. The marital adjustment of the parents showed no noticeable association with the behavior of either boys or girls when this factor alone was considered in relation to behavior problems.

Findings based on such single factors in the child's environment as the warmth of the mother, her nervous stability, or the marital adjustment of the parents were not as pronounced as the associations apparent when both the parental characteristics and the nursing situation were considered at the same time. In fact, the results of this study seem to indicate that the interaction of the nursing and parental factors are more important for the adjustment of the child than either the nursing situation or parental characteristics taken separately.

While the nursing situation by itself did not seem to relate significantly to later behavior, it became a variable of importance when considered in connection with parental attributes, the sex of the child, and differences between the experience of breast feeding and length of nursing as such.

The most pronounced maladjustment shown in any group in the study was among boys who were nursed (on breast or bottle) for a long period of time (15 months or longer) by a *cold* mother (distant, hostile, inexpressive of affection). Length of nursing, when considered apart from the personal characteristics of the mother doing the nursing, was not associated with any noticeable behavioral disturbances. Furthermore, boys who were nursed for a long period of time by a *warm* mother tended to be relatively free from behavioral difficulties. What became evident was the effects of experiencing *both* long nursing and a cold mother at the same time.

Extended nursing in our culture may be regarded as a sign of continuing dependency needs on the part of the child. The mother who accepts or fosters these dependency needs, but at the same time has feelings of rejection toward the child, is obviously ambivalent and providing an atmosphere of conflict for the child. Such a mother is perhaps not truly nurturant, but may use the dependence of the child as a basis for maintaining hostile control.

Dependence in the first years of life is not likely to be maladaptive if it is expressed and met within the context of genuine feelings of nurturance on the part of the mother. The boys in this sample who were long-nursed by a cold mother were, in effect, experiencing oversolicitousness and hostility at the same time. Too much from a mother who in reality is able to give only too little is likely to result in confusion for the child.

Long nursing (weaned from the breast or bottle at 16 months or later) as such showed no significant overall association with behavior problems for girls, as it did for boys. However, when the results of the interaction between length of nursing and the maternal nervous stability were considered, girls who had a relatively unstable mother had fewer behavior problems when they were nursed for a long period of time. A shorter total nursing period was the most favorable duration when the mother was more stable.

Possibly mothers unable to provide a generally stable atmosphere for their daughters are able to compensate by added solicitousness in the nursing area. The capacity of the girl to benefit from a longer period of nurturance through nursing may reflect cultural differences in our demands for independence from boys and girls. Girls may be able to receive reinforcement of dependency needs longer than boys without being subjected to conflicting expectations that they become more independent and aggressive. This, of course, is clearly speculative. Apparently, however, boys and girls experience length of nursing in different ways depending, in part, on variations in personal-social environment.

Breast Feeding and the Mother

What about the effects of breast feeding generally when considered along with the feelings of the mother doing the feeding? For boys, breast feeding did not appear to be significantly related to problem behavior even when considered in the context of mother-child relations at the time of nursing. Whether the mother was warm or cold in her feelings toward her son was not associated with noticeably different kinds of behavior. In other words, the interaction of breast feeding and the warmth of the mother was not significant except when length of nursing was taken into account.

Girls, however, developed fewer behavioral difficulties if breast fed by a warm mother. However, those whose mothers were distant, unfriendly, and inexpressive of affection did better if bottle fed.

It is not unreasonable to suppose that the mother who breast feeds her daughter without real warmth provides an ambivalent and potentially more disturbing environment for her—a situation similar to the one experienced by boys fed by a long nursing, cold mother. The close, intense relationship between mother and daughter implied in breast feeding apparently should be part of a more generally warm mother-child relationship in order to effect lasting psychological benefits for the child. Where technical nurturance represents only a formal expression of love or when it occurs with feelings of rejection, the resulting confusion for the child again appears to be associated with behavior problems.

Why boys were unfavorably affected by the *long-nursing* situation with a cold mother and girls by *breast feeding* with a cold mother is not readily apparent. The ambivalence present in both of these general conditions, however, is clear.

The fact that behavioral difficulties seem to be generated by the long nursing-cold mother experience of the boys in this study and the breast feeding-cold mother situation of the girls has some relevance for the "double bind" theory of Bateson and associates.[12] It also has implications for Harlow's[13] findings on the importance of cuddling.

The main ingredients of the double bind, as described by Bateson, consist of two or more people in a repeated experience from which one, the victim, has no escape. The victim receives a primary negative (or positive) injunction which is in conflict with a more abstract secondary injunction. Thus the boys in this study who experienced a long nursing period with a cold mother were caught in a relationship in which the mother was expressing two orders of message, one of which denied the other. Technically, the long nursing or the breast feeding expressed a formal manifestation of nurturance or love, which was contradicted by a communication of the mother's feelings of hostility and lack of closeness.

Harlow's early work suggests the possibility that the amount and kind of cuddling the infant receives are more important psychologically than the nursing experience. While some of the evidence from the study described here indicated that the warmth and nervous stability of the mother as single factors in the child's early experience were more important than the nursing situation, the pattern of both factors together, nursing and the mother's personality, seemed to be the most decisive influence.

Implications of the Study

The results of this study point to the dangers of making oversimplified recommendations in relation to specific child-rearing procedures without consideration of the family atmosphere in which these procedures are to take place. Breast feeding or long nursing are not efficacious *per se*. In each instance, we must ask who the nursing mother is and what the other relevant factors in the home environment are which impinge on the nursing experience of the child.

Further evidence supporting these observations may be gained from the study's findings in relation to thumb-sucking. Freud used thumb-sucking as a model for explaining the erogenous nature of the oral zone. As a result thumb-sucking has become a diagnostic sign for insufficient sucking satisfaction, disturbed emotional development, troubled mother-child relations, and a host of other ills. Levy, for example, has stated that the main cause of finger sucking is insufficient sucking at the breast or bottle.[14]

The greatest incidence of thumb-sucking in this study occurred among girls who were breast fed by mothers who had achieved a good marital adjustment and who were also judged better than average in regard to nervous stability. Not only are the results the reverse of what would be theoretically expected, but, again, the interaction of two factors, the breast feeding and the parental characteristics, was more significant than the effects of either variable considered separately.

Moreover, the results in this study and in two additional investigations based on large, representative samples of children, thumb-sucking was negatively correlated with other behavior problems in the pre-school period. The thumb-sucking girl tended to come from a breast-feeding, stable environment, and girls and boys who as preschoolers sucked their thumbs were less likely than others to have other behavior problems.

Perhaps the most important conclusions of this study relate to the several methodological considerations raised in the early part of this article. Apparently sex differences *are* an important factor in evaluating the behavioral correlates of the nursing experience. Also, the pattern of the child's nursing experience within the context of varying personal-social conditions seems to provide a more decisive view of the child's emotional adjustment than do single factors, be they the nursing experience or particular characteristics of the parents.

The zeal of some people in trying to foster breast feeding or a particular child-rearing technique may derive from an oversimplified interpretation of psychoanalytic theory or a long held idyllic picture of mother-infant oneness. It is perhaps wiser without more definitive knowledge to view nursing as one aspect of the total life space of the infant or child. While the results of this study must also be viewed with caution, they do seem clear enough to raise serious doubts about some of the current *ex cathedra* pronouncements which appear on the topic of breast feeding or baby nursing in general.

References

1. Bronfenbrenner, U.: Socialization and social class through time and space. *In* Readings in social psychology. (E. E. Maccoby et al., eds.) Holt, Rinehart, and Winston, New York. 1958.
2. Meyer, H. F.: Breast feeding in the United States: extent and possible trend. *Pediatrics,* July 1958.
3. Robertson, W. O.: Breast feeding practices: some implications of regional variation. *American Journal of Public Health,* July 1961.
4. White, Martha S.: Social class, child rearing practices, and child behavior. *American Sociological Review,* December 1957.
5. Bock, W. E.; Lawson E. D.; Yankauer, A.; Sussman, M. B.: Social class, maternal health, and child care. New York State Department of Health, Albany. 1957.
6. Macfarlane, Jean W.: Studies in child guidance. I. Methodology of data collection and organization. *Monographs of the Society for Research in Child Development,* 1938.
7. Levy, D. M.: Maternal overprotection. Columbia University Press, New York. 1943.
8. Peterson, G. H.; Spano F.: Breast feeding, maternal rejection, and child personality. *Character and Personality,* September 1941.
9. Sears, R. R.; Maccoby, E. E.; Levin H.: Patterns of child rearing. Row, Peterson and Co., New York. 1957.
10. Newton, N. R.; Newton, M.: Relationship of ability to breast feed and maternal attitudes toward breast feeding. *Journal of Pediactrics,* May 1950.
11. Heinstein, M.: Behavioral correlates of breast-bottle regimes under varying parent-infant relationships. *Monographs of the Society for Research in Child Development.* In press.
12. Bateson, G.; Jackson, D. D.; Haley, J.; Weakland, J.: Toward a theory of schizophrenia. *Behavioral Science,* October 1956.
13. Harlow, H. F.: The nature of love. *American Psychologist,* December 1958.
14. Levy, D. M.: Finger sucking from the psychiatric angle. *Child Development,* March 1937.

6. A Reinterpretation of the Direction of Effects in Studies of Socialization

Richard Q. Bell

It is not too surprising to find that most research on parent-child interaction has been directed to the question of effects of parents on children. The historian Palmer (1964) maintains that our political and social philosophy emerged in a period when there were many revolutionary or protorevolutionary movements ranging from the Carolinas to Sweden, movements directed not just against monarchical absolutism but against all constituted bodies such as parliaments, councils, assemblies, and magistracies. These institutions tended to be hereditary, either in theory or through firmly established practice. In taking a strong stand against hereditary determination of position in our society we have also stressed the malleability and susceptibility to improvement of the child. Although scientific research on parents and children is a fairly recent phenomenon, it still shows the primary influence of this broad social philosophy by emphasizing parents and educational institutions as determinants of human development.

Until recent years there have been very few findings which would indicate that this is not a fruitful approach. The prolonged helplessness of the human infant, in comparison to the early competence of some other animal infants, fits in with the picture of an organism designed to be taught and modified by the parent in the early years. It seems eminently plausible to visualize the human parent as the vehicle for the transmission of culture and the infant as simply the object of an acculturation process. The parent is the initial agent of culture, the child the object.

Because of this general view, it is often overlooked that even John Locke, to whom we are indebted for the concept of the infant as a tabula rasa, placed great emphasis in his advice to parents on early observation of congenital characteristics (Kessen, 1965, p. 67). Locke questioned the existence of innate ideas, not all innate characteristics. Currently, at least one major work on the socialization of the child has acknowledged that there are probably constitutional differences between children which affect behavior (Sears, Maccoby, & Levin, 1957, 454–455), and that the model of a unidirectional effect from parent to child is overdrawn, a fiction of convenience rather than belief (Sears et al., 1957, p. 141). The model was adopted in order to proceed with research, leaving the validity of the approach to be judged by the results.

From *Psychological Review*, 1968, **75**, 81–95. Copyright 1968 by the American Psychological Association and reproduced by permission.

This paper summarizes data indicating that a unidirectional approach is too imprecise and that another formulation is possible which would accommodate our social philosophy as well as new data from studies of man and other animals. Before proceeding, usage of two terms must be explained. Individual behavior sequences cannot be referred to as exclusively genetically or experientially determined. It is possible, however, to employ experimental operations in such a way that a *difference* between two groups or between two conditions applied to the same subjects can be attributed to genetic or experiential differences. Thus the terms *genetically, congenitally,* or *experientially determined* are abstractions derived from experimental operations. For brevity, a *congenital effect* will refer to both genetic and congenital determination.

The same consideration applies to the question of whether parent and child effects can be separated. In the ordinary interaction of any parent and child we can speak only of an event sequence. However, by experimental operations we can isolate parent effects and child effects. In the remainder of this paper a child or parent effect will refer to such a derivative of an experimental operation. No implication about origin of the behavior need be drawn in this case since such studies can take as their starting point any behavior which is available at the time in the repertoire of parent or child.

We must also keep in mind that demonstration of a child effect indicates only that it plays *some* role in parent behavior. The development of the parent behavior is not explained by such a demonstration. In the same vein, Epstein (1964) has pointed out relative to studies of learning that evidence of the modifiability of a response provides no explanation of its origin.

Recent Data Discordant with Parent-Effect Model

Discordant data at the human level are still meager. This is because most research efforts have been directed to the task of testing parent effects and have not always been designed so as to permit clear interpretation of "negative" results. It will be necessary to rely upon informal observations and data generated unintentionally.

Rheingold (1966, pp. 12-13) has pointed to a compelling fact observable under ordinary circumstances in any human group containing an infant. "The amount of attention and the number of responses directed to the infant are enormous—out of all proportion to his age, size, and accomplishments." The effect of the appearance of helplessness and the powerful stimulus of distress cries were also noted. "So aversive, especially to humans, is the crying of the infant that there is almost no effort we will not expend, no device we will not employ, to change a crying baby into a smiling one—or just a quiet one."

Studies of variations in parental behavior with different children provide one other kind of data discordant with a parent-effect model. A mother of identical schizophrenic quadruplets was found to be uniformly extreme in restrictiveness with her daughters but not uniform in affection when rated against a theoretical normal group (Schaefer, 1963). Yarrow (1963, pp. 109–110) has reported that the same foster mother showed differences in behavior with infants assigned to her at different times. In one particularly dramatic case extreme differences in maternal care existed for two infants of the same sex and age assigned to a foster mother at the same time. Characteristics of the infants appeared to have evoked very different behavior in this foster mother and in other members of her family.

Reports of lack of uniformity of behavior of parents towards their children are not confined to intensive case studies. Stott (1941) reported a correlation of only .22 between sibling reports of a positive or negative home environment. Lasko (1954, p. 111) correlated maternal characteristics across 44 sibling pairs and found that mothers were not consistent in affection but were in restrictiveness, a finding which is in agreement with the report on the quadruplets. In a parent-effect model, it is easy to explain differences between the behavior of two parents with the same child, but awkward to accommodate a difference in the behavior of one parent toward two children. The latter difficulty is due to the fact that the parent-effect model assumes a fixed and invariantly applied repertoire. The usual method of explaining differences in behavior of a parent with different children is to postulate effects associated with ordinal position or sex of siblings. The reports on infants in foster homes could not be explained this way.

Levy (1958, p. 8) was unable to find consistency in maternal greeting behavior when the infant was brought from the nursery for a feeding, until it was noted that this behavior was a function of the state of the infant. The present author carried out separate chi-square analyses of Levy's data for each of three successive observations. There were no differences on the initial observation, but for the second and third observations it was found that infants awake or awakening were greeted, whereas those asleep were not ($p < .01$; $p < .05$, respectively). Other data in the same volume support Levy's contention that specific maternal behavior could be accounted for more by the infant's behavior than by the mother's general "maternal attitude," whether the latter was estimated from interview material or from actual observation of her behavior. Another finding with a similar implication was reported by Hillenbrand (1965). The amount the infant consumed in breast-feeding during the newborn period was highly correlated with the number of weeks the mother continued feeding at the breast, whereas the latter measure showed no correlation with personality characteristics of the mother.

One other study at the human level is best accommodated by a bidirectional model (Bell, 1964). Scores on one parent-attitude scale have been found consistently higher in mothers of children with congenital defects than in mothers of normals. Differences between groups of parents were ascribed to the effects on parents of a limitation in coping ability associated with the congenital disorder in affected children.

Research on lower animals provides stronger evidence of the stimulating and selective effect of the young. A volume edited by Rheingold (1963) covers maternal behavior from the deer mouse to the baboon and provides a number of observations on the importance of the young in shaping interactions. An example is the report of two instances in which the clinging of rhesus infants fostered with nonlactating females induced maternal responsiveness and biochemically normal lactation (pp. 268–269). In other studies offspring effects have been manipulated experimentally. Lactation in the rat has been maintained for long periods by supplying new litters of pups; number and age of pups were effective parameters (Bruce, 1961). Licking and nest-building occurred when 1-day-old pups were presented to female mice without previous experience; short-term stimulus-specific decrements in the maternal response followed repeated presentation of 1-day-old pups, but recovery of response was shown to an older pup (Noirot, 1965). This study is the most recent in a series supporting the hypothesis that changes in the interest of the female mouse in the litter from birth to weaning depend mainly upon changes in stimuli coming from the young.

It has been shown by cross-fostering that pups from one strain of mice induced more retrieving and licking behavior than pups from another strain (Ressler, 1962). The open-field behavior of rat foster mothers has shown effects of the experience of rearing pups subjected to direct treatments such as shock (Dennenberg, 1963), or indirect treatments such as subjecting their true mothers to premating and gestational stress (Joffe, 1965).

In a classic study, Beach and Jaynes (1956) manipulated appearance and behavior of offspring so as to identify specific classes of stimuli controlling parent behavior. Visual, olfactory, tactile, thermal, and movement cues from rat pups were shown to be capable of inducing maternal retrieving, being effective individually and in combination.

It is evident from the foregoing brief review that students of animal behavior have been much more aware of offspring effects on parents than investigators of human parent-child interaction; this more comprehensive view of parent-offspring interaction may be a simple consequence of availability; all phases of development are accessible to direct observation and manipulation. It is also possible that our political and social philosophy has limited scientific outlook at the human more than the animal level. The animal mother is not seen as an agent of socialization, nor her offspring as a tabula rasa.

There are many implications of this research on animal behavior. For the present purpose two are most salient. If variations in offspring behavior affect animal parents from which we expect fairly rigid patterns, even greater effects would be expected on human parental behavior, which is presumably more plastic and susceptible to all classes of influence. The other point is brought out by the variety of offspring stimulus parameters being opened up by animal studies; it should not be difficult to accept the notion of offspring effects if we consider the fact that offspring are at least sources of stimuli. Some stimulus control of human parental behavior should be expected since we take for granted the general likelihood of finding stimulus control over behavior in general.[1]

[1]The author is indebted to Leon J. Yarrow for suggesting this point.

Modifiers of Parent Response

Congenital Determinants

Three propositions concerning congenital determinants of later behavior will be advanced in this section. Some studies of human subjects will be cited which provide relatively clear evidence. Only reasonable inferences can be made from others. All in all, these studies suggest but by no means document the propositions which are advanced concerning child effects. The present objective is to take the first steps toward developing an alternative to existing socialization theory. A limited scheme which is merely plausible and parsimonious will serve the purpose. Provisional acceptance of this scheme will make it possible to provide concrete illustrations of how some recent findings in the research literature may be reinterpreted.

It will first be assumed that there are congenital contributors to human assertiveness, which will be taken to mean maintenance of goal-directed behavior of high magnitude in the face of barriers. Reasoning, threat of withdrawal of love, and appeals to personal and social motives can all be used to arrest ongoing child behavior in excess of parental standards, providing the child is not extreme in assertiveness. With a child who is strongly assertive a parent may more often fall back on quick tangible reinforcement or nonreinforcement. At times when the child, the parent, or both are stressed, the parent falls back further to distraction, holding, frightening verbalization, and physical punishment. The foregoing effects on parent behavior also are considered likely to issue from the behavior of hyperactive, erratic, and unpredictable children, and it is assumed that there are congenital determinants of this kind of behavior as well.

It is further assumed that a different kind of behavior is shown by parents of children congenitally low in assertiveness, activity, or sensory-motor capability. Drawing attention to stimuli, rewarding an increase in behavior, urging, prompting, and demanding are examples of parent response to these child characteristics.

It is also assumed that there are congenital contributors to differences in person orientation. Children high in person orientation attend to the behavior of their parents and reinforce social responses emanating from them. Children low in person orientation induce less nurturance from parents, and their behavior is controlled less by variations in social response of parents. They are interested in physical activity and inanimate objects. Their stimulus characteristics primarily mobilize those elements in the parent nurturance repertoires pertaining to providing and withholding physical objects and activities. Since love-oriented control techniques are less useful with these children and material reinforcers cannot always be flexibly applied, their parents more frequently show further recourse to physical punishment.

Support for a congenital contribution to assertive behavior is seen in the finding that sex differences in socialization training are pronounced in primitive cultures in which large animals are hunted (Barry, Bacon, & Child, 1957). Furthermore, in all of the 224 primitive cultures surveyed by Murdock (1937), males were accorded roles involving fighting. Greater skeletal muscle development in males is probably an important factor, since even newborn males possess more muscle tissue, females more fat, relative to total body weight (Garn, 1958). It appears reasonable that some potential for use of muscles in physically assertive behavior can also be assumed. We would not expect the exclusive allocation of the fighting role to males if they possessed only greater skeletal muscle mass with no accompanying potential for use, or if there were equal distribution of this potential between the sexes. Males in our advanced societies do not carry spears, but it is improbable that our congenital dispositions have changed as rapidly as our cultural evolution. Even theoretical systems committed to the study of parent effects have acknowledged the probable existence of constitutional bases for sex differences in overt aggressiveness (Sears et al, 1957, p. 484).

One other line of evidence is from twin studies. Direct observation of monozygotic and dizygotic twins each month during the first year of life has shown significant heritability for an item from the Bayley Infant Behavior Profile labeled "goal directedness," which denotes absorption with a task until it is complete (Freedman, 1965). Vandenberg (1962) has pointed out that such twin contrasts in early infancy are more likely to detect genetic contributions than studies of children and adults because later social functioning shapes behavior in ways remote from the circumstances under which genetic selection took place. However, even in studies of school-age children which use the admittedly insensitive self-report questionnaires, significant heritability has been shown for groups of items interpreted as reflecting vigor (Vandenberg, 1962) and dominance (Gottesman, 1965).

Stronger evidence exists for a congenital contribution to person orientation; not only in the twin studies just cited but in several others summarized by Scarr (1965), heritability has been shown for social responsiveness or sociability, the findings cutting across age, sex, social class, and even cultural differences.

Some specific ways in which congenital factors may affect person orientation can be suggested on the basis of data from other studies. Schaffer and Emerson (1964) concluded that avoidance by some infants of being held, carried on the lap, stroked, or kissed was not accounted for by propensities of the mothers, but was due to the infant's restlessness and negative response to the restraint involved in these contacts. Infants who avoided contact showed lower intensity in later social contacts, though neither timing nor breadth of contacts was affected. There was a nonsignificant tendency for those who avoided early contacts to be males. The study is suggestive rather than conclusive because the sample of infants who avoided contacts was small.

Moss (1967) reports from day-long naturalistic observations in the home at 3 and 12 weeks that male infants were more irritable (crying, fussing), and slept less than females. This would mean that, on the average, the mother-son interaction was more one of physical caretaking, the mother being engaged in a variety of efforts to soothe males. Walters and Parke (1965) summarize evidence that the development of social response is relatively independent of the primary-drive reduction which might be expected to follow from such physical acts of care-taking. In fact, there are many reasons for expecting that greater irritability in the males would not favor development of social responses positively valued by parents (i.e., smiling, visual regard, noncrying vocalizations): (a) appearance of the mother at the time of crying could lead to an increase in the rate of crying, as reported for institutional infants by Etzel and Gewirtz (1967); (b) ministrations which follow the mother's appearance would necessarily contain some stimulation of an aversive nature, as in diaper changing or efforts to release ingested air, a point made by Rheingold (1966, p. 11); (c) nonaversive reinforcing elements in caretaking would be less likely to reinforce the infant's positively valued social responses since an irritable infant probably emits less of this behavior; (d) the mother would have less time available for purely social stimulation, and might simply wish to avoid the infant when he is quiet.

These possibilities are all consistent with Moss' (1967) finding that by the 12th week, mothers provided less stimulation of an interactional-social nature (imitation) for male than for female infants. It might also be argued that mothers imitated female infants more because of the earlier maturation of social responsiveness in females, an alternative explanation in congenital terms. Mothers could have begun differential sex-role training in social responsiveness sometime in the intervening period, but a ready explanation for initiating such training in just this period is not available. The data do not permit decisions on these different explanations, but the one selected for the present thesis seems at least as defensible as the others: Greater irritability in males led to less stimulation from mothers of the kind which should produce positively valued social responsiveness. This, in turn, may be extended developmentally using data from Bayley and Schaefer (1964, p. 44): Males were rated as less responsive to persons during 11 out of 12 developmental examinations between 10 and 36 months. Goodenough's (1957) report of sex differences in object and person orientation is typical of many other reports in the literature which indicate that males show less social orientation by the preschool period.

The research of Pasamanick, Robers, and Lilienfeld (1956) provides evidence that complications of pregnancy and delivery are associated with later behavior disorders of children, including hyperactive behavior, and that males are more frequently affected. The foregoing studies permit an inference that there is a congenital contributor to early response to social reinforcement. If hyperactive or restless infants do not respond as well as other infants to some of the early social reinforcers, it would be reasonable to expect that their later behavior would be controlled less adequately by use of love-oriented techniques which depend for their efficacy on the strength of the social bond. It could also be inferred that they would be less person-oriented, as a consequence of the less intense primary social bond.

Stechler (1964) lists a number of recent prospective studies which confirm the general validity of Pasamanick's approach, and reports his own finding that neonatal apnea was associated with low developmental quotients in the first 2 years of life. Higher irritability or crying during the newborn period and lower developmental quotients later in infancy have been reported for infants whose mothers reported fears or anxiety during pregnancy (Davids, Holden, & Gray, 1963; Ferreira, 1960; Ottinger & Simmons, 1964). We have already mentioned a study of congenital handicaps which limit sensory-motor development (Bell, 1964). Reports of congenital contributors to sensory-motor development are not limited to populations showing pathology. Kagan and Garn (1963) have reported that chest width measured from roentgenographic films of parents or their children is positively correlated with the children's perceptual-motor and language development in the preschool years.

To summarize, there is direct evidence of congenital factors contributing to two classes of child behavior which are likely to have very different effects on parents: impaired sensory-motor development, and behavior disorders involving hyperactivity. From twin studies there is evidence of a congenital contributor to person orientation and to facets of behavior which appear related to assertiveness. On the other hand, the evidence for congenital contributors to sex differences in person orientation and assertive behavior is mostly inferential. This is particularly true for assertive behavior: No relevant data on early development of sex differences could be located in the literature. In view of this, the arguments relative to assertiveness are merely advanced to indicate that congenital determination is at least reasonable. If we accept this, albeit provisionally, we can further assume that variation within the sexes on congenital grounds could also occur. Polygenetic rather than simple all-or-none determination would be favored by modern genetic theory.

Differentiation of Parent Response

Parents do not have fixed techniques for socializing children. They have a repertoire of actions to accomplish each objective. Furthermore, activation of elements in the repertoire requires both cultural pressures and stimulation from the object of acculturation. Characteristics that most infants and children share, such as helplessness, evoke responses.

Another major effect of the child is shown in the parent's selective performance of elements from the caretaking repertoire. It is assumed that there are hierarchies of actions, that different children induce responses from different parts of these hierarchies. Others escalate the actions of their parents so that at one time or another, or in sequence, the entire hierarchy relevant to a certain class of child behavior may be elicited. The child in turn reinforces or fails to reinforce the parent behavior which is evoked. The repertoire changes as a function of cultural demands and also as a result of stimulation and reinforcement received from the child.

Two types of parent control repertoires must be differentiated. *Upper-limit control behavior* reduces and redirects behavior of the child which exceeds parental standards of intensity, frequency, and competence for the child's age. *Lower-limit control behavior* stimulates child behavior which is below parental standards. In other words, parent control behavior, in a sense, is homeostatic relative to child behavior. To predict interaction in particular parent-child pairs it is necessary to know the behavior characteristics of the child, the cultural demands on the parent, and the parents' own individual assimilation of these demands into a set of expectations for the child. Nonetheless, for purposes of illustration we might say that the average parent would show an increase in upper-limit control behavior in response to excessive crying in the infant, or in response to impulsive, hyperactive, or overly competent or assertive behavior in the young child. These widely different behaviors are only considered similar with respect to their effect on upper-limit control. Parental lower-limit control behavior would be stimulated by lethargy in the infant, by low activity, overly inhibited behavior, and lack of competence in the young child. Again, these are different behaviors but are assumed to be similar in effect.

It is customary to observe or rate parental behavior without reference to stimulation provided by the young. When this is done, a parent showing extreme upper-limit behavior in several areas is likely to be described as "punitive," or "restrictive," one showing extreme lower-limit behavior as "intrusive," or "demanding." Both could be considered "controlling," but according to the present conceptual scheme designed to accommodate child effects, the history of preceding interaction sequences could be quite different. The need for differentiating these two types of control is indicated not only by the present theoretical considerations but also by the empirical findings that punitive and strict behavior is not correlated with intrusive and demanding behavior in parents of young children (Schaefer, 1959, p. 228).

Reinterpretation of Recent Literature

The child-effect system of explanation which has just been developed states that parent behavior is organized hierarchically within repertoires in the areas of social response and control. Reasonable bases exist for assuming that there are congenital contributors to child behaviors which *(a)* activate these repertoires, *(b)* affect the level of response within hierarchies, and *(c)* differentially reinforce parent behavior which has been evoked.

This system will be applied next to current findings in several major areas in which parent and experiential family effects on children have been given almost exclusive consideration. The findings in most cases are from recent studies which replicate or are consistent with previous studies, or in which results are more defensible than usual because of careful attention to sampling, procedural controls, and measurement. In most cases the authors of these papers were careful not to claim that causes and effects could be clearly differentiated. The question of direction of effects may be raised nonetheless, to ascertain whether the findings are relevant to the theory which motivated the research.

Though in the discussion which follows, the evidence is organized to support the validity of a child-to-parent effect, this should not be taken to mean that an "either-or" approach to the study of parent and child effects is preferred to an interactional view. This reinterpretation is only an expedient considered necessary to direct attention to the possibility of child effects. If this possibility is admitted we can then begin the task of thinking of parent *and* child effects. The primary goal of an expanded model of the socialization process is to uncover interactions of child and parent effects as well as main effects attributable to either source.

Lefkowitz, Walder, and Eron (1963) found in 8-year-olds that peer ratings of aggression were highest and parent reports of the child's use of confession lowest where use of physical punishment was reported by the parents. Bandura and Walters (1959) reported more physical punishment used in a group of male 15- to 16-year-old repeated offenders than in nondelinquents. One theory being tested in each case was that use of punishment in the home produces frustration and conflict or affords a model of aggression which in turn produces aggressive behavior in the child. An alternative explanation is that these children were congenitally assertive. Congenital assertiveness activated upper-limit control repertoires in parents and techniques within the repertoire were escalated toward physical punishment. Congenital hyperactivity could produce similar results.

Reviewing the area of moral development, Hoffman (1963) found consistent results in studies dealing with reaction to transgression. His interpretation was that an internalized moral orientation, indicated by confession, guilt, or reparation efforts, was fostered by an affectionate relation between the parent and child, in combination with disciplinary techniques which utilized this relation by appealing to the child's personal and social motives. One alternative explanation is that the children showing little internalization of a moral orientation were congenitally low in person orientation. Because of this their mothers were less affectionate and did not appeal to the child's personal or social values.

A study of sex-role development by Mussen and Rutherford (1963) reports findings which replicated those in a previous study. Boys 5–6 years old scoring high in masculinity on the IT test in comparison with lows, revealed high father nurturance, punishment, and power in doll play. A high power score indicated that father figures were both highly rewarding and punishing. These findings generously supported all major contending theories: developmental identification, defensive identification, and role-theory. A congenital explanation would be that the highs were more masculine in the sense that they showed lower person orientation and higher assertiveness. The father responded with affection because the son's assertiveness and interests in physical activity and toys were sex appropriate, reinforcing his own identification vicariously through his boy. Much as he felt affectionate toward his masculine boy he found he retreated to punishment frequently because the child, being assertive and less responsive to social stimuli, could not be controlled readily by love-oriented techniques.

In the area of intelligence, Bing (1963) found that mothers of children who showed higher verbal than spatial or numerical ability had a more close and demanding relation with their children both in interviews and observation situations than did mothers of children who showed discrepant nonverbal abilities. These findings confirmed the hypothesis that discrepant verbal ability is fostered by a close relation with a demanding and somewhat intrusive mother, discrepant nonverbal abilities being enhanced by allowing the child a considerable degree of freedom. An alternative explanation would be that the high-verbal children were high in person orientation and low in assertiveness. This is a reasonable combination of characteristics if one assumes that congenital determinants of assertiveness and person orientation are independent or at least not highly positively correlated. These children reinforced their mothers' social responses and elicited nurturant behavior. The resultant interaction intensified verbal expression because this is the primary channel of communication. The fact that these children were low in assertiveness led to lower-limit control behavior reflected in the mother's demanding and intrusive behavior.

Schaefer's (1959) summary of his own work and that of others indicates that a major portion of the variance in parent behavior can be accounted for under two dimensions described as love-hostility and autonomy-control. This is a useful finding, offering the possibility of descriptive parsimony, regardless of the question of direction of effects. However, the two-dimensional model might represent a system of effects of children on parents. The hostility extreme of the love-hostility dimension (strictness, punishment, perceiving the child as a burden) could be characterized as a parent upper-limit control pattern in response to overly assertive, unpredictable, or hyperactive behavior. The love extreme could reflect positive evaluation of children showing more modal behavior but not behavior extreme in the opposite direction.

In support of this we find in longitudinal data from the Berkeley Growth Study (Schaefer & Bayley, 1963) that calm children were evaluated positively by their mothers during the first 3 years. Children who were rapid and active were perceived as a burden during the first 15 months. The next set of measurements available for both mothers and children covered the period when the child was between 9 and 12 years. Mothers of children rated as rapid at this time were themselves rated as irritable and perceiving the child as a burden. No rating of calmness was available. A rating of the child's inactivity in this same period could not be considered a simple inverse of the activity rating made in the first 3 years, either from the standpoint of wording or correlation pattern across the sexes. If we assume that it primarily differentiated degree of inactivity running from the highly inactive to modal levels of activity, this rating becomes relevant to the autonomy versus control dimension.

The autonomy extreme of the autonomy-control dimension might reflect parents' granting autonomy to children who conform to parental expectations of capability and assertiveness. The control extreme (intrusiveness, anxiety, achievement demand, anxiety relative to the child's behavior and health) would be considered parental lower-limit control behavior in response to children low in assertiveness or sensory-motor capability. In support of this we find that mothers of male and female inactive children during the period 9–14 years were rated as intrusive and as high in achievement demand, but low in granting autonomy to the child. All relations cited from this study (Schaefer & Bayley, 1963) were consistent for both sexes and significant beyond the .05 level for combined male and female samples according to the present author's analysis of tabular material on pages 109–110 and 121–122. Data from earlier age periods could not be brought to bear on a child-effect interpretation of the autonomy-control dimension because of very differing relations between maternal and child behavior in mother-son versus mother-daughter pairs.

Social class differences in parent behavior may also be interpreted as influenced by child effects. According to Bronfenbrenner's (1958) analysis, middle-class parents show less use of physical punishment and more use of love-oriented techniques than lower-class parents. There was no clear evidence of a change in this finding in the period from 1932 to 1952, as there was for other child-rearing techniques. Complications of pregnancy and delivery are more frequent in the lower classes (Pasamanick & Knobloch, 1960), and on this basis we could expect more hyperactivity in children from lower-class samples. From the earlier discussions relative to hyperactivity we would expect to find in lower-class parents more upper-limit control behavior, of which physical punishment is a salient example, and less use of love-oriented techniques. It is clear that studies of social-class differences in the future should control for complications of pregnancy and delivery. Some class differences may be reduced in magnitude or altered qualitatively when the samples are made comparable with respect to complications of pregnancy and delivery.

Another area receiving considerable attention in the research literature is that of family structure effects such as birth order, sex of siblings, and family size and density. Data from several studies would support the assumption that differences in parent behavior with different children in the family may be primarily due to increased experience and change in availability to children as the family grows (Conners, 1963; Lasko, 1954; Waldrop & Bell, 1964). However, this does not make it possible to dismiss the possibility of child effects. Second- or later-born neonates show higher skin conductance than firstborn (Weller & Bell, 1965). There is collateral evidence that this indicates heightened arousal and greater maturity in this early period, though there is no information available on later development. Another paper summarizes data indicating that the physiology of pregnancy and delivery is quite different for the mother with her first versus later births (Bell, 1963), raising the possibility that some differences in parent behavior with first- versus later-born children may be a response to congenital differences in the child.

A similar child effect could be operative with increases in family size and density. Since greater dependency was found in preschool children coming from large families with short intervals between siblings it was assumed that these children were simply more deprived of maternal attention (Waldrop & Bell, 1964). While this may have been true in part, further study revealed that newborns from large dense families were more lethargic (Waldrop &

Bell, 1966). In this case information on later development was available and the finding was that measures of lethargy in the newborn period were correlated with later dependency. In short, there may be congenital factors operating in determining family structure effects, and credence cannot be given to an interpretation solely in terms of experiential factors until influences identifiable in pregnancy, delivery, and the newborn period are isolated.

Examples of Studies Difficult to Reinterpret

In contrast to these studies, there are others yielding data which could not be reinterpreted as a function of congenital effects contributed by the child. For example, there are studies which substitute experimenters for parents and assign children at random to experimental groups in which different "parental" treatment is administered. In one study, experimenters played the role of parents who did or did not control access to food and toy resources in familylike interactions with pre-school children (Bandura, Ross, & Ross, 1963): Children imitated parents who controlled resources. In a study of moral development, experimenters behaved with different groups of children in such a way as to create differences in the child's control over punishment and in the cognitive clarity of a task which preceded a contrived transgression (Aronfreed, 1963). Self-critical and reparative responses following transgression were maximized by prior cognitive clarity and child control. These studies used a flexible approach which can be applied to a wide variety of parent-effect parameters very rapidly. One limitation is that we do not obtain data on the cumulative effects of parents on children. The other problem is that of ownness. It is encouraging in this respect that Stevenson, Keen, and Knights (1963), in studies of social reinforcement with 4- and 5-year-olds, found effects common to fathers and male experimenters, and effects common to mothers and female experimenters. This reassures us that at least with young children it may be possible to produce results with experimenters similar to effects parents have on their own children.

One other approach involves experimental manipulation of the behavior of parents and measurement of the effects on children. This is an approach that is only slightly less flexible than the foregoing and can be carried out very rapidly. Merrill (1946) manipulated parent behavior by providing mothers in two matched groups with different feedback relative to the behavior of their children. As in the previous approach which substituted experimenters for parents, the possibility of pseudo-parent effects being produced by latent child effects is minimal where the children are assigned to experimental groups at random, or on the basis of some relevant matching variable. On the other hand, since the parent is present in the interaction, the child may respond in terms of past expectancies rather than to the manipulated behavior of the parent as such. This operates against obtaining differences in child behavior in different treatments, but where differences are obtained they can be interpreted as free of child effects.

Offspring effects can also be isolated. An example is provided in a summary of a series of studies carried out by Siegel (1963). Retardates aged 10 and 15 were classified into high- and low-verbal ability groups. Children in each group were then placed in brief interaction situations with adults who had had no previous contact with them. The adults were to assist children in learning how to assemble a puzzle. Generally, adult responses and questions with low-verbal children were more frequent but shorter and more redundant. Labeling children of similar verbal ability as high or low had no effect on the adult behavior. Support was provided for the hypothesis that linguistic level of children exerts a control over adult verbal behavior.

A second variant of the first design is suggested by the research of Yarrow (1963), already discussed, which took advantage of the assignment of young infants to foster mothers for temporary care while adoption procedures were pending. It is necessary only to measure infant characteristics prior to assignment to foster mothers and then make the assignment systematically so that each foster mother's behavior with at least two different kinds of infants could be measured.

One other approach would make it possible to obtain effects with natural parents. Clinicians frequently report that successful medication of children who are hyperactive and impulsive produces pronounced reactive changes in parent and even total family behavior. Addition of pre- and postmedication measures of parent-child and family interaction to a well-controlled study of drug effects should make it possible to evaluate this and other possible child effects.[2]

Other approaches have been mentioned in the introductory section of this paper (Bell, 1964; Levy, 1958). A detailed discussion of all possible research designs is beyond the scope of this paper, which is primarily concerned with a substantive question of how studies of socialization may be interpreted. This brief recapitulation of designs is to serve the purpose of emphasizing the fact that offspring and parent effects can be separately identified and experimentally manipulated. This will require less reliance on correlation studies of parent and child behavior upon which theories of socialization have been largely based up to the present. Even correlations obtained between parent and child behaviors from longitudinal studies offer no means of ascertaining the direction of effects, unless specially designed for the purpose. Kagan and Moss (1962) have pointed out that the problem of whether maternal hostility is a reaction to child aggression or vice versa is not solved by the demonstration of long-term relations between these maternal and child behaviors in follow-up studies.

References

Aronfreed, J. M. The effects of experimental socialization paradigms upon two moral responses to transgression. *Journal of Abnormal and Social Psychology,* 1963, **66,** 437–448.

[2]This adaptation of drug studies was suggested by Paul H . Wender.

Bandura, A., Ross, D., & Ross, S. A. A comparative test of the status envy, social power, and secondary reinforcement theories of identificatory learning. *Journal of Abnormal and Social Psychology,* 1963, **67,** 527–534.

Bandura, A., & Walters, R. H. *Adolescent aggression.* New York: Ronald Press, 1959.

Barry, H., III, Bacon, M. K,. & Child, I. L. A cross-cultural survey of some sex differences in socialization. *Journal of Abnormal and Social Psychology,* 1957, **55,** 327–332.

Bayley, N., & Schaefer, E. S. Correlations of maternal and child behaviors with the development of mental abilities: Data from the Berkeley Growth Study. *Monographs of the Society for Research in Child Development,* 1964, **29**(6, Whole No. 97).

Beach, F. A., & Jaynes, J. Studies of maternal retrieving in rats. III. Sensory cues involved in the lactating female's response to her young. *Behaviour,* 1956, **10,** 104–125.

Bell, R. Q. Some factors to be controlled in studies of behavior of newborns. *Biologia Neonatorum,* 1963, **5,** 200–214.

Bell, R. Q. The effect on the family of a limitation in coping ability in a child: A research approach and a finding. *Merrill-Palmer Quarterly,* 1964, **10,** 129–142.

Bing, E. Effect of childrearing practices on development of differential cognitive abilities. *Child Development,* 1963, **34,** 631–648.

Bronfenbrenner, U. Socialization and social class through time and space. In E. E. Maccoby, T. M. Newcomb, & E. L. Hartley (Eds.), *Readings in social psychology.* New York: Holt, Rinehart & Winston, 1958. Pp. 400–425.

Bruce, H. M. Observations on the suckling stimulus and lactation in the rat. *Journal of Reproduction and Fertility,* 1961, **2,** 17–34.

Conners, C. K. Birth order and needs for affiliation. *Journal of Personality,* 1963, **31,** 408–416.

Davids, A., Holden, R. H., & Gray, G. B. Maternal anxiety during pregnancy and adequacy of mother and child adjustment eight months following childbirth. *Child Development,* 1963, **34,** 993–1002.

Denenberg, V. H. Early experience and emotional development. *Scientific American,* 1963, **208,** 138–146.

Epstein, W. Experimental investigations of the genesis of visual space perception. *Psychological Bulletin,* 1964, **61,** 115–128.

Etzel, B., & Gewirtz, J. Experimental modification of caretaker-maintained high rate operant crying in a 6- and a 20-week-old infant *(Infans Tyrannotcarus). Journal of Experimental Child Psychology,* 1967, **5,** 303–317.

Ferreira, A. J. The pregnant woman's emotional attitude and its reflection on the newborn. *American Journal of Orthopsychiatry,* 1960, **30,** 553–561.

Freedman, D. G. Hereditary control of early social behavior. In B. M. Foss (Ed.), *Determinants of infant behaviour III.* New York: Wiley, 1965. Pp. 149–159.

Garn, S. M. Fat, body size, and growth in the newborn. *Human Biology,* 1958, **30,** 265–280.

Goodenough, F. W. Interest in persons as an aspect of sex difference in early years. *Genetic Psychology Monographs,* 1957, **55,** 287–323.

Gottesman, I. I. Genetic variance in adaptive personality traits. Paper presented at the 73rd annual convention of the American Psychological Association, September 1965, Chicago, Illinois.

Hillenbrand, E. D. The relationship of psychological, medical, and feeding variables to breast feeding. Unpublished master's thesis, George Washington University, 1965.

Hoffman, M. L. Childrearing practices and moral development: Generalizations from empirical research. *Child Development,* 1963, **34,** 295–318.

Joffe, J. M. Genotype and prenatal and premating stress interact to affect adult behavior in rats. *Science,* 1965, **150,** 1844–1845.

Kagan, J., & Garn, S. M. A constitutional correlate of early intellectual functioning. *Journal of Genetic Psychology,* 1963, **102,** 83–89.

Kagan, J., & Moss, H. A. *Birth to maturity.* New York: Wiley, 1962.

Kessen, W. (Ed.) *The child.* New York: Wiley, 1965.

Lasko, J. K. Parent behavior toward first and second children. *Genetic Psychology Monographs,* 1954, **49,** 97–137.

Lefkowitz, M. M., Walder, L. O., & Eron, L. D. Punishment, identification and aggression. *Merrill-Palmer Quarterly,* 1963, **9,** 159–174.

Levy, D. M. *Behavioral analysis: Analysis of clinical observations of behavior as applied to mother-newborn relationships.* New York: Thomas, 1958.

Merrill, B. A measurement of mother-child interaction. *Journal of Abnormal and Social Psychology,* 1946, **41,** 37–49.

Moss, H. A. Sex, age, and state as determinants of mother-infant interaction. *Merrill-Palmer Quarterly,* 1967, **13,** 19–36.

Murdock, G. P. Comparative data on the division of labor by sex. *Social Forces,* 1937, **15,** 551–553.

Mussen, P., & Rutherford, E. Parent-child relations and parental personality in relation to young children's sex-role preferences. *Child Development,* 1963, **34,** 589–607.

Noirot, E. Changes in responsiveness to young in the adult mouse. III. The effect of immediately preceding performances. *Behavior,* 1965, **24,** 318–325.

Ottinger, D. R., & Simmons, J. E. Behavior of human neonates and prenatal maternal anxiety. *Psychological Reports,* 1964, **14,** 391–394.

Palmer, R. R. *The age of the democratic revolution:* Vol. II. *The struggle.* Princeton: Princeton University Press, 1964.

Pasamanick, B., & Knobloch, H. Brain damage and reproductive casualty. *American Journal of Orthopsychiatry,* 1960, **30,** 298–305.

Pasamanick, B., Robers, M. E., & Lilienfeld, A. M. Pregnancy experience and the development of behavior disorders in children. *American Journal of Psychiatry,* 1956, **112,** 613–618.

Ressler, R. H. Parental handling in two strains of mice reared by foster parents. *Science,* 1962, **137,** 129–130.

Rheingold, H. L., (Ed.) *Maternal behavior in mammals.* New York: Wiley, 1963.

Rheingold, H. L. The development of social behavior in the human infant. In H. W. Stevenson (Ed.), Concept of development: A report of a conference commemorating the fortieth anniversary of the Institute of Child Development, University of Minnesota. *Monographs of the Society for Research in Child Development,* 1966, **31**(5, Whole No. 107).

Scarr, S. The inheritance of sociability. *American Psychologist,* 1965, **20,** 524. (Abstract)

Schaefer, E. A circumplex model for maternal behavior. *Journal of Abnormal and Social Psychology,* 1959, **59,** 226–235.

Schaefer, E. Parent-child interactional patterns and parental attitudes. In D. Rosenthal (Ed.), *The Genain quadruplets.* New York: Basic Books, 1963. Pp. 398–430.

Schaefer, E., & Bayley, N. Maternal behavior, child behavior, and their intercorrelations from infancy through adolescence. *Monographs of the Society for Research in Child Development,* 1963, **28**(3, Whole No. 87).

Schaffer, H. R., & Emerson, P. E. Patterns of response to physical contact in early human development. *Journal of Child Psychology and Psychiatry,* 1964, **5,** 1–13.

Sears, R. R., Maccoby, E. E., & Levin, H. *Patterns of child rearing.* Evanston, Ill.: Row, Peterson, 1957.

Siegel, G. M. Adult verbal behavior with retarded children labeled as "high" or "low" in verbal ability. *American Journal of Mental Deficiency,* 1963, **68,** 417–424.

Stechler, G. A longitudinal follow-up of neonatal apnea. *Child Development,* 1964, **35,** 333–348.

Stevenson, H. W., Keen, R., & Knights, R. M. Parents and strangers as reinforcing agents for children's performance. *Journal of Abnormal and Social Psychology,* 1963, **67,** 183–186.

Stott, L. H. Parent-adolescent adjustment: Its measurement and significance. *Character and Personality,* 1941, **10,** 140–150.

Vandenberg, S. G. The hereditary abilities study: Hereditary components in a psychological test battery. *American Journal of Human Genetics,* 1962, **14,** 220–237.

Waldrop, M., & Bell, R. Q. Relation of preschool dependency behavior to family size and density. *Child Development,* 1964, **35,** 1187–1195.

Waldrop, M., & Bell, R. Q. Effects of family size and density on newborn characteristics. *American Journal of Orthopsychiatry,* 1966, **36,** 544–550.

Walters, R. H., & Parke, R. D. The role of the distance receptors in the development of social responsiveness. In L. P. Lipsitt & C. C. Spiker (Eds.), *Advances in child development and behavior.* Vol. 2. New York: Academic Press, 1965. Pp. 59–96.

Weller, G. M. & Bell, R. Q. Basal skin conductance and neonatal state. *Child Development,* 1965, **36,** 647–657.

Yarrow, L. J. Research in dimensions of early maternal care. *Merrill-Palmer Quarterly,* 1963, **9,** 101–114.

Chapter Three

Race, Social Class, Intelligence, and Education

This chapter considers some of the major current controversies on the effects of race and social class on IQ and scholastic performance. Much of this controversy can be attributed to Jensen's (1969) highly provocative report, which presents a theory of racial differences in intellect and learning ability. As a result of his published findings, Jensen has been referred to as a racist and has provoked stormy outbursts from both laymen and professionals. However, many of the arguments advanced by Jensen have not been adequately refuted, and some of his statements may be valid. Following upon Jensen's work, Eysenck (1971) published a report attempting to show the racial differences he believes to exist in intellectual and learning ability between blacks and whites. In a somewhat related vein, Herrnstein (1971) has recently described possible caste differences in the United States that will be based on differences in innate intelligence. Herrnstein's argument is not that there are racial differences but that as opportunities become more equal and social class differences are gradually eliminated, the main factor that will determine an individual's attainments and position in society will be his innate intellectual ability. Herrnstein has done a skillful job of presenting a strong argument for his position. However, this position has also provoked considerable recent controversy and disagreement among both lay groups and professional academicians.

This chapter contains some of these men's views and also some of the critical responses to them. Moreover, we will find that some believe current notions about the deprived child are really myths—in other words, that many contemporary views held about so-called deprived children are unfounded and misleading. Related to this is the myth of intelligence testing; critics say that current-day approaches to IQ testing are unjustified and lead only to confusion rather than clarification.

Outcomes of Compensatory Education Programs

In a somewhat related vein are controversies concerning the outcomes of compensatory education programs such as Project Head Start. At first, Head Start was met with wide acclaim and support; programs such as these seemed bound to have beneficial effects on the intellectual development and academic attainments of lower-class children who were felt to suffer from lack of environmental stimulation during their earliest years. Thus, when these programs were initiated not too many years ago, many people regarded them as a panacea, and almost all agreed that they would lead to positive outcomes. However, after a few years of operation, evaluations of the outcomes of these programs have, in many instances, been negative and discouraging. That is, reports (see Hellmuth, 1970) indicate that no long-range benefits are derived from these special educational programs for lower-class children who are believed to be "deprived children."

Not only has Project Head Start been found wanting, but the U.S. Office of Economic Opportunity (OEO) has recently concluded that large educational development corporations (for example, Westinghouse Learning Corporation) are unable to teach children any better than regular school teachers. A recent statement in *Behavior Today* (1972) indicated that a report on the OEO's multi-million dollar trial venture in "performance contracting" has shown no significant gains resulting from this form of special education in comparison with traditional methods. This contract teaching was concerned with content areas similar to those studied in conventional school subjects (reading, writing, arithmetic), but used modern technology: programmed instruction, teaching machines, specially designed textbooks, and principles of operant conditioning.

The six large organizations that had accepted the government contracts to attempt to improve academic skills in individual students did so with the understanding that their fee would be proportionate to the amount of gain shown by their students. As a result of the negative findings from this experimental approach to education, four of the six contractors are reported to have given up the performance contracting business. These unanticipated findings of inability to improve students' performance even with special efforts on their behalf were obtained from large-scale evaluations conducted at 18 different sites where contractors had been plying their educational trade.

It was also reported that other experiments involving incentives to teacher groups (rewarding them for their students' academic gains) also suffered similar results, with findings of no significant improvement. According to the statement in *Behavior Today* (1972), the immediate impact was for the OEO to reconsider its role in attempting to break poverty cycles via educational approaches. It was felt that the biggest danger that might result from this unhappy experiment in compensatory education would be a return to the traditional tendency to blame the children for their underachievement and school failures. Even worse, it was feared that these results might encourage educators and legislators to accept the status quo placidly.

The Issues

Various theories and ideas have been offered to account for the lack of significant effects from these compensatory education programs, why any immediate gains evidenced by these children are found to disappear after a very short time. The papers that follow take conflicting sides of this controversy and show why some studies have led to positive findings and others to negative findings. Thus, Chapter Three is concerned specifically with issues pertaining to IQ, school failure, and special education; possible influences of race and social class will be considered in relation to each of these topics.

References

Behavior Today, 1972, **3** (6), 1.

Eysenck, H. J. *The IQ argument: Race, intelligence, and education.* New York: Library Press, 1971.

Hellmuth, J. (Ed.) *Disadvantaged child. Vol. 3. Compensatory education: A national debate.* New York: Brunner/Mazel, 1970.

Herrnstein, R. IQ. *Atlantic*, 1971, **228** (3), 44–64.

Jensen, A. R. How much can we boost IQ and scholastic achievement? *Harvard Educational Review*, 1969, **39**, 1–123.

7. Jensen's Views on Race, IQ, and Learning and Kagan's Evaluation of the Evidence

Anthony Davids

Arthur Jensen, an outstanding educational psychologist at the University of California, Berkeley, has proposed that social class and racial differences in IQ are largely genetic in origin (Jensen, 1969). In arriving at this theoretical position, Jensen analyzed masses of empirical and statistical evidence and presented his findings in a long scholarly report. However, its publication provoked bitter controversy, with subsequent published rebuttals and critiques, and articles and letters appearing in many of the country's leading magazines and newspapers.

Jensen's argument begins with the observation that recent efforts to increase IQ and achievement through programs of compensatory education have failed, thus suggesting that the premises underlying these efforts should be reexamined. He questions the central notion on which these educational programs have been based—that IQ differences are almost entirely determined by environmental influences and the cultural bias of IQ tests. He discusses the concept of "heritability" and analyzes several lines of evidence suggesting that genetic factors are much more important than environmental factors in producing IQ differences.

Jensen's analysis of environmental influences leads him to conclude that prenatal factors may well be the most critical environmental determinants of IQ. He then discusses evidence suggesting that environmental differences cannot account for social class and racial variations in intelligence, and they must be partially attributed to genetic differences.

Jensen's detailed examination of results obtained from educational programs for young children reveals that any changes in IQ produced by these programs have been quite small. The findings lead Jensen to conclude that environment acts as a "threshold variable." By this he means that extreme environmental deprivation can cause a child to perform below his genetic potential, but educational enrichment cannot push a child above that potential.

Jensen also proposes that there are two types of learning—labeled Level I (associative learning) and Level II (conceptual learning). He maintains that lower-class children learn in rote fashion (associative learning), while middle-class children are capable of conceptual learning. Actually, according to Jensen, all children are characterized by associative learning prior to age 5. This is mainly a mechanical, unthinking process, with the child automatically forming connections between stimuli and responses. This form of learning essentially involves a conditioning process, with application of positive and negative rewards leading to desired results from training, with no necessary involvement of thought or conceptualization. All young children are adept at this type of learning; there is no evidence of social-class differences.

Beyond 5 years of age, however, conceptual learning becomes more important; at this point, middle-class children begin to surpass those from lower social classes. This form of learning involves more complex cognitive activity mediating between stimuli and responses. Jensen gives the example of learning a list of words. With associative learning, the child learns the words in a rote, unorganized, unthinking fashion; with conceptual learning, the child groups the words on the basis of similarity, and when asked to recall the words does so in an organized fashion. In the first instance, each stimulus word is simply linked to a response, but in the second instance, conceptual activity (categorization) mediates between the two.

According to Jensen, middle-class children's superiority over lower-class children in conceptual learning is attributable to genetic inheritance. In keeping with this view, he proposes that lower-class children should probably receive a very different form of education than that appropriate for middle-class children. He concludes that educational attempts to boost IQ have been misdirected and recommends that the educational process focus on teaching more specific skills.

As stated earlier, Jensen's views did not meet with a warm response from either the academic community or the general public. The more commonly accepted view is that all children learn in the same way, although the content of what is learned may be influenced by social class. In a recent book concerned with poor children's intellect and education, Ginsburg (1972) comments " . . . there is little point in pursuing Jensen's ideas concerning heredity and environment, since his basic notion of social-class differences in conceptual and associative learning is so thoroughly misguided." Following a detailed examination of evidence cited by Jensen, Ginsburg (1972) concludes that " . . . Jensen's notions appear to be without empirical or theoretical foundation."

Jerome Kagan, a distinguished developmental psychologist, is also severely critical of the logic in Jensen's article. Kagan has presented evidence that IQ results obtained from conventional tests are not likely to reflect the actual intellectual potential of lower-class children (Kagan, 1969). According to Kagan, the two major fallacies in Jensen's work are (1) inappropriate generalization from within-family IQ differences to an argument that separate racial gene pools are necessarily different, and (2) the conclusion that IQ differences are genetically determined. Kagan reports that I. I. Gottesman, a leading behavioral geneticist, also questions the validity of Jensen's ideas. He cites Gottesman's (1968) conclusion that "The differences observed so far between whites and Negroes can hardly be accepted as sufficient evidence that with respect to intelligence the Negro American is genetically less endowed."

Kagan then presents evidence from new studies he believes cast doubt on the validity of Jensen's position. Longitudinal studies in Kagan's laboratory at Harvard have revealed that lower-class white children do not experience the same quality of mother-child interaction that occurs in middle-class white families. Lower-class mothers spend significantly less time in face-to-face vocalization and smiling with their infants, do not reward the young child's maturational progress, and do not enter into extended periods of play with the child. According to Kagan's theory of mental development, the absence of these specific experiences tends to retard mental growth and leads to lower scores on intelligence tests. He hypothesizes that black children's lower IQ scores result from early experiences that do not facilitate performance on IQ tests, partly because they do not understand the nature of the problems being presented on the test.

In support of this position, Kagan cites unpublished research by Francis Palmer, who administered mental tests to middle- and lower-class black children from Harlem. To counteract the likely possibility that many of the children would fail to appreciate the requirements of a testing situation, the examiners did not begin the testing until they felt certain the child was completely relaxed and knew what was expected of him. Few prior studies have devoted so much time to establishing rapport with the children being tested, and this study found very few significant differences in mental ability between lower- and middle-class children.

Kagan's concluding argument is that compensatory education programs have been neither adequately developed nor evaluated. Thus, he finds no basis for Jensen's suggestion that compensatory education is not likely to help black children. He maintains it is unreasonable to assume that compensatory education has failed merely because brief Head Start programs, organized on a crash basis, fail to produce stable increases in IQ scores. In this regard, Kagan states, "The flaws in this logic are overwhelming. It would be nonsense to assume that feeding animal protein to a seriously malnourished child for three days would lead to a permanent increase in his weight and height, if after 72 hours of steak and eggs he was sent back to his malnourished environment. It *may* be that compensatory education is of little value, but this idea has not been tested in any adequate way up to now [1969, p. 128]."

Finally, Kagan points out that genetic constitution of a population does not produce a specific level of mental ability; rather, it sets a range of mental ability. According to Kagan, learning to read, write, and do arithmetic are easy skills, well within the competence of all children who are not seriously brain damaged. Thus, he feels it erroneous to suggest that genetic differences between populations could be responsible for school failure. He concludes with the following admonition, "Ninety out of every 100 children, black, yellow, or white, are capable of adequate mastery of the intellectual requirements of our schools. Let us concentrate on the conditions that will allow this latent competence to be actualized with maximal ease [1969, p. 129]."

References

Ginsburg, H. *The myth of the deprived child.* Englewood Cliffs, N. J.: Prentice-Hall, 1972.

Gottesman, I.I. Biogenetics of race and class. In M. Deutsch, I. Katz, & A.R. Jensen (Eds.), *Social class, race, and psychological development.* New York: Holt, Rinehart & Winston, 1968.

Jensen, A.R. How much can we boost IQ and scholastic achievement? *Harvard Educational Review,* 1969, **39**, 1–123.

Kagan, J. Inadequate evidence and illogical conclusions. *Harvard Educational Review,* 1969, **39**, 126–129.

8. In the Dark: Reflections on Compensatory Education, 1960–1970

James F. Winschel

I

Seamen have a custom, when they meet a whale, to fling him out an empty tub by way of amusement, to divert him from laying violent hands upon the ship.

Jonathan Swift
Tale of a Tub (1704), Preface

Compensatory education may be a fraud perpetrated upon a poor and unsuspecting citizenry which has traditionally looked to education to lead it out of bondage. Compensatory education may be a hoax by which the politicians and educators of middle class America salve their consciences and maintain the status quo. Or compensatory education may be simply the best efforts of a politico-educational complex blinded in one eye by prejudice and in the other by do-goodness—both equally detrimental to the welfare of children and society. Because compensatory education has resulted in a rising tide of expectations among the poor, the Black, and the disadvantaged, its failure to achieve a noble end presents a danger to the very fabric of American education that cannot long be ignored. It is for this reason that the "National Debate on Compensatory Education" has been set in motion.

The 60's was a decade of paradox: hunger in the midst of plenty, strife in the struggle for peace, riots in the citadels of learning, and poverty the plague of prosperity. Youth in search of freedom imprisoned themselves with drugs, soldiers trained to kill refused to fight, and the recipients of public welfare refused to be everlastingly grateful.

It was an age of madness, too. A popular president was assassinated, the disciple of non-violence was murdered, and a promising politician—some would say a rare species—was cut down in a crime more absurd than monumental. "With all deliberate speed" meant endless delay, and the "war on poverty" seemed uncertain of victory as its goal. The invasion of privacy became a national concern, but with unremitting zeal educators demanded that teachers get into the homes of the poor to "see" how *they* lived.

The decade 1960–69 was an era in which the old truths were challenged as never before. The never-ending God was dead; patriotism lost its sheen; the dirty book was surpassed by the dirty movie—and both were accepted as mature art. The casually accepted prejudice inherent in the black list, black ball, black market, black sheep and black beard were exposed by a new concept, "Black is Beautiful." The Negro community would never again accept an inherent inferiority in social roles, education or intelligence. Statistics be damned; if education cannot deliver the promise of full equality under whatever name, then, as Larry Cuban (1967) has suggested, "the structure of education must be rethought and, ultimately, revised . . . (p. 220)." And while Cuban limited his observations to the education of inner city youth, it is likely that substantial changes in the education of the disadvantaged would be but a prelude to sweeping changes throughout public and private education. That these changes may be born on the edge of social chaos or in the shadow of political revolution, if not a foregone conclusion, is at least a sober and frightening possibility.

Christmas in Purgatory, The Manufacture of Madness, Biological Timebomb, God is Dead, and compensatory education. In the tide of our times one questions whether the latter was a sufficiently bold concept; the challenge seemed somehow to call for a greater imagination, a more splendid effort. As Jennings has stated,

> The continuing challenge, then, is to provide an education as various as the diversity of the country, which will allow the least advantaged, the most gifted, and the ordinary to grow together, to learn to communicate (and to have significant experiences and feelings and opinions to communicate), to be able to work and live in communities which are not merely tolerant of but genuinely hospitable to uniqueness and even to heresy. At the same time these communities must be capable of cherishing the ordinary and the commonplace. Unless this is achieved, we will be diminished as a nation. (1967, pp. 351–353)

To the extent that compensatory education was thought capable of achieving the above goals, it has failed; to the extent that it has been utilized to modify the dissidents and cool the scene, it has had the opposite effect. Contrary to widespread opinion, compensatory education was an unpretentious idea capable of modest success. Unfortunately, it has been puffed up beyond its potential and is now about to burst. In illustration of what has happened, Evline Omwake (1968) tells of attending an early conference in which the possibility of a head-start-like program was explored. The authorities agreed that such a program might help children to begin school with greater confidence and pleasure, but that school success in academic terms would not necessarily be promoted.

> In short, children themselves might indeed benefit but the elementary school would still face the problem of large numbers of poor learners. Now, three years later, it seems that new experiences, greater self-confidence, and a positive feeling about school are not considered sufficient reason for so expensive and elaborate a program; children must have made up for their deficiencies in academic skills and knowledge, as well.... This seems to be the result of adults being carried away by fantasies of their own magical powers... (1968, p. 539).

The problem, then, is that we have promised too much and in the promising have floundered upon the rising expectations of our clients. An examination of most compensatory education programs with their emphasis on guidance, reading and language development, parental and community involvement, modified curriculums and more adequately trained teachers suggests that we have nothing so very new to offer the disadvantaged learner. Certainly all of the preceding should be a part of any good educational program. Perhaps the problem lies in our having failed with many to do the ordinary with any extraordinary skill—and we have sought to hide our omissions behind labels: *the disadvantaged child* and *compensatory education.*

II

> Nothing is better calculated to drive men to desperation than when, in attempting to carry out beneficial reform, they find the whole world aligned against them. The more especially so if amongst those so aligned they discover men who had preached the same ideal, but now dreaded its concrete realization.
>
> Hewlett Johnson
> *The Soviet Power: The Socialist*
> *Sixth of the World* (1940)

Black is beautiful. What an improbable statement! Red is beautiful, or blue or green. One might even accept magenta or chartreuse. And while white is not exactly beautiful, it is at least pure and clean as they say "like the driven snow." *Don't give up the ship, Remember Pearl Harbor, Ask not what your country... , Yankee, go home!* One can sense in these the call to patriotism and pride, self-respect and duty. But "Black is Beautiful"? What can it possibly mean?

In one sense it stands as a powerful rejection of the 'melting pot' ideal. We had dreamed that groups of diverse background would relinquish most of their identifying characteristics in exchange for the American character. And while for many the image became reality, it was for the Negro only a mirage—a dream from which he was, with rare exception, systematically excluded. Having gloried in their success with a great flow of immigrants, our schools must now bear the responsibility for failure with twenty million black Americans. Black is beautiful because America allowed itself to be blinded by color, and in losing its vision must now adapt to new realities.

But Black is also beautiful because there is no alternative in cities which John Gardner described as "fragmented worlds of ignorance, fear and hostility, not communities, but encampments of strangers (Holmes, 1969, p. 200)." And it is beautiful because the seemingly inexhaustible patience of the Negro has worn thin, and a people long committed to non-violence grow restless amidst the patronage of their oppressors, tired of loving, determined not to emulate. It is because lynchings, murder, discrimination, poverty, ignorance and hate are ugly that Black is beautiful. In a larger sense it is because America is rather unpretty. "Our universities are in deep trouble," writes Peter Rossi. Our cities sink further into a morass of decay and anarchy, and our school systems fail both the society and the pupils they are supposed to serve (1969, p. 332)."

In reply to the new reality of color and pride in an oftentime sick society, the educational community shuddered briefly, labored timidly, and brought forth compensatory education. They said it was for the disadvantaged, the deprived, and the poor, but the target was unmistakably Black. Compensation in the educational process was to be an affluent society's payoff for two and a half centuries of exploitation and humiliation, the reward for a history of servitude and neglect. Compensatory education was to be carried out with a certain flair and rhetoric so as to disguise its basic quality, that of offering more of what hadn't worked in the past. A black author addressed himself to the problem:

> A number of panaceas, for instance, involve the assumption that quantitative inputs will effect qualitative outputs. Thus, one finds sincere attempts to fight cancer with corn plasters. The proponents of this view hold that we must sensitize the teachers, inject Negro history, reduce class size, and add some new services (but only when substantial outside pressure to do so is exerted). Where these initial attempts to patch up the system fail, schools can always fall back upon the processes of labeling and stigmatizing inner-city children as deviants either culturally, socially or emotionally, and thus placing them in "special" or "compensatory" programs. Then the children can be blamed, rather than the racism which permeates our educational institutions (Johnson, 1969, p. 244).

The problem, of course, is that compensatory education has attempted to solve the problems of racial and social class isolation in schools which are themselves isolated by race and class, staffed by teachers who have been systematically steeped in the passive acceptance of discrimination and underachievement, and led by an intellectual elite more committed to the rhetoric of democracy than to its practice. Label the child; parrot the cliche; accept the subtle prejudice; send your daughter to a private school, and advise the President on the "benign neglect" of things racial. It is this mixture that continues to nourish a growing separatism within the black community and may yet result in the tragedy of parallel social and political structures, color coded and competitively hostile.

The lesson America must learn is not that black is beautiful, but rather that "black is." The lesson is not without precedent, for white and black alike recognize that "white is." "White" is people, stupid and smart, good and bad, ugly and beautiful, some glorying in the history of their ancestors, but many unconcerned. Black is much the same, I think, and we should not be goaded into accepting slogans which are usually the first and most dramatic step in the cessation of thought and feeling. Schools have a dramatic task before them: to close the gap between races so that in education and in all other aspects of life *white is* and *black is* are replaced by *people are*. It is not a task for "compensatory education" with its division of learners and its inherent suggestion of inferiority, but rather for education, straightforward and not always exciting, unadulterated by qualifying terms no matter how glamorous.

A peaceful revolution within education may yet stave off the portents of human conflict which surround us. Action is called for which will rescue black children from schools which produce failure and white children from a world which gives acquiescence to the intolerable. Starkly before us—if we fail—is the prospect that "Black is Beautiful" may yet turn ugly.

III

The office of government is not to confer happiness, but to give men opportunity to work out happiness for themselves.

William Ellery Channing
*The Life and Character of
Napoleon Bonaparte*

War is too potent in the affairs of man to be left to the military; education too subject to control—with too great a portent for the manipulation of human beings—to be left in the hands of government. "What is needed," writes Joseph Durham, "is a massive reordering of social and political power so that education again becomes a national passion (1969, p. 22)." It is not a passion—personal, intimate, all-pervasive—because compulsory education has been imposed from without, and the individual, his family and community have increasingly lost any sense of its control or direction. Nowhere has this fact been more evident than among the poor.

The literature is replete with characteristics of the disadvantaged. Poverty, alienation, delinquency and low achievement are but a few. While accurate in varying degrees, these characteristics miss the essence of disadvantagement, which is a severe restriction on freedom of choice and freedom of response. Indeed educational disadvantagement might best be gauged by the extent, both in distance and degree, to which what is "good" for children has had its germination and received its direction from beyond the individual, his family and community. As the disadvantaged are those for whom others decide what is good, the educationally disadvantaged are those for whom others decide what is good education. It is apparent that, in whatever form, disadvantagement is the product of forces outside the individual, and that only change in the advantaged can alter the plight of the disadvantaged. The danger in compensatory education lies in focusing our efforts on the few when change is demanded of the many. To some extent it was recognition of this fact that led Durham to conclude, "The challenge is to relegate compensatory education to the museum of educational antiquities along with corporal punishment and the Lancastrian system (1962, p. 22)."

Public education today constitutes the nation's largest monopoly. Like all monopolies, it is in turn arrogant, rigid, paternalistic, and coercive. Like all monopolies, it is as much interested in perpetuating itself as in the welfare of its clients. More than that, self preservation is a tenet of its faith. Frightened by lawlessness, shamed by overt prejudice and discrimination, and chagrined at its low achieving products, public education spawned compensatory education. Then, in a subtle distortion of purpose, it offered the disadvantaged not merely equality of opportunity but equality of achievement as well. It is upon this shoal that compensation as an educational doctrine has run aground. Public education has not (probably cannot) deliver on its promise as the work of Coleman (1966), Durham (1969), Freeman (1969), Jensen (1969), and others have amply suggested.

We do not castigate compensatory education for its failure to improve in any dramatic way the education of the disadvantaged. Rather we question its implied promise to eliminate those differences in ability and achievement which are a part of the richness of a people no less than is the equality of opportunity, once attained, a part of the wealth of a nation. Of the differences in educational achievement among people Glazer wrote:

> History and social research convince me there are deep and enduring differences between various ethnic groups, in their educational achievement and in the broader cultural characteristics in which these differences are, I believe, rooted; that these differences cannot be simply associated with the immediate conditions under which these groups live, whether we define these conditions as being those of levels of poverty and exploitation, or prejudice and discrimination; and that if we are to have a decent society, men must learn to live with some measure of group difference in educational achievement, to tolerate them, and to accept in some degree the disproportion in the distribution of rewards that may flow from differences in educational achievement (1969, p. 187).

I believe we have to accept differences in ability and attainment if we are to live in harmony, one with another, or if we are to stave off the relentless pressures which accelerate us on the path to a faceless society.

In support of man's uniqueness Jennings writes:

> He can be dealt with as a statistic, but he will not behave like one. He can be usefully described by a stereotype, but in his recalcitrant uniqueness, he will not always perform in a fixed or general pattern (1967, p. 352).

In spite of this optimism, breakthroughs in biology have accelerated the prospects of genetic engineering and modern techniques of communication and persuasion leave one unaware of the erosion of free choice. Operant conditioning is hailed as a sometime savior, and the vision of a salivating dog is but a distant memory. Technology is placing in the impersonal hands of monolithic government and its increasingly beholden servant, public education, such potential for the destruction of individuality that new forms of education and new protections for the rights of man must be developed without delay.

A step in this direction might pattern itself upon the successful educational aspects of the popular G.I. Bill of Rights. Parents would be obligated or at least encouraged to purchase the educational process which best met their needs. Limited profits would be permitted and the purveyors of a shoddy process or a faulty product would at least now be more subject to judicial restraint and the loss of clientele. Sounder, more imaginative plans than the foregoing are even now being developed by individuals who are concerned with the disadvantaged and are disillusioned by the failures of compensatory education (see Jencks, 1968). As innovations begun with the least advantaged have invariably been incorporated into the broad spectrum of educational practice, so too can we expect these new forms to alter the face of education for all and thereby frustrate indefinitely the nightmares of Huxley and Orwell.

The quality of education offered minority group children has seldom met with widespread approbation. Second class schools, worn out teachers, and ineffective programs have been the lot of the disadvantaged child. These conditions exist in the face of herculean efforts to alter the pattern, largely because minority group parents have been denied their share of responsibility for making decisions pertinent to the education of children. There is among the poor an abiding faith in education which, if acknowledged, respected, and utilized can be a mainspring to the improvement of education for all.

As we move forward in this venture let us not speak of community control; such terms easily become the focal point of strife and dissensions. Let us think instead of involving people, black and white, rich and poor, ignorant and educated alike in a new passion for education. If we are successful, the need for compensatory education will indeed have been relegated to the "museum of educational antiquities." The goal, after all, is not one of equivalent people achieving equally, but rather of equal people achieving through equivalent opportunities. In the pursuit of this goal we will find safety from the oppression of government and honor in the quest for individuality.

IV

There is nothing on earth intended for innocent people so horrible as a school. To begin with, it is a prison. But it is in some respects more cruel than a prison. In a prison, for instance, you are not forced to read books by the wardens and the governor.... In prison they may torture your body, but they do not torture your brains.

Bernard Shaw
Parents and Children

It is difficult to find anyone to mourn the passing of the sixties. Perhaps the issues which divided society had been too finely honed, the conflicts brought too sharply into focus. Alienation was the prevailing mood of the country, and nowhere was this more apparent than in the disenchantment with the educational establishment evidenced by millions of miseducated Americans. Symbolic of this disillusionment, and occurring in disproportionately large numbers among the disadvantaged, was the school dropout.

While dropout may be descriptive of the final act, it fails miserably to convey the nature of the problem or the direction of its solution. Why did youth cut short their school experiences? At times dropouts were the end product of low expectations for achievement endemic to the teaching profession and directed extensively toward poor and minority group children. At other times students left because out-of-school experiences had promoted a degree of independence incompatible with continued educational servitude. In still other cases, dropping out was the student's ultimate refutation of an educational stratagem which presumed that all could achieve equally if only sufficient pressure or expertise was brought to bear upon the learner. This strategy resulted from a misreading of both compensatory education and civil rights. The attempt to equalize achievement, while sometimes instrumental in motivating teachers, inevitably ended in disappointment. Achievement could not be equalized.

The contribution of the school to the dropout problem stems from the long term inability of education to adjust curriculum and methodology to the 15% of youth that Havighurst and Stiles (1961) termed "the alienated group" and for whom schooling is an uncertain path to adulthood. As Strom succinctly stated,

> Every year a significant number of basically sound young Americans discover that they are not really wanted and that neither their teachers nor their curricular experiences seem to pay any attention to who they are, what they have and what they have not, and what they can do and what they cannot do. Instead, imposed upon them is a nonsensical experience which goes under the name of education (1966, p. 60).

It is an education in which children of the poor have been passive recipients and for which dropping out is often an escape from an oppression of body, mind and spirit. Rapid changes in society make tradition-bound schools irrelevant and foster among students a rejection of the school, its processes and control. It may be that we should speak of the school as dropout rather than the student. In its unresponsiveness to the demands of the poor, particularly the Blacks, for a greater say in decisions affecting their education, the school drops out of the child long before the student drops out of the school. One may at least postulate that the needed revisions of theory and practice which will preclude this happening cannot be accommodated within the present framework of compensatory education and must await more basic changes in the democratic structure—changes not only in education but in people as well.

In retrospect the ten years spanning 1960–69 was a decade of dropouts.

Spiraling divorce rates gave testimony to the marriage dropout, and decreased attendance figures sent paroxysms of holy reform through church leaders. College professors urged students to drop out and "turn on," and with the help of drugs they did so in alarming numbers; years of education had apparently given them little skill in "turning on" on their own. One nationally circulated publication captioned an idyllic picture of a dropout family as follows: "Refugees from affluence fled from the rat race into older, steadier rhythms (Life, Dec. 24, 1969, p. 25)." Surely millions of readers, fed up with the pressures of living and disillusioned in the quest for a good life, must have lingered upon that portrait with more than a tinge of envy. And of course, as school administrators across the country could testify, teachers also dropped out. One teacher in an urban Junior High School put it this way:

> I know the teachers in my school. Several of them are young and inexperienced, but they are also devoted and energetic. A large number are Negroes who have a special interest in these youngsters. And yet in the end, well-nigh every teacher, no matter who he is or why he is teaching, gives up and leaves the school or the profession altogether (Ornstein, 1965, p. 105).

Obviously, the scope of our problem is not confined to children who fail to complete school. The student dropout is only a manifestation of a larger social malady affecting the moral standards, mental health, and social welfare of a nation. To suggest remediation through compensation, whether within education or without, is a little like throwing a cork to a drowning man. It may be indicative of our good will, but the victim is going to go under.

Interestingly, the rate of dropouts among secondary school students has declined impressively in the last fifty years. Schreiber (1967) estimated that in 1964 two out of every three children who had entered 5th grade eight years earlier had graduated and that the trend is toward ever larger percentages. Open to conjecture, however, is whether these students remain in school because of more meaningful programs, or in the broadest sense benefit from the experience. Wasserman and Reimann (1969) have suggested that the "law" of competitive accreditation may be partially responsible for the school's holding power. This "law," in effect, denies entrance to the ladder of independent adulthood for those who have not been accredited at a high school level, regardless of the individual's potential for success or the idiocy of the program from which he withdrew. A kind of coercive retention takes place in which schools glory in their new found holding power at the same time they become overburdened with the psychological dropout, the student whose withdrawal is complete in all but body. It seems probable that students so retained will acquire a growing disrespect for the conventions of society and in so doing will develop a susceptibility to discontent, mayhem, and revolution. Indeed, forced feeding is the antithesis of education, and *argumentum baculinum*—the argument of the cudgel—even when subtly stated is little likely to solve the problems of disenchanted learners.

"The ultimate prevention of the school dropout and consequent conservation of human resources is quality education which takes into account the unique needs and characteristics of the individual student." So wrote then Commissioner of Education, James E. Allen, Jr. (1969, p. 8), aware, no doubt, that knowledge poorly taught and poorly learned is both the progenitor and sustainer of the dropout problem; aware, no doubt, that the multitude of causes which appear so voluminously in the professional literature are more excuse than cause; aware, no doubt, of education's attempt to attribute cause to factors outside itself and then to demonstrate its good will with a flurry of activity designed to smother the problem and obfuscate its origin. Lack of motivation and poor achievement attitudes may be a challenge to teaching, but they do not cause dropouts; poor education does that. Meaningful school retention, then, will not be the product of the numerous and sometimes imaginative plans sponsored by government and industry except as these are catalysts for an educational experience which preserves individuality, recognizes the right of self-determination, and promotes self-respect.

In January, 1968, approval of the Title VIII amendments to the Elementary and Secondary Education Act placed the federal government in the battle to improve education so as to reduce the number of children failing to complete their elementary and secondary schooling. In recognition of the complexity of the problem and the paucity of reliable information in this area, the Office of Education refrained from developing a model for funded programs. The uncertainties surrounding ameliorative efforts and the resistance of the problem to solutions have since been described by Kruger.

> Numerous studies and experimental programs have made it clear that no simple cause-and-effect relationship explains why some students leave school. No socioeconomic level, intelligence strata, physical classification, or ethnic group is immune from the problem. No panaceas have been discovered, and few situations are responsive to short term or inexpensive remedies (Kruger, 1969, p. 7).

Model projects under Title VIII have not been lacking in imagination. Sensitivity training for teachers (students are presumably already too sensitive), storefront schools (education purchased through involvement and hard work), curriculum innovations (students in one project learn academic skills by studying welfare programs), students paid to learn (presumably penalties for not learning are inappropriate as long as teachers who fail to teach go scot free) and home visitations by teachers (a subtle invasion of privacy often foisted upon the poor by halo wearing, spy prone educators) are only a few of the techniques sponsored by the Model Projects of Title VIII in what supporters and critics alike must recognize as a random search for solutions to the dropout problem. But then, even when questioning, one must recognize that problems are as often solved through the random as through the systematic, and that the problem of school dropouts is even now decreasing in size, if not intensity.

We are inclined to agree with Roy Wilkins who suggested that the ultimate objective of healthy schools in a wholesome society is to create love, "the kind of affection that endears us to our brothers, of whatever color they are and whatever language they speak (*The Urban Review*, 1969, p. 22)." Dropouts haven't been in love with schools, and schools haven't much loved them. It is a deficiency for which compensation is inadequate; the challenge is greater than that. . . .

References

Coleman, J. S. et al. *Equality of educational opportunity*. Washington, D.C.: Government Printing Office, 1966.

Commissioner Allen stresses importance of guidance in dropout programs. *American Education*, 1969, 5, 8.

Cuban, L. Cardozo project in urban teaching. *Education*, 1967, 88, 216–220.

Durham, J. T. Who needs it? Compensatory education. *Clearing House,* 1969, 44, 18–22.

Freeman, R. A. The alchemists in our public schools. In J. M. Ashbrook, *Congressional Record—extension of remarks*, April 24, 1969, E3374–E3381.

Glazer, N. Ethnic groups and education: towards the tolerance of difference. *The Journal of Negro Education*, 1969, 38, 187–195.

Havighurst, R. J. & Stiles, L. J. National policy for alienated youth. *Phi Delta Kappan*, 1961, 42, 283–291.

Holmes, E. C. A philosophical approach to the study of minority problems. *The Journal of Negro Education*, 1969, 38, 196–203.

Jencks, C. Private schools for black children. *New York Times Magazine*, Vol. 118, Pp. 30, 132–140 (November 3, 1968).

Jennings, F. G. Educational opportunities geared to diversity. In *The sixty-sixth Yearbook of the National Society for the Study of Education, Part I*. Chicago: The University of Chicago Press, 1967. Pp. 351–353.

Jensen, A. How much can we boost I.Q. and scholastic achievement? *Harvard Educational Review*, 1969, 39, 1–123.

Johnson, J. L. Special education and the inner city: a challenge for the future or another means for cooling the mark out? *The Journal of Special Education*, 1969, 3, 241–251.

Kruger, W. S. They don't have to drop out. *American Education,* 1969, 5, 7–8.

Life, The sweep of the '60s. 1969, 67, (26), 12–31 (December 24, 1969).

Omwake, E. Head start—measurable and immeasurable. In J. Hellmuth (Ed.), *Disadvantaged Child, Vol. II, Head Start and Early Intervention*. New York: Brunner/Mazel, Inc., 1968, Pp. 531–544.

Ornstein, A. C. Effective schools for "disadvantaged" children. *Journal of Secondary Education*, 1965, 40, 105–109.

Rossi, P. H. The education of failures or the failure of education? *The Journal of Negro Education*, 1969, 38, 324–333.

Schreiber, D. The school dropout. In *The sixty-sixth Yearbook of the National Society for the Study of Education, Part I*. Chicago: The University of Chicago Press, 1967. Pp. 211–236.

Strom, R. L. The school dropout and the family. In J. L. Frost & G. R. Hawkes (Eds.), *The disadvantaged child*. Boston: Houghton-Mifflin, 1966. Pp. 58–61.

Urban Review, The. Interview with Roy Wilkins. 1969, 3, (6), 16–23.

Wasserman, M. & Reimann, J. Student rebels vs. school defenders: a partisan account. *The Urban Review*, 1969, 4, 9–17.

9. Children in Poor Families: Myths and Realities

Elizabeth Herzog
Hylan Lewis

One of several pitfalls in efforts to separate fact from fiction about children is that today's realities often turn out to be tomorrow's myths—and today's myths sometimes turn out to be tomorrow's realities.

A former interpretation of the so-called Bowlby thesis, to cite one example, held that group care is inevitably damaging to a child under three, and this interpretation has been legalized in the refusal of some states to license establishments for group daytime care of children under three. Today, the government is supporting demonstrations of group care for infants and very small children in the belief that such programs will contribute to enriched cognitive and social development.

Not so many years ago, a number of experts appeared to regard a newborn child as a lovable lump of clay, wholly molded by experience and environment, and exercising no reciprocal effect upon his caretakers. Today, with a powerful assist from Lois Murphy, we regard child development as at least a two-way process, with the child an active agent influencing the behavior of parents and siblings.

A further source of discomfiture in trying to separate myths from realities is the fact that today and tomorrow are closer together than ever before. Tomorrow treads so closely on the heels of today that the speed of change itself has become one of our most critical and disconcerting factors. Meanwhile, the research explosion and the publication explosion make it harder than ever to keep informed about today, let alone getting ready for tomorrow. The world for which we are trying to help children prepare is a world that we ourselves do not know.

Moreover, we seem to have diminished confidence in our ability to cope with the world of today and to change it into a better tomorrow. Among the elements that make it unfamiliar and frightening are galloping technological progress, the resurgence of race conflict, the persistence and visibility of poverty—plus the simultaneous readiness of adults to admit the existence of these problems and of the young to blame their existence on the adults.

All these elements complicate the task of disentangling fact and fiction, myth and reality, especially for those who are committed to serving children. On the one hand, we cannot wait until all the answers are in, for the development of children does not wait. On the other hand, we cannot afford to

From *American Journal of Orthopsychiatry*, 1970, **40,** 375–387. Copyright © 1970, the American Orthopsychiatric Association, Inc. Reproduced by permission.

base large programs—or for that matter, small ones—on dubious premises. One safeguard, of course, is to recognize the need for eternal vigilance against premature acceptance of instant revelations, without demanding full credentials. Such vigilance is especially necessary in those concerned with treating children.

When we talk about treating children we mean intervening in behalf of children, trying to put them in a position to cope with their world better than we have coped with ours and to change it more effectively than we have done. One word for the fruits of such efforts is socialization. One result of developments in the society at large, and among those concerned with studying society, is a redefinition of socialization.

Under this redefinition, socialization is a continuing process, extending from the cradle to the grave. It involves the family but it also involves settings and institutions beyond the family. It may be that in no other time or place has the learning to adapt and to cope continued so late in life and been so difficult, demanding and important for adults. Among the propositions and assumptions especially important in relation to the socialization of children are those concerning family composition and functioning, and concerning the ethnic or class group of which the family is part.

Some Assumptions Stand Up

To avoid the implication that all generalizations and assumptions should be challenged, we will mention three that promise to look real even tomorrow—though of course no guarantee can be offered about day after tomorrow. Then we will consider some that we would define either as myths or as myth-ridden realities. Finally, we will try to suggest a few clues that can help to differentiate between propositions and assumptions that seem to stand up against evidence and those that do not.

A generalization that is at least as old as Plato concerns the importance of the early childhood years. Without discounting the human capacity for growth and change throughout life, we dare to predict that the foreseeable future is unlikely to redefine as myth the proposition that the early years are formative and important. At the moment, in fact, we seem to be giving increased recognition to the influence of the prenatal days and months and years.

Another proposition that seems likely to stand up concerns the value of involving a child's "significant others"—especially his parents—in activities designed to promote socialization and education. This is not to say that a child whose parents cannot or will not be involved must be given up as lost, but merely that active involvement of his family can help and failure to involve them can hinder. This proposition also receives more rather than less support from current theory, research, and social practice.

A third proposition that so far stands up is the cardinal contribution of adult firmness and warmth to the socialization process, with its corollary to the effect that either warmth or firmness is insufficient without the other.

This proposition, supported by theory, research, and day-by-day experience, seems unlikely to topple soon.

The list could be extended. There is less danger, however, in realities commonly regarded as realities than in fallacies commonly regarded as realities. Therefore it seems more fruitful to consider some of them. In doing so, it is useful to remember that a proposition or assumption which lacks any element of reality is relatively unlikely to achieve a successful masquerade. None of the propositions or assumptions we shall discuss is wholly contrary to fact. Each has elements of reality, yet each also contains elements of myth, and the net result is in our view closer to fallacy than to fact.

The Matriarchal Label

A concept that is already under scrutiny is "the culture of poverty," a subject too broad for full discussion here. Prominent in it, however, is a cluster of assumptions concerning family composition, especially the female-headed family. A conspicuous feature is the current habit of referring to the Negro family, especially the low-income Negro family, as matriarchal.

Perhaps the least of the problems associated with this label is that it happens to be inaccurate. A matriarchal society would accept matriarchy as natural, inevitable, and desirable. Moreover, it would include male roles that are accepted and respected. Yet the woman-headed central city Negro family is by no means regarded as an acceptable norm, either by the larger society or by the low-income Negro families themselves. On the contrary, the accepted ideal norm, in ghetto as in Gold Coast, is a stable marriage in which the man is the chief breadwinner, and the so-called Negro matriarchs are the first to decry the perfidy of the male who does not fulfill this role.[8] [19]

The term matriarchal as applied to the low-income Negro family reflects two assumptions: that in these families the woman is dominant and that her earning power is greater than the man's. Neither of these assumptions is strictly accurate although neither is flatly contrary to fact. According to the Bureau of Labor Statistics, women who have jobs earn less than men who have jobs, and this is as true of Negroes as of whites. Moreover, unemployment rates among Negro females are higher than among Negro males.[4] At the same time, it is true that in fatherless Negro families and in some two-parent families the woman is likely to be either the only or the main breadwinner. Accordingly, the assumption about earning capacity cannot be called either strictly true or strictly untrue.

The same ambiguous status attaches to the assumption about the woman's dominance. To a considerable extent (although by no means entirely) she dominates the child-rearing activities and responsibilities, but the same can be said about most American families. In fact a good deal of hand-wringing is devoted to the pervasiveness of women in the lives of middle-income and upper-income white children, and the ascribed effects of this pervasiveness. (On the split level, it is called momism. We seem to reserve the matriarchal label for ethnic minorities viewed across a social distance.)

To return to the inner city, breadwinning and child-rearing are not the only areas of life for the Negro mother. And in some other areas—sex relations, for example—women are not necessarily in the ascendancy. Elizabeth Bott points out that among working-class English families, women are dominant in some areas and men in others.[2] Cohen and Hodges have made the same point with regard to American working-class families, pointing out that "to describe the working-class family as both 'male-authoritarian' (or 'patriarchal') and as 'mother-centered' is not paradoxical. They are, indeed, both, depending upon the functional area which one is attending to."[5]

This kind of labeling has consequences. One is the tendency to perceive a group of people viewed across a social distance as homogeneous, forgetting the infinite variations among individuals within groups. Another is that dubious labeling and lumping promote the imputing of fallacious reasons for behavior. And programs and practice are based on the interpretation of reasons for behavior. What the policeman does on the beat, what the teacher does in the classroom, what the social worker does in relation to a client, reflects such interpretations. Misinterpretations contribute to ineffectiveness of social institutions and programs, and to mutual antagonisms.

The readiness to apply the matriarchal label may relate to the overriding value placed on money in our society. Because the woman is believed to have greater earning power than the male, it is assumed that she must be dominant. This tendency to equate the breadwinning function with dominance in the family may account for a recent reference by an American sociologist to the "matriarchal family" of early immigrants from the East European Jewish small town, the now defunct *shtetl* that still lives in memory and tradition.

In theory the *shtetl* was unqualifiedly patriarchal. In practice, one analysis has remarked that it would be hard to say whether there were more patriarchs or matriarchs in the *shtetl*.[32] It was true that the wife of a scholar was likely to be the family breadwinner, but this did not make her a matriarch. It was also true that in many—perhaps most—*shtetl* homes both wife and husband participated in earning a living. The area of learning and of spiritual values belonged to the man. The home was the domain of the woman. The market place was not sex-typed. It belonged to either or to both. But whether she supported the family or not, a woman was viewed as inherently inferior to a man, and his domain of learning and religion was rated as inherently superior, beyond her highest aspirations. That some women achieved domestic dominance illustrates the potency of informal structure and processes. It did not make the *shtetl* a matriarchy nor shake its patriarchal characteristics and self-image.

Like the imputed matriarchy of the *shtetl*, the alleged matriarchy of our urban ghetto has a mythical quality. A stable two-parent ghetto family is probably more patriarchal than its middle-class counterpart. Typically, the man is boss. A female-dominated or female-headed family is perceived as out of harmony with preferred norms, even though it may be a practical accomodation to economic realities—including welfare regulations.[8 12 13 20]

The Apathetic Stereotype

Under any label, a number of social-psychological traits have been attributed to the inner-city family. Some of these have already been reclassified as myths—for example, low educational aspirations for one's children. By now it has been demonstrated repeatedly that the mothers of the inner city have high educational aspirations for their children, even though their expectations may lag behind their aspirations.

Another imputed trait is apathy, but evidence continues to demonstrate that the much advertised apathy of the poor has been a situational response rather than an inherent trait. To some extent the response has been physical, a reaction to inadequate diet, fatigue, and disastrous physical environment. To some extent it has been a product of hopelessness and helplessness. Yet even before the physical situation is repaired, a considerable number of inner-city mothers have responded energetically to the possibility of active intervention in their own situations, through participating in school-related activities and in welfare rights organizations.

The assumption that apathy and indifference are group characteristics is challenged not only by the dramatic demonstrations against powerlessness and the growing demand for accountability of service institutions to local communities, but also by the less spectacular though equally important indications that many poor people will change their behavior, given new opportunities. One of these indications comes from the family planning field. The Growth of American Families study reported verbalized preference of the poor for small families—and that poor Negroes on the whole desired smaller families than did nonpoor whites.[31] Jaffe and Polgar,[11] among others, present evidence that the belief that the poor nevertheless resist family planning services because of "internalized maladaptive attitudes and values" related to the culture of poverty, is a myth of classic proportions. They add a wry example of the persistence of class myths regardless of the minority group to which they are applied. Margaret Sanger, they tell us, heard from physicians more than 50 years ago, a "distillation of middle-class wisdom" that carries a familiar ring today:

> They admonished her that "the people you're worrying about wouldn't use contraception if they had it; they breed like rabbits." The people she was then worrying about were mostly impoverished Jewish immigrants who adopted contraception as soon as it became available to them and whose descendants are today among the most faithful contraceptors in American society; when Mrs. Sanger was prosecuted for opening a clinic in Brooklyn, the district attorney told the jury that "the clinic was intended to do away with the Jews"![11]

Fatherless Families

It is, unfortunately, no myth that the proportion of fatherless families is very high in our inner cities. Even though the majority of inner-city children are in two-parent homes at any given time, a smaller proportion remain in the same two-parent home throughout their first 18 years. The relation of income to family composition is well documented but often forgotten. The frequency of one-parent families is inversely correlated with income. As Lefcowitz,[17] among others, has shown, the difference between income levels is more striking than the difference between whites and blacks with regard to proportion of broken homes. Our habit of reporting national statistics by color rather than by socioeconomic level often results in attributing to differences in ethnic background what are in fact class differences.

It would be contrary to nature as well as to theory to assume that absence of a father made no difference in a child's development or general well-being. Where theory sometimes departs from nature is in assuming that father absence always or usually results in serious behavioral, intellectual, or psychological impairment of a child.

In the past few years several social scientists have had occasion to review in detail research studies inquiring into the effects on children of growing up in fatherless homes. At least three independent reviews have come up with the same conclusions: that so far no firm evidence supports some familiar generalizations about specific adverse effects of father absence—for example, that father absence contributes directly to juvenile delinquency, poor school achievement and confused sex identity.[9 15 16]

Research evidence is slight and ambiguous concerning the association of these three problems with father absence, if analysis is limited to studies that have a control group and employ methods rated as reasonably sound. The familiar generalizations are, of course, supported by countless studies that lack control groups. When a review is limited to studies that meet these criteria, more do than do not indict the fatherless homes. However, the dissenting minority is much larger than is often assumed. Among 60 studies included in one review,[9] 24 reported a significant association between father absence and the problem under investigation, 20 reported no such association, and 16 arrived at conclusions too mixed or qualified to be counted clearly on either side.

This kind of referendum can hardly be accepted as proving a proposition. It does, however, indicate that some alleged effects of father absence are not to be taken for granted.

Studies focusing on juvenile delinquency show the same pattern noted for the whole group reviewed: the studies reporting a significant relation with father absence were fewer than the combined number of those that either reported the opposite or came to mixed and highly qualified conclusions.

One kind of qualification stemmed from the frequent conclusion that family discord and dissension (often a prelude to father absence) contributed more to juvenile delinquency than did father absence itself; and the occasional finding that delinquency was more frequent in children of unhappy unbroken homes than in children of harmonious and cohesive one-parent homes.

Evidence concerning poor school achievement on the part of father-absent boys is even less solid than that relating to juvenile delinquency, even more conflicting, and at least as much confounded by inadequate control for socioeconomic status. Overall, it provides no firm basis for saying that father absence reduces school achievement.

Research with regard to confused sex identity on the part of father-absent boys suffers from a cluster of technical problems, each of which is shared in some degree with other categories of father-absence research, but which in this category exhibit special strength and persistence. This problem cluster merits attention because of its severity and because it contributes to frequently invoked generalizations which influence ideas about appropriate programs and interventions.

Prominent among the problems in this cluster are inadequacy of measures and vulnerability of interpretations. Among other objections, scales of masculinity and femininity have been criticized repeatedly as class-bound, culture-bound and time-bound. Clark Vincent's[30] ingenious exercise with the California Personality Inventory revealed that boys scoring high on femininity and girls scoring low on femininity were rated more favorably than their matched comparisons on about two-thirds of the remaining 17 scales, although the differences fell short of statistical significance. For example, low-F girls were high on poise, ascendancy, and self-assurance; high-F boys were high on dominance, "capacity for status," and responsibility. But the femininity of the low-F girls was marred by failure to be afraid of thunderstorms or the dark, or to feel that they would "go to pieces," or to covet the career of librarian. The masculinity of the high-F boys was impaired by failure to feel like starting a fist fight, to want to drive a racing car, or to enjoy reading *Popular Mechanics.*

In any content area, studies of fatherless boys suffer from insufficient differentiation between temporary and continuing father absence and between honorific reasons or stigmatized reasons for the absence. They suffer too, as does so much research, from inadequate controls for socioeconomic status and—especially in studies of children in poverty—from confusing socioeconomic differences with color differences.

A further problem common to research in all areas, but especially to studies of masculine identity, is the tendency to derive large generalizations from small, unreplicated studies, and to apply these generalizations without regard to class or culture. The much-cited Norwegian study of father absence has been held up as demonstrating what can be expected for fatherless boys in Harlem, although the Norwegian subjects were sons of sailor officers, in the managerial class and experiencing recurrent absence and returns for socially approved reasons.[29] This kind of generalization is dubious in itself. It appears the more questionable in light of a careful replication in Italy that produced findings in flat contradiction to those obtained in Norway.[1]

What must be said about studies of the effects of father absence is that in no area do findings establish clear and conclusive evidence that specified adverse effects are significantly associated with father absence. At the same time, we lack clear and conclusive evidence that no significant association exists. Nevertheless, two propositions stand strong and solid. The first is that father absence is only one among an interacting complex of factors which mediate and condition its impact on a growing child.

The second solid proposition is that, even if eventually a significant association can be demonstrated between father absence and one of the adverse effects attributed to it, that impact is dwarfed by other factors in the interacting complex. Among these others are: the coping ability and individual makeup of the mother, especially her ability to give adequate mothering and supervision; the economic situation of the family; and community influences.

Predictions Based on Insufficient Evidence

A source of misleading generalizations about children—poor and non-poor—arises from overestimating the predictive value of psychological assessments made in childhood. Sometimes this involves failure to differentiate developmental lag from continuing deficit. Mischel,[22] for example, reported that at ages 8–10, father-absent children were less able or less ready than father-present children to defer gratification. However, this difference was not observed at ages 11–14.[23] One may question his interpretation of the earlier difference and still recognize that it was not present in slightly older children.

Longitudinal studies of children in two-parent homes reinforce warnings against accepting a psychological snapshot at one point in childhood as a portrait of the individual in adulthood. Jean MacFarlane has spelled out some of the reasons why predictions based on careful psychological assessment in childhood proved wrong more often than right, and erred more often in overpredicting than in underpredicting future problems. Among these reasons were overemphasis on indications of problem, overestimation of the durability of childhood behaviors and attitudes, underestimation of human potential for late development—especially the potential of a dependent person to develop confidence and strength, underestimation of the extent to which childhood trauma may, under certain circumstances and for certain individuals, function as maturity-inducing experience.[21]

Mussen,[24] after studying a selected sample of the subjects followed by MacFarlane and her colleagues, concluded that "the data from adult personality tests and impressionistic ratings, based on interview data . . . lend support to the hypothesis that the self-assurance and positive self-conceptions of the highly masculine subjects decreased after adolescence, while correlatively, the less masculine group changed in a favorable direction."

These examples are cited to illustrate the hazards of a snapshot approach that classifies a person's potential on the basis of observations or measures taken during childhood; and to illustrate the need for viewing such observations in context and in perspective, recognizing the human propensity for growth and change.

Equally unreliable are predictions based on early experiences generally agreed to be adverse to a child's development. Skodak and Skeels[27] have documented the capacity of deprived infants for dramatic intellectual growth and the development of social competence. Kadushin[14] has summarized the findings of a number of followup studies of children adopted or placed in foster homes after traumatic early experiences, commenting that "in each instance the children studied turned out to be more 'normal' and less 'maladjusted' than they had any right to be, given the traumata and insults to psyche that they experienced during early childhood." He disclaims any implication that neglect, abuse, and physical deprivation are not harmful. On the contrary, he points out that in each of the studies reviewed, "a more detailed contrast within the followup group invariably favors those subsets of children who were provided with a more benign environment prior to separation." He argues not for "a rejection of the generally accepted tenets but rather for recognition of at least the partial reversibility of the effects of deprivation."

A similar message is conveyed by studies that compare mentally ill patients with matched controls classified as "normal" and find in the normal group a surprising proportion who experienced childhood trauma, who came from broken homes, and who exhibit symptoms often classified as neurotic.[3] [26]

An important part of the message conveyed by these studies concerns the danger of singling out one trait or one circumstance as bad and assuming that it, in itself, will determine an individual's development. A number of investigators point up the inadvisability of thus singling out one culprit variable. For example, "it is the combination of many factors rather than any single one that exerts influence."[28] And again, "It is suggested that the patterning of life experiences may be more crucial than occurrence or absence of specific psychic stresses."[26]

A frequent response to such statements is, "Of course. Whoever said otherwise?" Yet the points we have brought out bear witness that many have said otherwise about many a culprit variable.

Intersection of Poverty and Blackness

Sweeping and dubious generalizations about individuals and families interlock with sweeping and dubious generalizations about groups—especially, in USA 1970, about the poor and the black.

The grinding intersection of poverty and blackness in our cities is producing rapid and dramatic changes in how the poor see themselves as well as in how they are seen. These changes are affecting the planning and distribution of services as well as their administration and control. Many of the very poor, as well as working-class and middle-class Negroes, indicate that they have learned and are prepared to act on what other segments have taken for granted: that whether and when the community will provide the tools of competence and more options for many poor families depends more upon how the community is organized, on how responsive and accountable its institutions are, than on how the poor behave.

A number of misconceptions persist about the interest and capacity of the poor to share in decision-making. Whether both the middle-class representatives and the poorer people in the ghetto share in decision-making has direct bearing on whether services are available, and on the quality of services for ghetto residents. In the resolution of the dispute in Newark over the location of the New Jersey College of Medicine and Dentistry, the college President, Dr. Cadmus, remarked that the uneducated contribute in a different way than the educated. "Moreover," he said, "I have never seen them try to intervene in areas in which they have no competence, such as medical school curriculums, or how to treat illness.... Only physicians can practice medicine. But the doctor has no exclusive rights in determining the economics of health services, the location of facilities, or the percentage of the gross national product that is to be allocated for the delivery of care. The professional has a voice, but he has much to learn from the consumer outside of his profession."[18]

The intersection of poverty and blackness has contributed heavily to the growth of the black power idea, which has the willed effect of sharpening the line between Negroes and whites and the coincidental effect of fostering mythology. It is actually the beginning of a design, and a variety of tentative, sometimes competing, formulas for letting Negroes and the poor exercise American options over their lives. According to an Indian student of race relations in Britain, "Those who possess power and actually wield it do not blazon the fact abroad. It is only those who *lack* power who are driven to the rhetoric of black power."[25]

Ironically, the most spectacular success of the idea to date is the rapid adoption and circulation of the word "black." This managed change of designations, the reasons for it, and the speed with which it has happened are without precedent.

Any idea that this rapid acceptance involves a meaningful concession is a delusion. There is a question as to how really consequential it is to whites that any significant Negro group insist (1) that Negroes be called something different, (2) that Negroes as self-conscious blacks wish to be separated, (3) that Negroes wish to achieve, by themselves, their equivalent of the shared American dream. It appears that these kinds of non-gut issues are readily conceded. However, the evidence is firm that when groups of Negroes and their spokesmen insist on larger shares in controlling the local institutions affecting their lives, the acceptance and acquiescence by whites have not been as easy, as quick, and as pervasive.

Caveats and Safeguards

The propensity of today's verity to become tomorrow's fallacy poses problems for practitioners and program planners as well as for researchers. Neither the propensity nor the problems are likely to evaporate. However, the examples we have cited suggest a few clues that can alert us to the kinds of assertions and generalities which are more likely than not to be associated with myths. In place of a formal summary, we would like to line up these clues in the form of a few caveats and safeguards.

The first one is: beware the single-barrel approach. Those who plan and carry out treatment of children in poverty would be well advised to be skeptical about programs and interventions geared to a single factor.

This overriding theme has a number of variations. One concerns what we have called the culprit variable—that is, a single trait or circumstance arraigned as damaging to children, in and of itself. The propositions hailed as verities yesterday and redefined as fallacies today tend to involve a culprit variable which in the end is perceived as only one in a complex of interacting factors. This was the case with the working mother. Ten years ago, research investigators and program planners were asking how much harm it did to a child to have his mother gainfully employed outside the home. Today there is impressive consensus that a mother's outside employment is not in itself the critical variable. The view is rather that the impact on the child depends on a great many other things which, in turn, are affected by each other. These include the mother's individual makeup and temperament, her physical stamina, her attitude toward working or not working, the child's perception of why she has a job, the child's age, sex, and special needs, and above all the arrangements she is able to make for his supervision while she is away from home.[7] [10] A similar shift from single variable to interacting complex seems to have occurred with regard to antecedents of mental illness. An analogous sequence seems to be in process with regard to the effects of father absence. In each of these instances, it might be remarked, socioeconomic status is a salient element in the interacting complex.

Another variation on the single-barreled theme involves what we have called the snapshot approach—that is, the assumption that test scores or observations taken at a single point in childhood can, in themselves, be accepted as demonstrating either the presence or the absence of lifelong problems. Again, it is necessary to allow for the interaction of other traits and life circumstances, and for the growth and change of an individual through time—a development that will be influenced not only by what happens to him but also by his own individual history and makeup; and to allow for the individual's impact on his environment as well as for the impact of his environment on him.

Yet another variation involves the single-factor panacea—for example, the attempt to avert later school deficiencies by preschool programs of cognitive enrichment alone. In this context Gordon[6] points out that "in general, the emphasis in attempts to provide relevant education has tended to shift back and forth between a stress on cognitive achievement or development and an emphasis on socialization or 'development of the whole child,' with few attempts to focus on both simultaneously in an integrated manner. At the same time, emerging research is beginning to make more respectable a renewed emphasis on affective ... processes in learning." And he adds that "this new research is complemented in the political sphere by a greater demand for participation, which is generally considered to result in changed motivation and attitude."

One safeguard against the single-barreled fallacy is supported by feeling as well as by thought. Most of us experience a revulsion that is emotional as well as rational against consigning a whole category of children to the classification incurable or unhelpable. To conclude that children probably cannot be educated adequately if their parents are not involved, or that they probably cannot develop into competent human beings if their father has left the home, is unpalatable to say the least. And in this case, as in some others, the violation of feeling is also a misreading of evidence. Program planners and practitioners have a right to resist that kind of generalization. They have a right because the impact of any single trait or circumstance will be mediated and conditioned by a complex of other interacting factors. And they have an obligation to resist such generalizations because no group is homogeneous, and within-group variations are often as great as or greater than between-group variations.

A different caveat concerns the confusion of socioeconomic and ethnic factors. The current emphasis on social and racial considerations adds to the old danger of mistaking effects that are primarily due to socioeconomic factors for effects that are primarily due to cultural factors. For example, if assertions about the characteristics of black children in poverty are based on confusing the results of poverty with the results of race, attempts to alleviate disadvantage are likely to miss their mark.

Our final "beware" concerns generalizations that categorically deny the capacity for change in individuals and groups, lumped in a single category. We have mentioned, for example, underestimation of the extent to which adults can move from apathy to effective participation, which influences program design and individual treatment and the way they are carried out. This has to do with the ability of adult family members to help or to hinder the socialization of children as well as with the quality of their community participation.

We have harped on these points because we believe that some generalizations and assumptions which will be recognized as myths tomorrow are hurting today.

References

1. Ancona, L., Cesa-Bianchi, M., and Bocquet, F. 1963. Identification with the father in the absence of a paternal model. Archivio di Psicologia, Neurologia e Psichiatria.
2. Bott, E. 1957. Family and Social Network. Tavistock Publications, London.
3. Brockway, A., et al. 1954. The use of a control population in neuropsychiatric research: psychiatric, psychological, and EEG evaluation of a heterogeneous sample. Amer. J. Psychiat. 111:248–262.
4. Bureau of Labor Statistics. 1966. The Negro in the United States—Their Economic and Social Situation. Bull. 1511, U. S. Dept. of Labor. U. S. Govt. Printing Off., Washington.
5. Cohen, A., and Hodges, H. 1963. Lower blue-collar-class characteristics. Soc. Prob. 10:303–333.
6. Gordon, E. 1968–1969. Decentralization and educational reform. IRCD Bull. 4 & 5:1–5.
7. Herzog, E. 1960. Children of Working Mothers. Children's Bureau Pub. 382, Welfare Admin., U. S. Dept. of HEW. U. S. Govt. Printing Off., Washington.

8. Herzog, E. 1967. About the Poor: Some Facts and Some Fictions. Children's Bureau Pub. 451, Social and Rehabilitation Service, U. S. Dept. of HEW. U. S. Govt. Printing Off., Washington.
9. Herzog, E., and Sudia, C. 1970. Children in fatherless families. *In* Review of Child Development Research, Vol. 3, B. Caldwell and H. Ricciutti, eds. Society for Research in Child Development. In Press.
10. Hoffman, L. 1960. Effects of the employment of mothers on parental power relations and the division of household tasks. Mar. and Fam. Liv. 22:27–35.
11. Jaffe, F., and Polgar, S. 1968. Family planning and public policy: is the "culture of poverty" the new cop-out? J. Mar. and the Fam. 30:228–235.
12. Jeffers, C. 1966. Three Generations—Case Materials for Low Income Urban Living, Communicating Research on the Urban Poor, CROSS-TELL, Health and Welfare Council of the National Capital Area, Washington.
13. Jeffers, C. 1967. Living Poor. Ann Arbor Publishers, Ann Arbor, Mich.
14. Kadushin, A. 1967. Reversibility of trauma: a followup study of children adopted when older. Soc. Work. 12:22–33.
15. Kadushin, A. 1968. Single parent adoptions—an overview and some relevant research. Paper presented at Northwest Regional Conference, Child Welfare League of America.
16. Kohlberg, L. 1966. A cognitive-developmental analysis of children's sex-role concepts and attitudes. *In* The Development of Sex Differences, E. Maccoby, ed. Stanford Univ. Press, Stanford, Calif: 82–173.
17. Lefcowitz, M. 1965. Poverty and Negro-White family structures. Background paper for White House Conference: To Fulfill These Rights.
18. Lesparre, M. 1968. Interaction with the inner city: an interview with Robert R. Cadmus, M.D. Hospitals. 42:54–58.
19. Lewis, H. 1960. The changing Negro family. *In* The Nation's Children, Vol. 1: The Family and Social Change, E. Ginzberg, ed. Columbia Univ. Press, New York.
20. Lewis, H. 1967. Culture, class and family life among low-income urban Negroes. *In* Employment, Race and Poverty, A. Ross, ed. Harcourt, Brace and World, New York.
21. MacFarlane, J. 1963. From infancy to adulthood. Childhood Educ.: 83–89.
22. Mischel, W. 1958. Preference for delayed reinforcement: an experimental study of a cultural observation. J. Abnorm. and Soc. Psychol. 56:57–61.
23. Mischel, W. 1961. Father-absence and delay of gratification: cross-cultural comparisons. J. Abnorm. and Soc. Psychol. 63: 116–124.
24. Mussen, P. 1962. Long-term consequents of masculinity of interests in adolescence. J. Consult. Psychol. 26.
25. Nandy, D. 1967. Black power: fallacies of parity. Lecture delivered at the Institute of Race Relations, London. Mimeo.
26. Schofield, W., and Balian, L. 1959. A comparative study of the personal histories of schizophrenic and nonpsychiatric patients. J. Abnorm. and Soc. Psychol. 59:216–225.
27. Skeels, H. 1965. Effects of adoption on children from institutions. Children. 12:33–34.
28. Stone, R., and Schlamp, F. 1965. Characteristics associated with receipt or nonreceipt of financial aid from welfare agencies: an exploratory study. Welfare in Review, 3:1–11.
29. Tiller, P. 1958. Father absence and personality development in children of sailor families. Nordisk Psykologi's Monographs, Series 9. Oslo, Bokhjørnet.
30. Vincent, C. 1966. Implications of changes in male-female role expectations for interpreting M-F scores. J. Mar. and the Fam. 28:196–199.
31. Whelpton, P., Campbell, A., and Patterson, J. 1966. Fertility and Family Planning in the United States. Princeton Univ. Press, Princeton, N. J.
32. Zborowski, M., and Herzog, E. 1952. Life is with People: The Jewish Littletown of Eastern Europe. International Universities Press, New York.

Part II

Types of Childhood Psychopathology

Chapter Four

Childhood Neurosis
with Emphasis on School Phobia

This book considers several different types of childhood disorders, including neurosis, behavior (conduct) disorder, hyperkinesis, mental retardation, and psychosis. Chapter Four focuses on childhood neurosis, with special emphasis on school phobia. Before considering this topic, however, let us mention some basic differences among the categories of abnormality known as neurosis, behavior disorder, and psychosis.

Although there are many complex differentiating criteria, the essential differences can be stated quite simply. A person suffering from a neurosis mainly takes his difficulties out on himself. He is agitated, nervous, unhappy, and distraught, but does not directly hurt others. Moreover, the neurotic is well aware of reality and, if anything, overly concerned about his personal and social maladjustment. A person with a behavior disorder tends to "act out" against the world around him. He engages in behaviors that get him into difficulty with family, schools, employers, police, and other guardians of society. While usually knowing the difference between right and wrong, this type of person's characteristic way of handling emotional difficulties is to engage in some form of socially unacceptable behavior. The psychotic individual shows a break with reality, perceiving the environment in a distorted fashion and reacting in bizarre ways that are markedly different from most people in the society. Disorganization of thought and behavior, with inability to take care of oneself, are fundamental features of psychotic adjustment.

The essential characteristic of neurosis is the presence of disabling anxiety. Most theorists and clinicians regard anxiety as the key concept in attempting to understand neurotic behavior. White (1964) has developed a theory of conflict in which all neurotic symptoms are seen as resulting from attempts to defend against anxiety. On the basis of the concepts of anxiety and defense, White accounts for the vast variety of abnormal behaviors evidenced by people who suffer from neurosis.

In the early stages of his theorizing, Freud believed that repression of unacceptable sexual and aggressive impulses generated anxiety and led to neurosis in the adult patients treated in his private practice in Vienna. At a later stage in the formulation of this theory, Freud altered his view and then believed that anxiety led to repression. In other words, because the person felt anxious, he tended to repress (exclude from conscious awareness) all thoughts, memories, and feelings that were associated with the anxiety-provoking experience. Most theorists who have written on this topic in recent years have been strongly influenced by Freud's conceptualizations, and it is commonly agreed that anxiety is the root of neurotic symptoms. The abnormal behaviors shown by neurotic individuals are indications of the kinds of techniques they have developed in attempting to cope with or avoid the feelings of anxiety that threaten to overwhelm them.

Types of Childhood Neurosis

Several distinguishable types of neurosis are seen in adult patients, and some of them are also found in disturbed children. The three main types are: hysteria, obsessive-compulsive neurosis, and phobia.

Hysteria

While there is voluminous literature on the topic of hysteria in adults, relatively little has been written on this specific neurotic disorder in children. The symptomatic behaviors include tendencies to be overdramatic, overaffective, and highly suggestible. These traits, to a pathological degree, are more characteristic of girls than boys and are often accompanied by seductive behavior. One form of this disorder is known as conversion hysteria, in which some part of the body becomes functionally inoperative even though there is no physical abnormality. At the adult level, classic examples are the singer or actor who suddenly loses his voice and the writer or painter who becomes unable to hold a pencil or brush in his hand. In these instances, the anxiety is believed to become converted to a particular body organ that will serve to prevent the person from having to face anxiety-provoking situations.

In young children these types of disorders are more apt to affect bodily functions such as eating and toileting. Actually, in very young children it is common to observe behaviors and personality traits that would be signs of hysterical neurosis if found in adults. That is, it is normal for children to be highly emotional, suggestible, and over-reactive to mild frustration. Although hysterical adults may appear sophisticated on the surface, these childlike tendencies and behaviors are easily provoked.

One subvariety of a hysterical symptom in children appears in the form ot tics that involve excessive involuntary movements of parts of the body (eye-blinking, facial twitch, stereotyped gestures, jerky movements of arms or legs). All of these abnormal behaviors are believed to be symptomatic of the disturbing anxiety with which the child is struggling to cope.

Obsessive-Compulsive Neurosis

This type of neurosis is characterized by thoughts or ideas the child cannot keep out of his mind and/or behavior he feels he must repeat in a ritualistic manner. With this form of neurotic disorder, the person seems to be continually reminded of the very thought that is disturbing to him, but he cannot avoid thinking about. These obsessional thoughts are often accompanied by compulsive behaviors which are usually of two types. Some appear to represent precautionary behaviors designed to prevent certain occurrences (checking the locks on all doors and windows) and others seem to symbolize acts of atonement (touching certain objects a required number of times, washing the hands excessively and according to a set procedure).

It is quite normal for all children to show some degree of obsessive thinking and compulsive behavior in the course of development. For example, children set rituals for themselves such as touching every picket on a fence or carefully avoiding stepping on cracks in the sidewalk. These behaviors become neurotic when they reach a point of becoming extremely upsetting and anxiety provoking if they cannot be carried out. At this point, the abnormal behaviors are being used to defend against anxiety; when they fail, the child becomes panic-stricken.

Phobias

Phobias involve a morbid fear or dread of particular objects, people, animals, or places. If the object or event in question is truly frightening or threatening, we do not call fear of it a phobia; for example, fear of a vicious dog in the neighborhood, fear of a bully who physically abuses the child, or unwillingness to swim to a distant point he is afraid he cannot reach are not indications of phobic behavior. That is, to the extent that fears and anxieties have a basis in reality, they are not signs of neurosis. However, when the feared object is actually non-threatening (a tame, affectionate dog) or non-dangerous (water in a shallow swimming pool), yet the child is extremely terrified to approach it, then we are faced with the problem of a childhood phobia. Usually the child is preoccupied with the object or situation he so greatly fears. Thus, phobias are characterized by the degree of anxiety (bordering on panic), the irrationality of the fear, and the obsessional quality of the dread.

In Freudian theory, the phobia is believed to represent a psychological defense against socially unacceptable internal impulses. Freud's (1909) classic case of Little Hans was used to demonstrate the operation of sexual strivings and unconscious motivation in a 5-year-old boy with a phobia of horses. This case exemplified the unresolved Oedipal conflict that Freud believed formed the basis for much neurotic symptom formation in males. Freud wrote that Little Hans wanted to sleep with his mother and, consequently, felt considerable hostility toward his father whose presence prevented this sexualized mother-child relationship. According to Freud's theorizing, the little boy not only hated his father but also feared him, and because of this felt great anxiety lest his father castrate him. In order to resolve this conflict situation, the child displaced his hostility and fear onto horses and thus developed a phobia of them. In other words, since the child could not express his strong negative feelings toward his father and was terribly anxious as a result of this family conflict situation, he displaced these feelings onto horses. By avoiding horses he was able to avoid his repressed conflicts and anxiety.

Proponents of a learning theory formulation of phobic behaviors do not agree with Freud's account of the dynamics in the case of Little Hans. They prefer to view it as a case of learning and have presented evidence that Little Hans had actually been frightened by horses prior to developing his phobia. The classic case of Peter, who was conditioned by Watson and Rayner (1920) to fear a white rat strictly through the application of principles and procedures of classical conditioning, demonstrated very clearly how a phobia could be acquired. That is, by pairing a very loud, startling noise with the presentation of a white rat, this little boy soon learned to fear the presence of the animal. Not only did he acquire fear of this particular animal, but he also came to be afraid of a wide variety of white furry objects, demonstrating the learning of a phobia.

Thus there are conflicting theories of the acquisition of phobias with the psychodynamic school maintaining that phobias result from unconscious, unresolved, sexual and aggressive conflicts encountered in the process of psychosexual development. According to the learning theory formulation, the irrational ideas and phobic behaviors are learned by exactly the same procedures as all other behaviors that are acquired in the course of socialization. In the remainder of this section we will focus on school phobia to exemplify some of the most important current problems and issues in the area of childhood neurosis.

School Phobia

Recent years have witnessed an increasing interest in school phobia, and while considerable literature has been devoted to this topic, several important issues remain unresolved. Here we will introduce the subject of school phobia, the relevant literature, and the most pressing issues.

Definition

School phobia is generally defined as refusal to attend school based on unwarranted fear of the school and/or inappropriate anxiety about leaving home. Eisenberg (1958) has presented the following definition: "Partial or total inability to go to school that results from an irrational dread of some aspect of the school situation." This definition emphasizes the irrational aspect of the disorder, and the general definition includes the stipulation that the time not spent in school be spent at home. These definitions thus include features that differentiate between school phobia and truancy. In both instances, the child avoids going to school, but the phobic child does so because he suffers intense anxiety in the school situation and feels much more comfortable at home, while the truant is a child who deliberately avoids both school and home in order to engage in activities he finds more enjoyable.

Hersov (1960a) conducted a comprehensive study comparing children with school phobia to those who were truants. As with several other British investigators, Hersov uses the term "school refusal" to designate children who are more commonly diagnosed as showing school phobia. The following factors were found to be characteristic of truancy but *not* of school refusal: absence of father, inconsistent discipline, enuresis, lying, stealing, wandering from home, and diagnosis of conduct disorder. These findings indicate that several personality and social factors clearly distinguish between these two groups of children who do not attend school but for quite different reasons.

Within the category of school phobia (or school refusal), Hersov (1960b) identified three subtypes of family relationships. Type 1 is characterized by an over-indulgent mother, a passive father, and a child who is demanding at home and timid at school. Type 2 is characterized by an over-controlling mother, a passive father, and a child who is obedient at home and timid at school. While both of these subtypes are characterized by a passive father and timid child at school, the third subtype is quite different in these respects. In Type 3 there is an over-indulgent mother, but a firm father, and a child who is willful at home and friendly at school. These differing kinds of family dynamics are highly relevant to any attempt to understand the etiology (causes) of school phobia.

Coolidge, Hahn, and Peck (1957) have been concerned with whether school phobia indicates a neurotic crisis or a way of life. Their studies uncovered several characteristics that differentiate between what they term a "neurotic" type and a "characterological" type. Many of these differential characteristics have been summarized by Kennedy (1965). Characteristics of the neurotic type are: present occurrence the first episode; onset occurs on Monday, following complaints of illness; child is concerned about death and about mother's health; parents are well adjusted and responsive to professional help. The characterological type is distinguished by: recurring episodes; occurs more often in older children; death theme and health of mother is not an issue; poor communication between parents; father has a character disorder and mother is neurotic; parents are very difficult to work with.

Another way of classifying school phobias is in terms of acute versus chronic. The acute form fits with the Coolidge et al. neurotic type, in which the psychological disturbances appear quite suddenly and are limited to anxiety about attending school. These children tend to function adequately in other areas of life, with their neurotic anxiety focused on a school phobia. The chronic form is more in keeping with the Coolidge et al. characterological type, with the phobia developing gradually (incipient onset) and the disturbed personality-functioning showing up in other areas of social interaction.

Incidence

There are no exact, up-to-date figures available on the incidence of school phobia. These figures are greatly influenced by the criteria used in defining this disorder and by the facilities available for diagnosis and treatment. It is recognized, however, that school phobia has appeared with increasing frequency in recent years. Eisenberg (1958) noted that in an 8-year period at the children's psychiatric service at Johns Hopkins Hospital, the incidence increased from 3 cases per thousand to 17 cases per thousand. Kahn and Nursten (1962) have estimated school refusal in the general school population to be as high as 8 percent.

While boys outnumber girls for most types of abnormalities treated in child guidance clinics, school phobias tend to be somewhat more common in girls. Most often the difficulty appears in the elementary school years, although sometimes the school phobia does not present itself until secondary school. One published report (Hodgman & Braiman, 1965) has described "college phobia," which shows many similarities to the childhood phobia. However, school phobia is usually regarded as more of a problem with preadolescent youngsters than with any other age group.

While one might think that school phobia would appear most often in children of lower intellectual ability, this is not the case. Instead, this form of neurotic behavior is found in children at all intellectual levels—often in those who are very bright. Interestingly, children who are classified as showing so-called learning disabilities do not usually refuse to attend school. Thus, it is not the child who is destined to school failure who seems to acquire a school phobia, but rather the child who is sufficiently intelligent to do good work but who is unable to do so because of the unbearable anxiety engendered by the school setting.

Etiology

Just as with other types of phobia, in attempting to understand the causes of school phobia one can look to psychodynamic theory or to learning theory. The general psychodynamic explanation is in terms of a basically disturbed child interacting with disturbed parents.

In attempting to understand specific dynamics involved in the role of the mother, it has been said that in many cases the mothers of school-phobic children have never resolved dependency relations with their own mothers. They were led to feel inadequate and incompetent by their mothers; when they have children of their own, they tend to be unduly fearful and compensate by being overprotective. One particularly troublesome area for these mothers is their unresolved neurotic conflicts about aggression, thus making it difficult for them to discipline their children even when necessary. In general, they tend to identify with the child heaping upon him the love and security they feel they never received from their own parents.

Usually the mother is a good provider for the child during the earliest formative years but unknowingly lays the foundation for later maladjustment. When the child is confronted by frustrations in school and/or prefers to remain in the comfortable, undemanding home situation, the mother is quick to support this infantile withdrawal reaction. She agrees that the school setting is ominous and readily goes along with the child's complaints of headache or stomach pain or some other vague physical ailment calling for tender loving care. In this regard, an excellent paper written from a pediatrician's viewpoint (Schmitt, 1971) refers to school phobia as "the great imitator." By this he means that pediatricians often see cases of school phobia before they are so diagnosed. Schmitt points out that before these children ever reach the psychiatrist or psychologist, they are usually brought to the pediatrician because they are supposedly physically ill. Rarely do the parents even mention school refusal at this point because, as Schmitt states, " . . . they merely assume that everyone knows a 'sick child' doesn't belong in school. Only a heartless mother would force such a child to go to school."

While the mother is most often seen as the culprit in this particular childhood disorder, the father is also believed to play an important role in some cases. In general, this negative contribution stems from the father's failure to counteract the mother's overprotective, infantilizing approach and by helping to make her feel incompetent. Two types of paternal personalities have been described as contributing factors (Weiner, 1970). One type consists of men who are passive and dependent with a weak sense of masculine identification. They possess needs and motives very similar to their wives' and are equally overprotective of their children. The second type of father is markedly different, exemplifying masculinity in the extreme, with considerable involvement in work and hobbies, but little interest in happenings in the home situation. This type of father is often so uninvolved with both his wife and child that he is unaware of the school phobia until it has reached the stage of requiring professional attention. He then tends to become furious with his incompetent wife and disgusted with his ineffectual child—reactions that serve only to intensify the family psychopathology.

It should be noted that not all psychodynamic theorists accept the concept of "separation anxiety" as being fundamental to understanding of school phobia. For example, Leventhal and Sills (1964) reject this theory on the ground that very often the school phobic child is able to function independently of the mother in other areas of behavior. According to these investigators, the fundamental underlying problem in school phobia is an unrealistic self-image. During the early formative years, the child develops an unrealistically positive self-concept, regarding himself as exceptionally competent and admired for his outstanding achievements. When he encounters frustration and unrewarding situations in school, being forced to accept failure in the face of competition with peers, the child develops behaviors that enable him to avoid attending school. Thus the formulation of a school phobia.

Most behavior therapists have accepted the separation anxiety theory of school phobia. However, in place of unresolved emotional conflicts resulting from traumatic experiences in psychosexual development, the behaviorists use concepts and principles derived from learning theory. While the learning theory approach also emphasizes mother-child relations in accounting for the acquisition of school phobia, there is much more reliance on such concepts as positive and negative reward, instrumental acts, stimulus generalization, and discrimination learning. From this viewpoint, school phobia can result from any of the following factors: early learning that separation from mother can be dangerous and that home is a safe refuge from threat; insufficient rewards attained in school; and actual traumatic, anxiety-arousing experiences encountered in the school situation. It is evident that the psychodynamic and the learning theory approaches share many common views pertaining to the genesis of school phobia.

Treatment and Prognosis

The psychodynamic approach emphasizes the necessity of treating the parent-child relationship through a process of psychotherapy. However, psychotherapists disagree; some maintain that parent and child must be treated independently, and others argue for family therapy, in which parents and child are seen together. A related issue on which psychodynamic therapists have not shown complete agreement pertains to the desirability of returning the child to school as soon as possible. Some therapists believe that it is first essential to establish psychotherapeutic relationships with the mother and child, helping them both to resolve their emotional problems before encouraging the child to return to school. On the other hand, most psychodynamic therapists who have written on this topic believe that the very first consideration is to get the child back to school, using whatever methods may be necessary short of physical coercion. Interestingly, positive results have been obtained from both approaches—those emphasizing "insight" into the problem and deferring return to school as well as those stressing early return as the primary consideration.

With young children and early intervention, Waldfogel, Tessman, and Hahn (1959) found that in 25 out of 26 cases, school attendance resumed within a few weeks. Follow-up study showed that of those children who had received psychotherapy, a very high percentage were still free of symptoms, while only 3 of 11 cases who had received no therapeutic treatment were symptom-free at the time of the subsequent assessment.

Rodriguez, Rodriguez, and Eisenberg (1959) reported that 70 percent of phobic children seen in brief psychotherapy resumed regular school attendance. An interesting observation from this study, however, was that significant improvement occurred in almost 90 percent of the children who were under 11 years of age at the onset of the school phobia, while comparable improvement was found in only 36 percent of older children. Thus, this study reveals both the efficacy of brief, rapid treatment and the differential effectiveness in favor of younger children.

Kennedy (1965) also reported great success in rapid treatment of school phobia. He restricted his treatment program to children who were diagnosed as the "neurotic crisis type" and found that this type could be differentiated from other types of school phobia on the basis of ten symptoms. The rapid treatment program was presented in six steps that extended over a three-day period. The essential components in this program were good professional public relations, avoidance of emphasis on somatic complaints, forced school attendance, structured interview with the parents, brief interview with the child, and follow-up evaluation of the outcome. According to Kennedy, all 50 cases treated by this procedure responded with complete remission of school phobia symptoms, and a follow-up study revealed no evidence of substitute symptoms.

Behavior therapists have also obtained good results using techniques requiring rapid return to school. Garvey and Hegrenes (1966) instituted a program of systematic desensitization with a boy who had previously received six months of conventional psychotherapy, gradually forcing the child to approach the school setting. Although this boy had established a positive relationship with his psychotherapist and seemed to be showing improved general adjustment, his school phobia showed no improvement under the conventional therapeutic regime. Following only 20 sessions of desensitization, however, he resumed regular class attendance. Even more impressive, a two-year follow-up study revealed no subsequent signs of phobia. A study reported by Lazarus, Davison, and Polefka (1965), using classical and operant conditioning procedures, also showed remarkable improvement in a 9-year-old school-phobic boy, with complete success evidenced at the time of follow-up assessment almost a year later.

I studied the baffling case of a boy named Patrick, who was placed in a residential treatment center at 10 years of age because of severe depression, frequent temper tantrums, and school phobia (Davids, 1972). This seriously disturbed youngster had been raised by a neurotic mother in an unusually close and pathological relationship, with several traumatic experiences related to separation from the mother. During two years of residential treatment, Patrick received intensive psychotherapy, milieu therapy, and special education in the school at the treatment center. He showed noteworthy gains in all areas of functioning and was transferred to a halfway house for a transitional period prior to returning to the community. Although no specific attempt had been made to treat his school phobia during the two years of psychodynamic treatment, it was assumed that his abnormality would show improvement along with gains in other areas.

All boys living in the halfway house were expected to attend public school. However, after attending classes for the first three days of school in the fall, Patrick developed severe signs of agitation, anxiety, and depression, and he absolutely refused to attend school. He was taken there forcibly, but acted out in such bizarre ways that he had to be removed. Special allowances were then made for him, and he was permitted to attend classes at the treatment center and continued to receive psychotherapy while living in the halfway house. He was eventually discharged, following three years of intensive therapeutic treatment, showing general improvement but still school phobic. Follow-up study a year later revealed that this youngster followed exactly the same pattern when again confronted with attending regular public school. He went to classes for three days and then, the following Monday, refused to attend. No amount of coercion by the mother or stepfather could get Patrick to enter the school building, and the Juvenile Court eventually ordered him to a state mental hospital for observation. The outcome was enrollment in a day-care program at the hospital, where he successfully studied academic subjects at his expected grade level while living at home.

In terms of treating the problem of school phobia, this case must certainly be viewed as an utter failure. One can only wonder whether some form of behavior therapy (desensitization, counter-conditioning, systematic application of positive and negative rewards) might have successfully treated this disorder. Published findings suggest this is a very likely possibility. Of course, it may be that therapists, of whatever bent, are prone to publish reports of their successes, with the more perplexing and discouraging cases remaining quietly in their files.

The Issues

There appears to be ample evidence that various types of treatment have proven effective in helping children and parents cope with problems of school phobia. However, not all treatment programs have met with success, and professionals disagree on several important issues pertaining to diagnosis and treatment of school-phobic children and their parents. Some of these controversial issues are considered in the papers that follow. The importance of early return to school is emphasized by Leon Eisenberg, but contraindicated by Richard S. Greenbaum, who maintains that deferred return does not necessarily have negative consequences. According to Greenbaum, it is much more important to establish a secure therapeutic relationship with the child first. Eisenberg also considers whether the phobic child actually fears school or is primarily afraid to leave home.

While this introduction and accompanying papers are designed to provide the reader with considerable understanding of school phobia, Chapters Nine and Ten, devoted to the topics of psychotherapy and behavior therapy, also discuss the theory and treatment of phobias.

References

Coolidge, J. C., Hahn, P. B., & Peck, A. L. School phobia: Neurotic crisis or way of life? *American Journal of Orthopsychiatry,* 1957, **27,** 296–306.

Davids, A. *Abnormal children and youth: Therapy and research.* New York: Wiley-Interscience, 1972.

Eisenberg, L. School phobia: A study in the communication of anxiety. *American Journal of Psychiatry,* 1958, **114,** 712–718.

Freud, S. Analysis of a phobia in a five-year-old boy (1909). In J. Strachey (Ed.), *The standard edition of the complete psychological works of Sigmund Freud.* Vol. 10. London: Hogarth Press, 1955.

Garvey, W. P., & Hegrenes, J. R. Desensitization techniques in the treatment of school phobia. *American Journal of Orthopsychiatry,* 1966, **36,** 147–152.

Hersov, L. A. Persistent nonattendance at school. *Journal of Child Psychology and Psychiatry,* 1960, **1,** 130–136. (a)

Hersov, L. A. Refusal to go to school. *Journal of Child Psychology and Psychiatry,* 1960, **1,** 137–145. (b)

Hodgman, C. H., & Braiman, A. "College phobia": School refusal in university students. *American Journal of Psychiatry,* 1965, **121,** 801–805.

Kahn, J. H. & Nursten, J. P. School refusal: A comprehensive review of school phobia and other failures of school attendance. *American Journal of Orthopsychiatry,* 1962, **22,** 707–718.

Kennedy, W. A. School phobia: Rapid treatment of fifty cases. *Journal of Abnormal Psychology,* 1965, **70,** 285–289.

Lazarus, A. A., Davison, G. C., & Polefka, D. A. Classical and operant factors in the treatment of school phobia. *Journal of Abnormal Psychology,* 1965, **70,** 225–229.

Leventhal, T., & Sills, M. Self-image in school phobia. *American Journal of Orthopsychiatry,* 1964, **34,** 685–695.

Rodriguez, A., Rodriguez, M., & Eisenberg, L. The outcome of school phobia: A follow-up study based on 41 cases. *American Journal of Psychiatry,* 1959, **116,** 540–544.

Schmitt, B. D. School phobia—the great imitator: A pediatrician's viewpoint. *Pediatrics,* 1971, **48,** 433–441.

Waldfogel, S., Tessman, E., & Hahn, P. B. A program for early intervention in school phobia. *American Journal of Orthopsychiatry,* 1959, **29,** 321–332.

Watson, J. B., & Rayner, R. Conditioned emotional reactions. *Journal of Experimental Psychology,* 1920, **31,** 1–14.

Weiner, I. B. *Psychological disturbance in adolescence.* New York: Wiley-Interscience, 1970.

White, R. W. *The abnormal personality.* New York: Ronald, 1964.

10. School Phobia: A Study in the Communication of Anxiety

Leon Eisenberg

Psychiatric efforts to understand the meaning and genesis of neurotic behavior begin with the painstaking task of reconstructing a reliable version of the patient's previous life history from the accounts he and his relatives provide. We soon learn—as Freud disconcertingly discovered—that the emotional involvement of the participants distorts the very process of anamnesis. This leads us to attend to the behavior of the patient and his relatives toward the psychiatrist. The sample of behavior in the office, termed transference or parataxis, is presumed to be representative of other interpersonal transactions, though it is clearly a very special kind of interpersonal relationship, not immediately equivalent to any other. Both of these sources, case history and interview, valuable though they are, fail to provide the direct data of observation that might verify or contradict the dynamic hypotheses we erect to account for the origin of disturbed behavior. We are in search of the specific patterns of verbal and non-verbal communication *within the family unit* that give rise to the patient's symptoms.

It may be of interest, therefore, to report direct observations of parent-child interaction that bear directly upon the source of a particular syndrome of neurotic behavior: school phobia. The mode of relationship was available for study at the very juncture when the symptoms were *in statu nascendi:* the moment of separation. The drama could be seen as it unfolded rather than having to be reconstructed from the incomplete and colored versions offered by the actors in terms of their experience of it and their attitudes toward the auditor. In this way recurrent psychotherapeutic encounters with parental ambivalence were thrown into bold relief by observation of the critical role it played in the interaction between parent and child. The communication patterns that could be significantly related to the onset and perseverance of this specific syndrome may be pertinent to an understanding of the origins of neurotic behavior in children.

The Clinical Problem

Children with school phobia are coming to psychiatric attention with increasing frequency. In a survey of the last 4,000 admissions to our clinic, the incidence was noted to have risen from 3 cases per 1,000 to 17 cases per 1,000 over the last 8 years. It is difficult to ascertain whether this reflects a real change in incidence or merely in recognition and referral from physi-

From *American Journal of Psychiatry*, 1958, **114**, 712–718. Copyright 1958 by the American Psychiatric Association. Reproduced by permission.

cians and school authorities, the latter hypothesis representing the more likely explanation. Presumably, in former years such problems were handled by the truant officer or the children were made invalids at home by certificate of the family physician.

At the outset of this discussion, it is essential that school phobia be distinguished from the far more common problem of truancy. The truant, as a rule, has been an indifferent student. He cuts classes on the sly and spends his time *away from home,* frequently for antisocial purposes. He is likely to be a rebel against authority and usually stems from the lower socioeconomic strata of the community.

The phobic child, on the other hand, urgently communicates to his parents his inability to go to school and is usually unwilling to leave home at all during school hours. Most commonly, he is of average or better intellectual endowment and has done well academically prior to the onset of his neurotic symptoms. His difficulty may present itself frankly as fear of attending school or may be thinly disguised as abdominal pain, nausea and vomiting, syncope—or the fear of nausea or syncope in school. Frequently the child is unable to specify what he fears. At times, if pressed, he may offer a rationalization of his behavior in terms of a strict teacher or principal, unfriendly classmates or the danger of failing. The incidents that may be blamed for provoking the reaction do not differ in kind or intensity from those most children experience at some time during the course of schooling. Moreover, the correction of the apparent difficulty by change of classroom, reassurance of passing, etc. is conspicuously unsuccessful in resolving the problem. In general, the longer the period of absence from school before therapeutic intervention is attempted, the more difficult treatment becomes.

Systematic study of these children reveals that, almost without exception, the basic fear is not of attending school, but of leaving mother or, less commonly, father. Johnson and her collaborators (1, 2) have suggested, therefore, that these cases be classified as separation anxiety and that the term school phobia be discarded. We have no argument with the contention that this group of cases constitutes a clinical variant of separation anxiety (3). The older term, however, has not only the merits of historical priority and wide clinical usage, but as well the useful function of serving to emphasize clinical symptomatology that must be the first target of therapeutic efforts. That is, the key to successful treatment lies in insistence on an early return to school for older children or the introduction to a therapeutic nursery school for the younger; left at home, the patient is further isolated from his peers, multiplies his anxiety about returning, is trapped in the vortex of family pathology and is reinforced to persist in infantile maneuvering by the "success" of his efforts.

Sources of the Clinical Data

The findings to be summarized are based upon 2 groups of patients, totaling 26 cases. The first group comprised 11 children, 6 boys and 5 girls, of pre-school age, who were treated for separation problems at the Children's Guild, a specialized nursery school for emotionally disturbed children. The second group, 7 boys and 3 girls in elementary and 3 boys and 2 girls in junior high or high school, were studied in outpatient therapy, mostly at the Children's Psychiatric Service. On each of the patients, a thorough initial psychiatric evaluation was performed; in most cases, supplementary information was obtained during the course of psychotherapy. In the children attending nursery, careful observations were made of the behavior of child and mother during the initial period when mother was invited to be present and particularly during the transitional period when separation was accomplished. As we became aware of the significance of the interaction patterns that were noted in the younger group, we were alerted to waiting room behavior before and after therapeutic interviews and inquired more closely about parental actions during efforts to get children to school.

While the specific problems in no two families were identical nor were precisely the same behavior patterns exhibited during the moments of separation, an intense ambivalent relationship between parent and child was present in every case, with separation as difficult for the parent as for the child. In 24 of the cases, the nuclear problem for the child lay in his relationship to his mother, in 2 to his father. There would seem to be little purpose in statistical enumeration; rather, illustrative case synopses and representative anecdotes of separation behavior will be presented as exemplary of the dynamic factors evident in each case, but in varying intensity.

Parent-Child Interaction during Separation

During his first days at the Guild, the typical child remained in close physical proximity to his mother. Attracted to group activities despite himself, he could be seen oscillating toward and away from the play area. As he began to look less and less in his mother's direction and to enter tentatively into the nursery program, his mother was noted to move from her now peripheral position in order to occupy a seat closer to her child. The umbilical cord evidently pulled at both ends! Periodically the mother intruded herself into the child's awareness on the pretext of wiping his nose, checking his toilet needs, etc., each such venture being followed by his temporary withdrawal from the group—much to her dismay.

As trial separations were begun by having the mother move into an adjacent room after telling her child, several mothers jeopardized a previously successful transition by finding it "necessary" to return to the play area. When the director suggested actual departure, the mothers responded with an admixture of indecisiveness, apprehension and resentment. One anguished mother, literally led out by the hand, commented, "The least I can do is keep my feet moving." Another bid her twins goodbye with many reassurances of her early return. They played on unconcerned. She stopped again at the door to assure them they had nothing to fear. They glanced up but played on. Having gotten her coat, she made a third curtain speech in a tremulous voice, "Don't be afraid. Mommy will be back. Please don't cry." This time one of the twins got the cue and cried till she left. Another mother, after two farewells without responsive anguish in her daughter, turned to the teacher bitterly, "How do you like that! She doesn't even seem to care!" A fourth mother, tearing herself away from a whining daughter, took her departure with this parting shot, *"Miss Sally* (the teacher) says I *have* to go." Once gone, the mothers spent an unhappy hour or two, returned almost invariably before the time agreed upon and greeted their children effusively with unsolicited reassurances and anxious questioning about how they had fared.

In dealing with the school aged children, similar, though usually more subtle, phenomena were evident. On the first clinic visit, the psychiatrist might be told in the child's presence "you won't be able to get him to leave me." At that very moment, mother would tighten her grip on the child's hand or about his shoulder. During the interview, she was constantly on the alert for the sound of his voice or footsteps. If he did enter to ascertain her whereabouts, she was conspicuously ineffectual in getting him to leave. When mother and child had to be seen together, she answered for him and constantly catered to his demands, although in an exasperated fashion. A Binet under these circumstances would likely result in a composite I.Q. for the two!

We, of course, were not able to observe the actual school going behavior but obtained accounts dynamically equivalent to what had been observed in the nursery setting. One father reported during the course of treatment that on the day his son had agreed to begin his return to school, his mother wondered aloud whether it might not be wiser to wait a day since it was raining and he might catch cold. When the youngster insisted he should keep to his agreement, the mother suggested she consult his father. Called at his office, the father responded with an exasperated "of course he should go!" Whereupon, the mother turned to the patient and stated, "Your father thinks it's raining too hard." Another mother reported that her son, who had finally been gotten back to school for a week, had been absent the 3 days prior to the clinic visit because he lacked rubbers and there had been a heavy snow. This seemed not unreasonable until we learned from the patient that he had been out sledding each of those 3 days!

In one of the two cases where the father played the cardinal role, the following description was offered by his wife. When the morning for return to school arrived, the patient responded with his customary complaints of nausea and abdominal pain. After a few incoherent attempts to insist that his son must go, his father broke into tears, shouted "My God, I can't do it" and tore off to the bathroom to vomit. When the mother called me at 7:30 a.m., in a state of considerable agitation herself, I could hear the lamentation of the men in the family in the background. In the second case, the father was so distressed by his son's morning behavior that he had to be excused from his legal duties, couldn't eat and spent an agitated day—all this at a time when the patient was contentedly watching television at home.

The Parents

Without exception, the mothers were anxious, and ambivalent. Each gave a history of a poor relationship with her own mother; most were currently in the throes of a struggle to escape the overprotective domination of a mother or mother-in-law who visited daily, insisted on frequent phone calls and was constantly critical. Pregnancy had usually been regarded as a mixed blessing; childbirth was feared. The infant had been surrounded by apprehensive oversolicitude and had never been trusted to babysitters, at least outside the immediate family. As the child ventured forth from his home, he was constantly warned of hazards. As one mother phrased it, "I thought it was better to frighten my Joey than to lose him."

The dynamic forces in the mother-child relationship were quite complex. Several of the mothers had responded with primary overprotection to a child who had been a late arrival after many sterile years. Others saw the child in terms of their own pathetically unhappy childhood and reexperienced with each of the child's tears remembered moments of loneliness and misunderstanding. But, inevitably, the children's strivings for independence and self-gratification led to feelings of personal rejection and reactive hostility. "After all I've given her! How can she treat me like this?" was a typical expression.

Lacking emotional fulfillment in their marital relationships, many of these mothers turned to their children. On the one hand, the marriage yielding little, the child had to be both child and lover. On the other, he was resented as the hostage by whose presence the mother felt trapped. This anger, prominent in most cases, led to reactive guilt and secondary overprotection. These mothers could not let themselves experience the resentment normally aroused by difficult behavior and consequently had difficulty in setting limits. As the child, accustomed to having every whim gratified, finally drove her to exasperation, her explosion, disproportionate to the precipitating incident, would lead via guilt to another cycle of overindulgence and latent resentment.

Dependent and anxious as these mothers were, they found little support from their husbands. We found no instances of overt infidelity, but many of the fathers were more strongly wedded to occupational interests than to their wives. They tended to be more effective with the children when they troubled to take an interest, but usually confined themselves to disgruntled criticisms of their wives' inadequacies. Of the two fathers mentioned earlier, one had suffered from an unusually sadistic relationship with his own father and was attempting to provide and, at the same time, experience vicariously through his son, the kind of fathering he had missed and still searched for. His efforts to spare his son any unhappiness had been accelerated by a mild attack of poliomyelitis in the boy. The other father, as far as could be determined from a brief contact, had been tremendously affected by the sudden death of his own brother at 17, for which he felt responsible.

Parental Attitudes Toward Therapy

The ambivalent attitudes so evident between parent and child overflowed into relationships with the psychiatrist, the case worker and the teachers. One unusually blatant example may serve to dramatize the ever present rivalry between these mothers and those to whom they appealed for help to wean their children away from them.

> Mrs. L., "devoted" to her own hypochondriacal mother whom she feared to leave lest "something happen to her," married late in life a pleasant but ineffectual husband whom she completely dominated. Successful as a career woman, she commented, "I never thought I wanted marriage or children. Now I can't even think of leaving them." She reported her daughter's lack of interest in the nursery with evident satisfaction and did her best to insure that the school would have little special to offer by duplicating games and equipment at home. She told the nursery director one day, "You know my daughter really doesn't like you very much. In fact, the only nice thing she says is that you have a nice complexion." At this point, she leaned over, scrutinized the director's face, and added, "And I don't see what's so nice about *that*!"

Whereas advice was sought with an imploring and almost desperate air, it was usually received with, "and what do I do when that doesn't work?" There can be little doubt that this anticipation of failure effectively undercut whatever measures might have been taken. That the overdependence of the child had positive values for the mother was often pointed up by the disappointment and even resentment shown to the therapist when the child made strides out on his own.

The Children

Without exception, these children were of normal or superior intelligence. Those with prior school attendance had not been singled out by school authorities as deviant in any way. Their parents described them as having been sensitive to change, even as infants, and as fearful of new situations. Yet, pathetic and frightened as they might appear on arrival when separation was first attempted, they became remarkably free from anxiety once the therapist had won their confidence, usually in the first interview. In the younger children, intrinsic psychiatric disturbance was far less prominent than neurosis in their parents. The one significant exception was a child who conformed to Mahler's description of a symbiotic psychosis(4). In the adolescents, intrafamilial pathology had been translated into intrapsychic.

An element of infantile manipulation, at times more prominent than anxiety, was evident in the child's behavior. Richard, at 3½, had so successfully trained his mother that the merest cloud of dissatisfaction lowering over his face would send her into frantic activity to offset an impending tantrum. Eddie, at 10, needed only to whine and his father would purchase gifts beyond his means. Lisa, 6, was clearly involved in a vendetta of punishment for her mother's sin of leaving her for a vacation. Wendy, 3, had learned to arouse guilt and anxiety in her mother, who had been hospitalized twice, once post-partum, with the deliberate comment "you liked to go to the hospital" whenever mother attempted to leave. Arlene, 8, went to school without a murmur when staying at her grandmother's house but couldn't be budged from her mother's.

There would seem to be a line of demarcation, however, at about the junior high school level. The 5 adolescents were, as a group, far more disturbed. In this we agree with Suttenfield(5). Kathy, 15, tied to a chronically anxious mother, developed a fear of fainting at school or in crowds and retreated to a symbiotic relationship essential to both; interestingly, her mother had quit high school herself for the very same reason. Fear so strong as to overcome the need for conformity and the striving for independence in the adolescent implies a greater degree of illness than it does in the younger child who is normally more dependent. One might suppose that the chronic action of the forces we have identified in the families of the younger children had ultimately warped personality growth beyond the hope of ready change.

The Pattern of Symptom Formation

The configuration of psychic forces that generates separation anxiety has the following attributes. There is a background of overdependence on the mother (or father) almost consciously fostered by the parent in response to her needs rather than the child's. At the same time, the child's parasitic clinging is resented by the mother as it impinges on her own freedom of movement. Superimposed is hostility toward the child stemming from sources not in immediate awareness: the child as an image of a resented husband, as bond to a unwanted marriage, as symbol of a hated sibling, etc. Secondary to this is guilt and compensatory overprotection. The child responds as well to the rejection he can sense as to the indulgence in which he luxuriates.

This supersaturated atmosphere is precipitated out by some transitory situation which arouses anxiety: illness, change of school, harsh word from a teacher, etc. At a time when the support of firm handling is needed, the child's anxiety is multiplied by the sight of a distraught and decompensated parent. Maternal apprehension makes quavering the voice and tremulous the gestures that accompany empty verbal assurance. It is as if the children are told by nonverbal communication that what lies ahead is even more frightening than they had dared think—a kind of *folie à deux.*

The child's symptoms are comprehensible as the response to contradictory verbal and behavioral clues. He is told that he must go at the same time that he is shown he dare not; he is told that he is loved at the same time that his needs are lost in the morass of his mother's. The mother is unwittingly sabotaging her own ostensible goals as she struggles in the relentless grip of ambivalent feelings. The child, in response to felt hostility, strikes back by displaying the behavior that he senses will be most disconcerting to her. Anxiety is aroused when the latent (behavioral) cue to the child is rejection or fear; manipulation is activated when the latent cue is the possibility of gratification. The contradiction between words and behavior in the transactions between mother and child is the catalytic agent in generating separation anxiety. The history of early sensitivity to change in these children as infants suggests that an intrinsic anxiety proneness may exist which renders them more susceptible to the acquisition of these patterns. Certainly, they are not exhibited by all children who may grow up in dynamically similar family situations.

Treatment

The therapeutic corollary to this conception of the genesis of symptom formation is an insistance on early return to school. At the initial psychiatric consultation—made if necessary on an emergency basis for the school-aged child—an attempt is made to identify the etiologic factors and to assess the degree of sickness in family members. The parents are given the reassurance that the prognosis is relatively good and the main dynamic features they are deemed capable of assimilating are pointed out. A program for rapid return to school is outlined. Often this can be negotiated with the child once it is made clear to him that school attendance is prescribed by law and that the issue is not whether he will return but how and when. If necessary, he may be permitted to begin by spending his day in the principal's or counsellor's office or by having his mother attend class with him, but he must in any event be in the school building(6). We have, on occasion, when a thorough trial of other methods has failed, gone so far as to schedule a hearing in juvenile court—which did not have to take place—in order to shore up ineffectual parents. One father, indeed, decided on his own to call in police officers to convince his son (and himself) that he meant business. Once return has been achieved, therapy continues with the family in order to eradicate underlying pathological attitudes. Obviously, these strictures do not apply to the pre-school child for whom a nursery program can be introduced gradually on an elective basis.

Our results confirm the practicability of this plan. Not one child has been precipitated into panic or has gone into psychic decompensation as some might have expected. Ten of the 11 pre-school children and 10 of the 10 elementary school children have returned to and are still in school. Results have been far less impressive in the junior high and high school groups. Only 1 or possibly 2 are now attending school regularly; the remaining 2 have been in and out and as of this moment have a questionable outlook; 1 is definitely a therapeutic failure.

These results contrast with a situation uncovered in a recent survey of children in Baltimore on home teaching for medical reasons(7). Of 108 children taught by visiting teachers, 8 elementary school pupils were discovered to be on medical certificates for school phobia. Consequently, no effort had been made to insist on attendance. All had been out for at least 1 year and one as long as 3 years. This points to the unwisdom of recommending home teaching which makes the situation far too comfortable for the whole family and removes a major motivation for change. By accepting the apparent inability of the child to attend as a real inability, it reinforces his regression.

The insistence on attendance, on the other hand, conveys to the child our confident expectation that he can accept and carry through a responsibility appropriate to his age.

The objection may be raised that we have produced a symptomatic cure but have not touched the basic issues. It is essential that the paralyzing force of the school phobia on the child's whole life be recognized. The symptom itself serves to isolate him from normal experience and makes further psychological growth almost impossible. If we do no more than check this central symptom, we have nonetheless done a great deal. Furthermore, we have been impressed with the liberating role of this accomplishment in opening avenues for rapid progress in both child and parents in subsequent treatment. The psychiatric task is, of course, not complete when return is accomplished, though it is sometimes so regarded by the parents. Every effort should be made to follow through with family oriented treatment.

Summary

School phobia has been shown to be a variant of separation anxiety. Direct observations of transactions between parents and children at the time of separation have been presented. Key dynamic factors have been identified and the mode of symptom formation has been outlined as a paradigm for the genesis of neurotic behavior. The outcome of a treatment program has been reported in validation of the theoretical conception of the nature and genesis of the disorder.

References

1. Estes, H. R., Haylett, C. H., and Johnson, A.M.: Am. J. Psychotherapy, 10:682, 1956.
2. Johnson, A.M., *et al.*: Am. J. Orthopsychiat., 11:702, 1941.
3. Kanner, L.: Child Psychiatry. 3rd Ed. Springfield: C. C Thomas, 1957.
4. Mahler, M. S.: Psychoanalyt. Stud. Child, 7:286, 1952.
5. Suttenfield. V.: Am. J. Orthopsychiat., 24:368, 1954.
6. Klein, E.: Psychoanalyt. Stud. Child. 1:263, 1945.
7. Hardy, J. B. Personal Communication.

11. Treatment of School Phobias— Theory and Practice

Richard S. Greenbaum

The concept is prevalent that the treatment of choice in cases of school phobia is to return the child to school as soon as possible on any level he can sustain. This theory is based on the premise that if the child does not remain in contact with the school, a regression will routinely occur which will extend or intensify the phobia. If this happens, the less sick child will take longer to get better and the marginal patient may be pushed to the point where his recovery will be imperiled. This paper will present evidence to the effect that, in the cases seen by the author, no regression took place in those patients not in contact with the school. The theoretic constructs underlying the whole problem of the school phobic will be considered in terms of the treatment of phobias in general and school phobias in particular and the future of the children who have suffered from school phobias in relation to the nature and the degree of treatment. Also to be considered is the relationship of the symptom to other symptoms and to the culture in general. All this theory will be integrated with the available evidence and certain conclusions will be presented concerning the treatment of the child and his family.

It is necessary at the outset to distinguish between the learned and the "defensive" phobias and their respective treatments. A learned phobia can occur in one of two ways. A parent or parent surrogate can teach a fear to a child, either directly or by acting as a model in the child's development. Such phobias are usually overcome by a combination of reassurance, graduated contact with the feared object, and some insight into the fact that just because the parent fears something, it is not dangerous per se. A learned phobia can also come about as a result of some traumatic experience with an object that is not ordinarily dangerous and was not previously feared. Such phobias are usually overcome by closely facing the feared object or situation. For example, if a person is thrown from a horse, the treatment of choice is to get back on a horse and ride (without getting thrown this time). A "defensive" phobia is one in which the patient represses certain dangerous or painful affects and attempts to avoid stimulation of these thoughts by avoiding objects and situations associated with the unacceptable ideation or its previous stimulation, or likely to stimulate it currently. School phobias fit into this category.

From *American Journal of Psychotherapy*, 1964, **18**, 616–634. Copyright 1964 by the Association for the Advancement of Psychotherapy. Reproduced by permission.

History

In considering the concepts underlying the treatment of children with school phobias, I want to begin with a survey of the general principles of the treatment of "defensive" phobias. In the case of Hans (1), Freud discussed many of the principles underlying the development of phobic reactions, including both the recognition of a phobia as a way of warding off unacceptable feelings and the danger of proliferation of the phobia. His general concept of treatment at that time was that of helping the patient face the unconscious feelings, thus eliminating the need for defensive displacement of these feelings. The problem of proliferation was conceptualized in later years by Alexander (2), who wrote, "The phobia is an attempt to localize the anxiety in a single situation while keeping the ego from recognizing the real unresolved conflict and touching it. Localized anxiety often gives way to a gradually spreading anxiety and multiple problems develop." The phobia was seen as likely to spread when the initial phobia did not achieve its goal of suppressing the anxiety by limiting the ego's freedom (3), that is, the projection did not succeed in its attempt to render quiescent the patient's instinctual drives. When this happened, additional phobias developed and continued to do so until equilibrium was reached between the impulses and the ego. If the instincts were too strong or the ego too weak, then proliferation would take place. On the other hand, if the phobia did have the effect of reducing the anxiety either by limiting the patient's activities so that he did not have to face the anxiety provoking situations, or by providing an adequate defense for warding off the impulses, then a condition of stasis was reached and the phobic patient functioned well, but in a more restricted way.

The general principles of treating phobic patients are to establish a psychotherapeutic relationship and to encourage the flow of unconscious material (except when the phobias are a defense against a psychotic break). If the patient is unable to face the feared situation on his own, the therapist intervenes to the degree necessary to help the patient face the situation. This principle was initially postulated by Freud (4). He noted that his patients were having difficulty in facing the feared or phobic object on their own initiative. He felt that it was necessary to deviate from the technique of passivity and to intervene actively to help the patient face the phobic object. The basis for this was his perception that only when the patient could "go it alone and struggle with the anxiety ... only when this has been attained by the physician's recommendations [can] the associations and memories ... come into the patient's mind allowing the phobia to be solved." This was an act that took place late in therapy to stimulate the production of associations and which was necessary only where the patient did not face the phobic situation on his own. Other authors suggested other reasons for therapeutic intervention. Ivey (5) advocated the use of the developed transference to instruct the patient not to give into the symptom any longer as a method of attempting to limit the spread of the phobia. Many have suggested that facing the object gradually has the effect of desensitizing the person to the object.

Many people advocate treating school phobias differently than other phobias, in that they feel the child suffering from a school phobia should be pressed to face the phobic situation, that is, go to school at the onset of the therapeutic contact. Published evidence supporting this principle appears based on a single case of regression when the child was not rapidly returned to school. In 1945 Klein (6) originated the concept that there was a need for early return on any level the child could sustain, namely, visiting the school for ten minutes a day, sitting in a class with his parents, and so on. After noting that attempts to force the child back harshly could only intensify the anxiety, he stated that, based on his experience, "Not getting the child back has almost equally bad results. If the child remains out of school for a while, there is a quick development of primitive regressive fears, in young children of an oral character, in older ones of a paranoid nature simulating schizophrenia." Hence, he recommended brief psychotherapy based on psychoanalytic insight to bring about a recession of the acute phase and prolonged therapy to treat the underlying problem. In his study, he reported on seven patients. Of these, five were returned to school rapidly. Two were out for some length of time; of these two, regression occurred in one case.

The concept of early return was heartily endorsed by many. Eisenberg (7) felt that early return was necessary since complications might arise as a result of being out of school. For example, the child's fears concerning the school work he is missing, and embarrassment at facing his peers and teacher, the secondary gain of getting extra attention at home, the acceptance by others of his fears (of school) as being real, and the fact that the child's being at home feeds the neurotic family pattern which led to the development of the neurosis in the first place. Suttenfield (8) felt that early return was necessary to help the phobia from becoming fixed. Other advocates of early return for the same or unstated reasons include Sperling (9) and Spock (10) with his important influence on the thinking of the lay public. None of the above authors reported any cases in treatment that either regressed or had any other malevolent experiences while the patient was out of school.

Some authors disagree with this approach of attempting to get the child back as soon as possible. Kahn and Nursten (11) point out some of the dangers of attempting to force the psychotic or near psychotic child back to school. They note that such attempts, if successful, are likely to be interpreted by the patient's family to mean that since "the child is acting normal, he is normal." Talbot (12) expresses some reservations about pressing for an immediate return. Naturally, there are all shades of opinion in between.

The success of a psychotherapeutic process may be assessed in a number of ways. Among the criteria relevant to the treatment of school phobias, the literature considers three. First consideration is whether the child returned to school or not. Rodriguez (13), in a study of 41 cases, reported that about 70 per cent returned to school when attempts were made to use the principle of rapid return. When divided by age, 87 per cent of those under eleven years returned, but only 36 per cent of those over eleven got back to school. He concluded that the older children were sicker. In Klein's (6) original study, all the children returned to school regardless of age or treatment procedure.

Second, the literature considers the performance in school of those children who do return. Two studies (14, 15) report that children treated by the principle of rapid return remain symptom free for at least a period of 18 months to two years. Coolidge (16) reports that among such children successfully treated in this way before adolescence, namely, by getting the child back to school as soon as the strongest member of the family was ready to effect this return, some difficulty was evident during adolescence; 34 out of 47 children showed either moderate or severe limitations in meeting the developmental problems endemic to the adolescent period. These children showed evidence of difficulty in the areas of social relationships and heterosexual adjustments. Many did less well academically after return than before the onset of the symptom.

Third, the literature considers the future life adjustment of these children. Warren (17) reported on 16 children who had not returned to school after treatment as outpatients, and were then seen for treatment in an inpatient unit. He felt that these children were no sicker than those who did not reach his unit and that their referral was purely fortuitous. Seven other children who were sicker were screened out of the study group. When followed up between the ages of eighteen and twenty-two, of the 16 children seen, 10 showed marked to severe pathology.

All the above-mentioned children had been treated; thus on a theoretic basis, the outlook for the untreated ones should prove even more dismal. Takagi (18) reported on 32 cases. He noted that many of these youngsters appeared to be autistic or schizophrenic, necessitating residential treatment. Kahn and Nursten (11) have suggested that the unsuccessfully handled person with a school phobia is one who breaks down when faced with a separation experience later in life, such as going away to college or entering the armed services. Davy (19) in a study of break-down among university students away from home, noted that 50 per cent of them had experienced earlier psychotic or psychotic-like breaks, which was interpreted to indicate the presence of separation anxiety in most of the cases. In general, it would appear that rapid return tends to get the younger children back, but not the older ones, and that the majority of the children who get back do well for a few years but do not sustain themselves well when they get older.

Some inference may be drawn concerning the future adjustments from the length of time the child spends in treatment. As school phobias are deep-seated and complex problems, the longer the time spent in treatment, the greater the likelihood of resolution of the underlying conflict. In a treatment program based on a principle of rapid return and a continuation of therapy after return, Rodriguez (13) reports that of 41 patients, only seven had had as much as six months of treatment. Of the remaining 34 patients, 32 had less than 13 sessions. It appears that sympton suppression is often about as far as treatment goes with this approach. The article gives no information as to the relationship between the length of treatment and the timing of the return to school, but it is clearly inferred that treatment does not continue for any extended period of time following the return to school. Suttenfield (8) had much more success in keeping her patients in treatment after their return to school. A rapid return to school may not preclude resolution of the underlying conflict, but it does appear to seriously reduce the chances of staying in treatment long enough to do so.

Criticism of the Literature

The evidence in the literature upon which the concept of rapid return is based is meager. The theoretic foundation for such a concept is questionable. Forcing a defensively phobic person to face and deal with the feared objective cannot "cure" or bring about a resolution of the conflict of which the fear is symptomatic. This is patently obvious. If the child with a school phobia suffers from conflicting impulses regarding mother, forcing the child to return to school will not resolve his underlying problems with the maternal figure. However, forcing him can have one of a variety of consequences. In rapid return, in effect, the first attempt to handle the problem consists of "an appeal to give in to the superego and reality demands and would amount to an overpowering of the ego" (20). If he uses this approach, the therapist is involved in committing one of the cardinal errors of treatment, namely, siding with reality against the symptom. Of course, the intensification of the feeling of guilt may work like a hypnotic command directed against the symptom and the symptom may be suppressed and symptom removal effected. Then the child would return to school, but the likelihood of future adjustment problems would increase. Often the pressure results in an increase in regression, clinging to the mother, and overt separation anxiety. The literature does not indicate this, for such negatively responding children would be included among those who do not return to school in three out of ten cases, according to Rodriguez (13).

If the support offered by the therapist plus the therapist's injunctions added to the superego forces already operative are not enough to bring about symptom suppression, the phobia may spread to include the therapist (20). This would preclude future as well as present therapy for the patient. Then the child would not only remain out of school, but would never get better unless he were lucky enough to have a "spontaneous recovery." Since the reasons for treating school phobias differently than other phobias are to prevent a proliferation, a regression, or both, it is well to be aware of the danger of exacerbation of the symptoms by the very treatment advocated to prevent it. In theory, early return would seem to bring about a greater danger of symptom increase than allowing the phobic defense to function.

It is generally agreed that the school phobia has a separation anxiety at its base. The child is angry toward the mother, dependent upon her, and is concerned that the angry wishes will come true. This anger is not experienced as a conscious phenomenon; it is repressed, and it is repressed because it is unacceptable to the child. Usually its lack of acceptability as a conscious thought is based upon the threat it poses to the dependency needs and a feeling that it is wrong and dangerous to have such wishes. This in turn is a function of the presence of some magic thinking, specifically, a concern that the wishes may come true and a strong concept of what is proper or acceptable ideation. That ideation is an application of a general sense of right and wrong, that is, these children have strong superegos or the precursors thereof (21). Indications of this are quite evident in the pre-phobic behavior. The children usually do well in school before the phobia sets in, that is, they study, get good grades, and do not get into any trouble. Their conduct grades are customarily above average. They are, in short, rather guilt-ridden children who try to do the right thing. As getting back to school is the right thing for a child to do, they are anxious to get back to school and quite willing to do so on their own initiative when they are free of gross anxiety. It is this very sense of guilt that results in their getting back to school in such large numbers when the therapist's authority is added to that of the parents, and when the terror is slightly reduced by the therapist.

The pressure placed on a child to get back to school is enormous. Usually the teacher, the parents, the visiting teacher or truant officer, the family physician, friends, relatives, and neighborhood manipulators have all tried to get the child back before the child is brought to the therapist. In the case of no other phobia is this sort of pressure put on the patient. No one has ever, to my knowledge, threatened claustrophobic patients with jail if they did not take the elevator, yet the literature (7) reports just such threats being made if the child does not get back to school. In the author's own experience, children have been committed to the local institution for delinquents for refusal to attend school due to a school phobia. The child, concerned with what others think, is anxious to get back as proof that he is getting better and that he is not too different from the other children. It hardly seems necessary for the therapist to add to all of these pressures. In school phobias, unlike other phobias, the therapist may feel confident that pressure will be placed on the patient to face the phobic situation without any activity on his part.

Certain other divergencies from established principles appear in the writings of the advocates of rapid return. For one thing, other diagnostic features do not appear to be seriously considered. The advocates of early return maintain that this is desirable on the basis of the symptom, that it is the way to treat all children with school phobias. This is so, presumably, regardless of whether the child is psychotic, a borderline case, or neurotic. It is well recognized that school phobics encompass all three (11).

As far as the psychotic or borderline children are concerned, the often commented upon symbiotic nature of the syndrome (22) points up another violation of basic tenets. The theory of treatment of psychotic symbiotic relationships is summarized by Mahler (23) who says, "Separation as an individual entity can only be promoted very cautiously in the case of the symbiotic child." Rapid return of such children violates this principle.

The criticism of lack of sufficient flexibility in handling various nosologic categories can equally be applied to the handling of individual differences. Getting everyone back as rapidly as possible is a principle that does not consider the question of what this means in the individual case. It is generally considered advantageous to the patient to allow him to utilize his own resources to solve the problem. In the case of school phobias, this is usually possible. To the degree that it serves the patient's over-all interests to feel that he has overcome his difficulties due to his own efforts, thus allowing him to experience success realistically and to develop strength and confidence in his future ability to handle stressful situations—it is to the patient's benefit to determine the timing of the return as a function of his own therapy.

There is no generally accepted theoretic construct for the principle of rapid return. Klein (6) advocates it for one reason, Eisenberg (7) for a number of other reasons and Suttenfield (8) for still other ones.

The next point is not a criticism of the theory of rapid return, but of an outgrowth of the theory. Unfortunately, the theory of rapid return has been seriously misinterpreted. The result of this misinterpretation is that many people active in working with children in the organized structure of society feel that the way to treat children with school phobias is simply to get them back to school. Return to school has, in some parts of the country, become a substitute for treatment. Only those who do not get back are referred for therapy. The consequences of this approach are likely to be disastrous for the child. It is most important that this misconception be clarified.

The literature does not report on certain crucial matters, such as how many, if any, of the children who were rapidly returned break down later in life, what happens to the 30 percent who do not return to school as a result of therapeutic pressure and, of course, there is no controlled study of matched cases treated by rapid return and orthodox technique to compare the results. We are therefore left with an inferential comparison, that is, one between different study groups. In this case the groups are those treated by the principle of rapid return as reported in the literature discussed above and the group reported on in this paper.

Current Study

In the current study nine children were referred for treatment of school phobias. Unsuccessful efforts had been made to force all of them back to school by their parents, teachers, and others in the community. One of the children, on examination, turned out to be a boy who was attempting to handle some castration threats within the home by controlling the environment. He was returned to school rapidly and referred elsewhere for therapy. The remaining eight children were suffering from a true school phobia. Four of them were boys and four were girls. In age, at the time of referral, they were, reading upwards from birth, seven, eight, eight, eleven, eleven, fourteen, fourteen years of age. Nosologically, three patients were depressed, one was schizophrenic with paranoid trends, one was a borderline schizophrenic, and the other three were neurotic. All but one, the borderline, had good ego strength.

Ego strength is a term without clearly quantifiable referents. It is evaluated in terms of a standard which is relative and somewhat shifting and its prime referent is in the individual and collective experience of therapists. What constitutes good ego strength varies with the age and culture of the patient. Ego strength is also assessed in terms of the nosologic classification of the patient. It is usually assessed in terms of the evidence relevant to the ego's ability to retain its coherence under stressful conditions. This ability has been labeled by Hartman (24) as its "secondary autonomy." Where there is well-developed secondary autonomy of the ego, the boundaries between the id and the ego and the boundaries between the ego and the environment are fairly well defined. Considering school phobias in this light is done most easily if each nosologic category is separately examined.

The projective testing of the neurotic group on the Rorschach showed that the deep unconscious thoughts are without gross deviation of expected form perception, even when the patients are pressed for limits. Such a pattern is associated with good reality perception, a sign of ego strength. The death wishes in these children are well repressed and experienced only as overconcern, an indication of good boundaries between the id and the ego. The children did well in school before the phobic outbreak, indicating the ability to select stimuli from the environment, maintain the integrity of an idea and initiate and complete a task. All of these are signs of good boundaries between the ego and the environment. Relations with peers were good, demonstrating the existence of a behavior pattern of a nature appropriate to the child's psychosocial development. This implies drive control and a tolerance for stress, both of which require adequate ego mechanisms.

The depressed patients showed their strength in their lack of extreme withdrawal and the absence of overt suicidal ideation or behavior. These indicate good repression and good drive neutralization. On the environmental side of the ego, these children showed the same strength as did the neurotic group. The strength of the ego relative to the depression was such that in no case was all activity inhibited nor were there any manic outbursts, that is to say, mood swings were well contained.

The psychotic child had weaker ego boundaries than the depressed or the neurotic children. Reality perception was more distorted, stimuli more misinterpreted, the unconscious nearer the surface and the identity weaker. He distantiated himself from others and peer relations were more superficial. Within the limits of the greater pathology, and with it as a referent, he showed signs of strength. On the Rorschach, the deviant responses were followed by good ones. He was able to maintain the integrity of his ideas. He was able to limit his perceptual distortions to the point where he could, except for going to school, function well in a social situation. That is to say, the barriers between the ego and the id were quite weak but the barriers between the ego and the environment were fairly strong. This resulted in an ambulant psychotic state in which the schizophrenic process was well masked to the unsophisticated.

The borderline child had a weak ego structure, chronically disrupted by sporadically increasing anxieties. All had the separation anxiety noted by others and all suffered from some degree of depression, as has been noted by Agras (25).

The children were seen in private outpatient psychotherapy at least once a week, and in some cases two or three times a week. They were all told that as part of their treatment, they were to decide when to return to school. This decision would be made together with their therapist and they were not to return to school until it had been made. Return here was explained as meaning getting back full time and staying after they returned. The program for return could be graduated over a two-week period. Return was explained to the parents and the children as a question of the balance of the relative strength of some conflicting feelings which could only be realistically assessed in the following terms—as a step along the way to getting better which would take place when the desire to get back outweighed the fears of separation. In spite of what they were told, both parents and children looked upon return to school as the measure of success or failure of treatment, but it was hoped that the above statements helped to place this viewpoint in a more appropriate perspective.

In order to simplify the problems of return to school, it was suggested to the parents that tutoring be provided so that when the child was ready to return, he could do so at grade level. The parents were helped to understand that these were very unhappy children and that whatever might be done to make them happy should be done, provided that it in no way threatened the parental authority and control. Where there was a conflict between the two, it was explained that this should be resolved in favor of establishing or maintaining parental control. In practice, this worked out to mean that the children were expected to obey their parents, do some chores around the house, keep up with their studies and do whatever the other children in the neighborhood did after school and when school was not in session. In the cases where control was a problem, the parents were helped to understand that control of a child was best established in concrete areas where parental success is guaranteed and where the therapist's role is less active. Having the child do chores around the house or having the parents go out in the evening in spite of the child's protests appeared to be the best places to begin. The parents were encouraged to help the child with separation experiences by such procedures as going out at night, and leaving the child with a baby sitter or going away for week ends. If the parents had difficulty in doing this, their own feelings in the matter were examined. The children took this separation well.

Results

Of the eight patients, seven returned to school. The eighth was an over-all failure in treatment. One of the patients treated successfully did regress, but the regression took place while she was in school. For six of the seven patients who returned to school, the return followed shortly after the expression and analysis of the anger toward mother. In the seventh case, there was some delay between the expression of anger toward mother and the patient's return to school. In all cases, the analysis of the need to achieve was begun before the return and dealt with in detail after the patient returned and was able to consider achievement in terms of school grades. The depressed feelings tended to come out next, with the sexual feelings coming out last, usually some time after the return to school. In the younger children, the sexual feelings did not always emerge to the degree that the therapist felt was desirable. It has been suggested that younger school phobics may be returned to treatment during adolescence (16) and this would certainly prove wise in those cases where preadolescents have terminated treatment without exploring the sexual components of their pathology.

All of the children did well academically after returning to school. They have done fairly well in their social life, two of them having been elected to receive school honors by their fellow students. Two of the adolescents have made a good heterosexual adjustment, another one finds excuses to avoid dating too often.

All the children who were above the age of eleven when they returned to school, and one who was under eleven have been able to sustain extended voluntary separation experiences with no visible stress. They either went out of town to stay at a sleep-away camp or visited relatives without their parents being present for a period of two weeks or longer. The younger children did not have such an opportunity.

In all cases the patients remained in treatment after their return to school. One child who returned to school after four months was withdrawn from treatment by his parents two months later. The other children have had at least ten months of treatment after they returned to school and in none of these cases has treatment been terminated without resolution of the underlying neurosis.

The child who was a treatment failure and the one who regressed both warrant a closer look. The treatment failed in the case of a fourteen-year-old girl. Unlike the others, she was not referred for treatment at the onset of the symptoms. Instead, she had been committed to the local county home for delinquents for a period of five months for truancy, the truancy being due to her phobic condition. She was released in June and the following September was unable to return to school. She was examined independently by two other therapists who recommended that she be forced back to school. It was at this point that she came to the author's attention. She evidenced enormous difficulty in accepting the patient role, for she had become phobic about therapists. To complicate the picture further, her parents withdrew her from treatment twice when the pressures were reduced, the first time during the summer vacation, the second time when she temporarily returned to school as a flight from problems. This parental pattern was unacceptable and the case was closed. However, the generalization of the phobia to the therapist was seen as the primary cause of the lack of success.

The child who regressed was a ten-year-old girl diagnosed as a borderline psychotic who differed from the other children with school phobia in that they were strong representatives of their particular type of pathology and she was not. She was having some difficulty in going to school, but was in more or less regular attendance. The separation difficulty had been the subject of some discussion in her therapy. One day, about a year after treatment was started, she experienced a traumatic incident in school. Her finger was broken and she was unable to call her mother or see a doctor until after school was over for the day. This occurred as a result of a series of misunderstandings. At this point, the regression took place. She developed a marked school phobia and it rapidly extended itself. She was treated as the other children reported in the study group were treated and returned to school after ten months.

She appeared to be undergoing a negative therapeutic reaction. Although the literature on such processes does not suggest that they are precipitated by trauma, the other features of this case seem to fit the pattern. In general, the negative therapeutic reaction is a phenomenon of the later stages of therapy. A patient who is doing well suddenly regresses either due to an unconscious need for self-punishment, or a need to retain omnipotence, which leads to the patient's inability to sustain the benefits of his therapeutic gains. As has been noted, regression during the early stages of treatment of phobias is usually due to the lack of establishment of equilibrium. Regression may usually be assumed to occur in the weaker personality structure, that is, the atypical school phobic. Such regression would then appear to be unrelated to contact with school in any predictable way.

Children treated by the principle of allowing the child to decide when to return as part of the therapeutic process actually returned to school in a higher percentage (85%) than did those where the therapist attempted to get them back rapidly (70%). They remained in treatment longer and in general did better in school academically and in peer relations than those returned more rapidly. They made good progress in therapy. They sustained other separation experiences without undue difficulty. In no case did regression appear while the child was out of contact with the school, nor did the phobia become a fixed pattern which resisted responding to routine therapeutic progress.

Discussion

The good results obtained in these cases appear to be related to certain qualities of the person who develops the school phobia as a symptom. Prognosis formed on the basis of a symptom are dangerous because they do not consider so many aspects of the total situation. However, school phobics need to do well and have the ability to start and finish a task, as their good previous school grades attest. They have a strong sense of right and wrong, a tendency to internalize problems, are embarrassed and unhappy about their symptom and have good ego strength; all qualities which make a person a suitable candidate for psychotherapy. Hence the high recovery rate.

The reason that such a high percentage of these children remain in therapy appears to be due to two things. One is that the patient and the parents are able to experience a real change as a result of therapy before the child gets back to school and in areas seemingly unrelated to the problem of school attendance. Secondly, as has been noted, there is a symbiotic process at work here. The child is obeying an unconscious wish of the mother in remaining at home. The mother's unconscious wish is handled overtly by discussing her feelings in the matter. Covertly, the mother's needs to have somebody to depend upon become transferred from the child to the therapist. This serves to make the mother reluctant to terminate the child's therapy. None of the above phenomena occur if the child is returned to school rapidly.

The future of these children deserves the closest scrutiny. The goal of therapy is not only to solve the immediate conflict and remove the disabling symptom, but also to provide the patient with strength and techniques for meeting future stresses. As has been noted in the survey of the literature, the future prospects of these children are not too hopeful. One sign of this may be the greater pathology reported in the older children. It is possible that the school phobia of the older child may be due to a process that has been fulminating over the years as a result of the child having been forced back to school with the basic problem untouched. This is a factor to be considered in addition to the characterologic ones noted by Coolidge (25); and the sexual components which become so overwhelming in the adolescent should also be noted.

Reichenberg (26) has suggested that these children may move in yet another direction. When returned to school without resolution of the basic conflict, such children tend to become increasingly autistic, to move into the realm of their own fantasy. The effects of this development are dependent upon the prephobic personality structure, the severity of the threats used to effect the return to school, and the degree to which the child becomes autistic. Where the pressure is extreme in relation to the ego strength, we might observe the schizophrenic break recorded by Davy (19), or a break followed by recovery and sealing up. This could leave the child without good functioning in the academic situation, that is, a schizophrenic nonlearner. Such children are characterized by politeness, effort, and intelligent appearance in school and no one can understand why they cannot learn until a clinical examination reveals the basic underlying psychotic process. Where the effect is minimal, we get the child who functions in school academically below his intellectual capacity, like the children mentioned by Coolidge (16). The consistency of early separation difficulties in those children who are polite, hard-working, bright, and in trouble academically is astonishing when one asks the parents about this problem. Many of them represent *masked school phobias.*

Another possibility is for these children to develop psychosomatic reactions. Lewis (27) has pointed out that one of the prerequisites for the development of such a reaction is to be in a stressful situation and to be unable to leave it due to some counterforce. As school phobias are normally accompanied by some somatic reaction, usually nausea and vomiting in the morning, the pathways for psychosomatic patterns have already been established at the time of the onset of the symptom. If the child is returned to school and the underlying problem is not resolved, then the child is in a chronically stressful situation brought about by internal and external authority forces. A regression to primary process and somatic expression of the stress become decided possibilities, with chronic somatic reactions the final result.

If a child should return to school rapidly and remain in treatment, with the therapist able to retain his normal role, there is every reason to believe that therapy will proceed successfully. This is certainly an easier situation socially for the child and the family. Keeping the child out of school for some time confronts the therapist and the patient with the problem of attempting to effect a return at grade level. Where attendance is marginal, it would appear advantageous to make efforts to maintain the child in school. Where it is feasible without interfering with the therapeutic process, it should certainly be considered.

The dire consequences usually attributed to the lack of contact with the school did not appear in the cases reported in this study, leading to the conclusion that there is no need to get the sicker child back to school to avoid a regression; other factors then become more important in evaluating a case to ascertain the timing of the return. Return to school serves its optimal purpose when fitted properly into a therapeutic program aimed at resolving the child's basic problem. The timing of the return, according to this principle, must be determined by its relationship to the child's internal processes. Early return would then be the treatment of choice only in those cases where the child's progress in therapy would not suffer as a result of it and where the child's readiness to handle the social situation is such that the difference between the demands of the school situation—academic, social and sexual—and the child's readiness to meet them is not too great.

Relation to Other Personality Features

Separation anxiety appears in the first instance as a normal maturational factor in the form of "infantile separation anxiety" (28). The school phobic represents a more complex form of this anxiety, but at the core lies the infantile concern. Such separation anxiety, similarly heightened by fixation or regression, also characterizes agoraphobia. In many ways, the relationship between school phobias and agoraphobia is marked. Etiologically, both are characterized by an inability to leave home, based in part upon a concern that an unconscious death wish toward a parent may come true (29, 30). As a concomitant of this aspect of the pathology, in both syndromes the patient is able to enter the feared place if accompanied by a parent or a parent surrogate.

Both syndromes have sexual components. The difference between school phobia and agoraphobia lies mainly in the ability of the school phobic to leave home, unaccompanied, to go any place from which he may return to his home any time he wants to without it being considered abnormal. When regression takes place in a school phobic, then the behavior becomes more like that of a true agoraphobic. One basis for the difference between the two appears to be in the pregenital nature of the school phobia. The younger school phobic usually has sexual conflicts, but due to his age, the feelings are not very intense. The adolescent school phobic has intense sexual feelings, but due to his immaturity they never reach genital level, or if they do, the onset of anxiety results in a rapid regression. This shows up later in his difficulties in heterosexual relations. The sexual components of agoraphobia are well known (2, 3, 29, 30). The pregenital nature of these in school phobics, the relatively good ego strength, and the cultural factors involved in school attendance all appear to provide the basis for permitting the school phobic greater mobility. It is postulated that school phobia is a culturally determined pregenital space phobia etiologically similar to agoraphobia in older persons.

Sexuality on a more mature level in school phobics appears to enter into the picture only in terms of denied homosexual stimulation. This usually occurs in the dressing and showering associated with physical education, where the stimulation is overt. Adolescent school phobics often have difficulty here and usually ask to be excused from this activity if they return to school before working out this problem.

Other factors also enter into the use of the school as a focus of projection. Foremost among these is that when one is young there are not too many things to be phobic about which involve enforced separation from the parents; in fact school is really the only one. School and the movies are the only situations customarily found wherein the child cannot go home when he wants to without it being considered abnormal behavior. If these children are concerned over achievement, as they almost always are, with their strong concepts of right and wrong, then the school is the only place where all the anxiety can be focused. As one might expect, they are usually anxious about going to the movies without a parent, unless the movie is within walking distance of the home.

Basis for Rapid Return

The treatment procedures advocated in this paper are quite orthodox. In view of this, one wonders about the widespread acceptance of the principle of early return. Three factors appear to be involved. Since such principles of "action before insight" apply to this degree only to school phobias, one basis for them may lie in the therapists' feelings about school. In all Western societies, school is the most formalized, the most rigid and the most concrete way in which society organizes behavior in relation to children. Concurrently, school attendance and achievement represent an important aspect, both temporally and effectively, of the child's social growth. The events taking place associated with school and the child's reaction to these events have great bearing upon his ego development. Interruption of school thus simultaneously breaks the progression of social and psychosexual development in the child by removing him from the normal channels of such development and at the same time attacks the stability of one of society's most uncritically accepted strictures, to wit, the desirability of a child going to school. One result is to provoke a reaction from those whose unconscious orientation is toward preserving the stability of the structure.

We therapists are a product of this system. Therapists are highly educated people, individuals who value education in themselves and others. As a group, we are people who expect our children to go to school, go to college, and do well while in attendance. Not only are academic values of importance to us but so is being law abiding. The law maintains that a child must attend school. It is easy to accept what our unconscious tells us is right, especially where it is reinforced with all the pressures of contemporary society. While the well-trained therapist will have handled in his own analysis his need to be omnipotent, his need to do what others cannot do and his need to impress with rapid solutions to the problems, he is unlikely to have handled his feelings about his patients being in school.

Further support for the principle of rapid return comes from the concept of "brief therapy." While such techniques are of unquestioned value in certain circumstances, the reports concerning the future of children with school phobias suggest that they do not serve the patient's best interests in most cases of this nature.

Last, the idea of placing the child in a healthy environment makes the therapists feel that there is merit in rapid return. It is axiomatic in therapy, especially with children, that the extratherapeutic environment is important and often crucial in determining the course, effectiveness, and outcome of treatment. There is usually no question but that the school offers a healthier situation to function in than does the home. In addition, school offers opportunities for development in areas not available in the home. However, if the child is psychologically sealed off from these benefits and reacts to being in school by becoming more anxious and more autistic, then the healthier environment is not serving the child's needs. An environment that is realistically better by objective standards does not aid in treatment if the patient's response to being placed in such environment is an increase in terror.

Although the lay public may confuse the traumatic phobias with those due to displaced anxiety and may feel that getting the child back to school is like getting the rider back on the horse that has thrown him, the trained therapist appreciates the difference. Attempts to treat them in a similar manner are, in the last analysis, probably due to therapist's screening through himself the demands of the society in which he was raised and in which he practices.

Summary

This paper has considered the problem of the treatment of children with school phobias in terms of evidence and theory concerned with returning the children to school rapidly in contrast to allowing the child to determine the timing of return as part of his treatment. The theory that the child will regress if not in continuous contact with the school was not substantiated in the cases described. In fact, the only case of regression was observed while the child was in contact with the school. In most cases, there are advantages in not having children return too early, in the direction of a more favorable outlook for continued and successful treatment. The future of unsuccessfully treated children and those not treated at all was discussed, as well as the syndrome of the masked school phobia. The relationship between school phobia and agoraphobia was pointed out. The basis of treating school phobias differently than other syndromes was analyzed. School phobias must be differentiated from other types of neurotic school refusal. The essence of the paper is that school phobias should be treated like any other pathologic condition not subject to social censure. When these children get better, they get back to school without any difficulty.

References

1. Freud, S. Analysis of a Phobia in a Five Year Old Boy. In *Collected Papers,* Volume 3, Hogarth Press, London, 1925.
2. Alexander, F. *Fundamentals of Psychoanalysis.* W. W. Norton, New York, 1948, p. 217.
3. Fenichel, O. *The Psychoanalytic Theory of Neurosis.* W. W. Norton, New York, 1945, p. 210.
4. Freud, S. Turnings in the Ways of Psychoanalytic Theory. In *Collected Papers,* Volume 2, Hogarth Press, London, 1925.
5. Ivey, E. P. Recent Advances in Psychiatric Diagnosis and Treatment of Phobias. *Am. J. Psychother.,* 13: 35, 1959.
6. Klein, E. The Reluctance to Go to School. In *Psychoanalytic Study of the Child,* Volume 1, 1945, p. 263.
7. Eisenberg, L. The Pediatric Management of School Phobia. *J. Pediat.,* 55: 758, 1959.
8. Suttenfield, V. School Phobia: A Study of Five Cases. *Am. J. Orthopsychiat.,* 24: 368, 1954.
9. Sperling, M. Analytic First Aid in School Phobias. *Psychoanal. Quart.,* 30: 504, 1961.
10. Spock, B. *Baby and Child Care.* Pocketbooks, New York, 1946.
11. Kahn, J. H. and Nursten, J. P. School Refusal: A Comprehensive View of School Phobia. *Am. J. Orthopsychiat.,* 32: 707, 1962.
12. Talbot, M. Panic in School Phobia. *Am. J. Orthopsychiat.,* 27: 286, 1957.
13. Rodriguez, A., Rodriguez, M., and Eisenberg, L. The Outcome of School Phobia *Am. J. Psychiat.,* 116: 540, 1959.
14. Waldfogel, S., as cited in Rodriguez, A. (See 13).
15. Glaser, K. Problems in School Attendance, *Pediatrics,* 55: 758, 1959.
16. Coolidge, J. C., Brodie, R. and Feeney, B. *Workshop on Treatment of School Phobia.* Paper presented at the 40th annual meeting of the American Orthopsychiatric Association, Washington, D. C., 1963.
17. Warren, W. Some Relationships between the Psychiatry of Children and Adults. *J. Ment. Sci,* 106: 815, 1960.
18. Tagaki, R. School Phobia. *Acta Paedopsychiat.,* 30: 135, 1963.
19. Davy, B. W. The Sources and Prevention of Mental Ill Health in University Students. *Proc. Roy. Soc. Med.,* 53: 26, 1960.
20. Bornstein, B. Analysis of a Phobic Child. In *Psychoanalytic Study of the Child,* Volume 3–4, 1949, p. 181.

21. Coolidge, J. C., E. Tessman, S. Waldfogel and M. L. Willer. Patterns of Aggression in School Phobia. In *Psychoanalytic Study of the Child,* Volume 17, 1962, p. 319.
22. Johnson A. M., E. F. Falstein, S. A. Szurek, and M. Svendsen. School Phobia. *Am. J. Orthopsychiat.,* 11: 702, 1941.
23. Mahler, M. S. On Childhood Psychosis and Schizophrenia. In *Psychoanalytic Study of the Child,* Volume 7, 1952, p. 286.
24. Hartman, H. Mutual Influences in the Development of the Ego and Id. In *Psychoanalytic Study of the Child,* Volume 7, 1952, p. 9.
25. Coolidge, J. C., M. L. Willer, E. Tessman and S. Waldfogel. School Phobia in Adolescence. *Am. J. Orthopsychiat.,* 30: 599, 1960.
26. Reichenberg, N. Personal communication.
27. Lewis, W. C. Early Defenses and Percursors. *Int. J. Psycho-Anal.,* 44, 132, 1963.
28. Benjamin, J. D. Developmental Observations Relating to the Theory of Anxiety. Reported by Rubinfine, D. L., *J. Amer. Psychoanal. Ass.,* 7, 561, 1959.
29. Fromm-Reichman, F. *Psychoanalytic Remarks on the Clinical Significance of Hostility in Psychoanalysis and Psychotherapy.* University of Chicago Press, 1959.
30. Deutsch, H. The Genesis of Agoraphobia. *Int. J. Psycho-Anal.,* 10, 128, 1929.

Chapter Five

Juvenile Delinquency

Juvenile delinquency represents a major problem area in the United States today. Defined as the violation of legally established codes of conduct, delinquent acts range from relatively minor misbehaviors to serious crimes against persons and property. Often there is an aggressive or destructive aspect to the delinquent behavior, although sometimes it merely involves failure to comply with society's demands (for example, not going to school) or taking for one's own what rightfully belongs to others (as in petty theft, car stealing, or armed robbery).

All of these forms of delinquent behavior are rampant today and are frightening and disturbing. It is commonly accepted that certain sections of most large cities are unsafe after dark. Public places that a few years ago were attractive settings for leisurely walking, relaxing, and enjoying the scenery are now off-limits or known danger spots for the pedestrian (especially one who is alone, old, or relatively weak). When the persons who do the threatening, stealing, or physical attacking are legally minors, the antisocial activity is termed "delinquent behavior."

Prevalence

In view of the many and varied forms that delinquency can take, it is impossible to derive accurate figures indicating its prevalence. However, government reports show that each year more than two percent of the population between 10 and 17 years of age appears in juvenile courts, and the percentage is increasing steadily. The available figures show very definitely that boys and lower-class youngsters are more likely to be arrested and prosecuted for delinquent behaviors than are girls and middle- or upper-class youths.

It is a well-known fact that only a very small proportion of delinquent acts are recorded or legally punished. In a study conducted many years ago, Porterfield (1943) compared the previous delinquent behaviors admitted by college students with those found in known delinquent youths. That is, college students recalled and admitted the kinds of unsocialized behaviors they had performed in their previous years, and these were compared with the behaviors for which other youngsters were referred to juvenile courts. Porterfield found no differences either in the type or severity of delinquent acts among these two very different groups of subjects. The only significant differences in their delinquent acts were that the college students had committed their delinquent acts less frequently and had not been apprehended for them.

More recent findings relevant to understanding this phenomenon known as "hidden delinquency" were presented by Offer, Sabshin, and Marcus (1965). These investigators reported a very high prevalence of delinquent acts among middle-class, suburban adolescents who had not been identified as demonstrating any form of problem behavior. This finding of delinquent acts in 75 percent of the "normal" youngsters and other similar reports of unusually high rates of hidden (undetected) delinquency have led some observers to conclude that in the normal course of psychosocial development, almost all adolescents engage in certain activities that would be labeled "delinquent" if brought to public attention.

Types and Determinants

While some investigators have tended to treat juvenile delinquency as involving a homogeneous form of psychopathology, it is now widely recognized that this broadly defined legal category actually consists of several subcategories of behavior and determinants. Three main types identified with great consistency and recently described by Quay (1972) are: (1) the unsocialized, aggressive, rebellious delinquent; (2) the neurotic delinquent, with anxiety, depression, and related emotional problems; and (3) the socialized delinquent who accepts and adjusts to the social values of a delinquent subculture. It has been suggested that the unsocialized aggressive type is associated with parental rejection, the neurotic type with parental overcontrol, and the socialized type with parental neglect and permissiveness.

In an excellent treatise on problems of adolescence, Weiner (1970) gives detailed consideration to sociological and psychological determinants of delinquent behavior. He discusses the following dichotomies that help to clarify understanding of various determinants: (1) adaptive versus maladaptive; (2) social versus solitary; and (3) lower-class versus middle-class. Adaptive delinquency is defined as motivated, goal-directed behavior involving learning from experience; while maladaptive delinquency consists of frustration-induced behavior that is rigid, stereotyped, and resistant to punishment. Several large-scale research projects have utilized this distinction, referring to those who show the adaptive behaviors as socialized delinquents and labeling the maladaptives as unsocialized aggressive children. These studies suggest that youngsters in the unsocialized aggressive category have experienced maternal rejection from infancy or very early childhood, while the socialized delinquents were more apt to have experienced inadequate parental care at a later stage in childhood.

The socialized delinquent collaborates with others to commit criminal acts that are endorsed by his subculture and earn him status within it, whereas the solitary delinquent acts alone and for private reasons, engaging in criminal activities that are usually unacceptable in his social milieu. It is believed that the social delinquent tends to be psychologically normal, sharing antisocial values within his cultural group, while the solitary delinquent is more likely to be psychologically disturbed.

Weiner, as others before him, points out that delinquent behavior has been studied and interpreted primarily as a lower-class phenomenon, with very little research devoted to delinquency among middle-class youth. When comparisons are made, the tendency is to regard adaptive-social delinquency as largely characteristic of lower-class youngsters and maladaptive-solitary delinquency as more typical of middle- and upper-class youth. Kvaraceus and Miller (1959) state that since delinquency is much less likely to be "norm violating" in lower-class groups, it is less likely to be indicative of emotional disturbance. When middle- or upper-class children become involved in delinquent activity, according to Kvaraceus and Miller, they are much more apt to be emotionally disturbed. In fact, these investigators maintain that the greatest portion of the delinquent population consists of emotionally normal lower-class youngsters. It seems, however, that this conception is oversimplified, and there is probably a much greater degree of overlap in the kinds of delinquency evidenced by children reared under different socioeconomic conditions.

Physique and Delinquency

While many clinicians and theorists have emphasized the importance of social and psychological factors, other investigators have focused on possible physical components that might contribute to delinquency. A leading figure in this regard is William Sheldon, who is the most influential modern proponent of "constitutional psychology." Sheldon is famous for having established the system of somatotyping, in which a person's physique is judged in terms of three components: ectomorphy, mesomorphy, and endomorphy. Essentially, ectomorphy represents the thin, fragile physique; mesomorphy the muscular, athletic physique; and endormorphy the round, soft physique. Sheldon developed a system whereby any individual can be categorized according to his relative standing on each of these three basic components of physique.

Along with these classifications of body-build, Sheldon developed a system for rating temperament (personality) using the three categories of cerebrotonia, somatotonia, and viscerotonia. Each of these components is represented by certain personality traits. For example, cerebrotonics tend to be quiet, withdrawn, restrained, thoughtful, and solitary. Somatotonics tend to be aggressive, active, adventuresome, and dominant. Viscerotonics tend to be friendly, outgoing, relaxed, and sociable. Through an extensive program of research, Sheldon demonstrated noteworthy association between the components of physique and behavior. More specifically, the general findings show statistically significant association between ectomorphy and cerebrotonia, mesomorphy and somatotonia, and endomorphy and viscerotonia. These studies showing relationships between measures of body-build and ratings of personality characteristics were conducted with such varied groups as male and female college students and patients in mental hospitals.

For present purposes, Sheldon's (1949) most relevant research was an eight-year study of delinquent youth. A relatively large number of boys who had been institutionalized in a treatment facility in Massachusetts were studied both for measures of physique and for psychiatric ratings of their personality traits. Also analyzed were their detailed life histories, including information about the boys' intellectual and academic performance, family background, and types of delinquent activities in which they engaged. A major finding from this research program was an obviously greater amount of mesomorphy among the delinquents than in groups of normal males studied previously. There was also noticeably less evidence of ectomorphy among these delinquent boys. This research led Sheldon to conclude that there are not only important differences in physique between delinquents and normal college students but there are also physical and temperamental differences among various subgroups of delinquents. These conclusions were supported by findings of association between physique and delinquency reported by Glueck and Glueck (1956).

Sheldon's theory places heavy emphasis on the importance of constitutional (hereditary) factors as possible sources of delinquent behaviors. However, there are those who believe that even if delinquents do tend to be athletic in body-build and aggressive in temperament, these findings can be better accounted for in terms of social learning than on the basis of inherited constitution. From the kind of research conducted by Sheldon and by Glueck and Glueck, it is not possible to answer questions regarding cause-and-effect relationships. One might argue from the data that delinquents have inherited predispositions toward aggressive acting-out against others, but it is equally plausible that because one is well-built, athletic, and physically strong he learns to impose himself on others.

Prediction of Delinquency

A comprehensive study of antecedents of delinquency by Conger, Miller, and Walsmith (1965) showed that personality characteristics of future delinquents differed from those of non-delinquents even in the early school years. These differences were found after other factors—such as sex, social class, intelligence, and ethnic-group membership—had been controlled through a matching technique. This well-designed investigation demonstrated that intelligence and social-class background had to be taken into account in order to comprehend fully the personality differences between delinquents and non-delinquents. In the period from kindergarten to the third grade, the future delinquents, as a group, manifested less acceptable social behavior, more academic difficulty, and greater incidence of emotional disturbance.

Among their numerous publications on this topic, Glueck and Glueck (1950, 1952, 1959) have described procedures for predicting delinquency. They developed prediction tables based on factors in the family and social background plus measures of character, temperament, and personality derived from psychological tests and psychiatric interviews. On the basis of extensive research, these investigators concluded that the "social prediction score" could make an early identification of future delinquents with a surprising degree of accuracy (that is, 9 out of 10 correctly identified at age 6).

The Glueck social prediction tables have been revised over the years and used with considerable success by other investigators. Craig and Glick (1963) followed a large number of boys from age 5 to 17 and found that social factors were more important than personality factors in predicting delinquency. Utilizing the three factors of discipline by the father, supervision by the mother, and cohesiveness of the family, Craig and Glick reported 85 percent accuracy in predicting future delinquency. These findings led the investigators to conclude that eradicating family pathology and enriching family life is the primary step needed in prevention of delinquency.

Traditional Psychotherapeutic Treatment

While there are disagreements about the etiology (causes) of delinquency, there is unanimous agreement that psychotherapeutic treatment of most delinquents is extremely difficult. Here we will not present an extensive review of the literature but merely state that a high rate of failure is consistently reported by clinicians who attempt individual psychotherapy with delinquents and by research projects that study the effectiveness of therapeutic programs for delinquents. A basic premise in psychotherapeutic work with disturbed people is that the individual must be personally motivated in order for the therapy to have any beneficial effects. Traditionally, it has been felt that many delinquents are not consciously dissatisfied with their personality make-up and are reluctant to consider inadequacies in themselves. Therefore, they seldom seek change in their motivation or behavior and are hesitant to enter a relationship with a professional psychotherapist such as a psychologist, psychiatrist, or social worker.

Experimenter-Subject Psychotherapy

An extremely interesting paper by Slack (1960) describes an original method designed to introduce "unreachable" cases to psychotherapy. In connection with a research project in Cambridge, Massachusetts, Slack found that delinquent youths were very reluctant to be tested by a clinical psychologist or to talk about themselves in therapeutically oriented interviews. Slack, who was a rather uninhibited, unusual, likeable, and creative psychologist happened on the idea of hiring the delinquent youths to serve as paid subjects in his investigations; that is, rather than requesting that they take psychological tests and be interviewed about their backgrounds and personalities, Slack offered to pay them for serving as subjects in his laboratory. Many of these delinquent boys seized the opportunity to be paid for doing the "stupid" things this psychologist was interested in and were happy to come to his office to smoke his cigarettes, drink Cokes, talk into the tape recorder, and be paid for their time. There was certainly nothing to be ashamed about in this routine. One could even brag to friends about this strange but nice doctor who was willing to pay good money just to hear kids talk into his tape recorder. Anyone could easily see that this was very different than willingly talking to a therapist about one's personal and social difficulties.

Interestingly, however, many of these delinquent youths were unknowingly forming a therapeutic relationship with the psychologist. After his experiment ceased and there were no longer research funds to pay the boys for their time, some continued to stop by voluntarily to visit the psychologist and often talked with him about their problems. It was reported that this innovative approach to therapy led to positive long-range results with many of these youngsters.

Comprehensive Vocationally Oriented Psychotherapy

Noting that "traditional approaches to treatment of adolescent delinquent boys have frequently been unsuccessful," Massimo and Shore (1963, 1967) developed a new treatment technique for lower-class boys. This approach attempts to integrate the three services of vocational placement, remedial education, and psychotherapy by using a single practitioner, experienced in all three areas, who can offer whatever help is needed at a given time. The initial study involved 20 white lower-class delinquent boys who had just withdrawn or been suspended from school. They were randomly divided into two groups, one participating in the intensive 10-month treatment program and the other not participating. This demonstration program proved highly effective in bringing about therapeutic changes on many levels—academic areas, personality aspects (self-image, attitude toward authority, control of aggression), and overt behavior (legal status and job history). A follow-up study revealed that the boys who had participated in this program continued to show positive changes two and three years after treatment was terminated, while the untreated group deteriorated during that time.

Alternatives to Institutionalization

Recent reports have indicated that several states are considering doing away with traditional institutions for delinquents. The appalling statistics on recidivism (repeat offenses and incarcerations) among delinquents today provide ample evidence that current institutional training and treatment rarely lead to improved behavior. In fact, it is commonly believed that what first offenders actually learn in most training schools and other types of large institutions for delinquents is to think and act more like the older, experienced delinquents who serve as their models in such settings.

Massachusetts announced plans to close the large, old institutions for delinquents and replace them with group homes in which delinquents would continue to live in close contact with the community while undergoing therapeutic treatment, special educational experiences, and vocational training. Recent newspaper accounts have indicated that Rhode Island is also seriously considering the possibility of placing delinquents in such treatment homes instead of in the state training school that seems to be a continual trouble spot for all concerned. Hiring currently unemployed people to serve as foster parents for delinquents was also mentioned. Since it now costs about $10,000 per year to institutionalize each delinquent youth, and since many respectable, sincere, and capable people are now unemployed and receiving funds in the form of welfare, it seems that this experimental approach to helping delinquents may well prove to be a very worthwhile investment. It is believed and hoped that these radical departures from traditional institutionalization will lead to decreased recidivism and prevent neophyte delinquents from pursuing a life of crime.

The Issues

From this review of material selected from the vast literature on delinquency, it should be apparent that biological, psychological, and sociological factors all play a role in the etiology of delinquency. In a recent book, Cortes and Gatti (1972) present a comprehensive "biopsychosocial theory" of delinquency and crime. According to this theory, "Criminal and delinquent behavior are the result of a negative imbalance within the individual in the interaction between (a) the expressive forces of his psychological and biological characteristics, and (b) the normative forces of familial, religious, and sociocultural factors."

Of the many problems and issues in this broad field encompassed by the above theoretical formulation, we will here focus on (1) social class factors, (2) inadequacies of traditional approaches to "treatment," and (3) an innovative approach that has met with some success. In the first paper, David Elkind discusses the neglected problem of middle-class delinquency. He maintains that the usually poor results obtained from attempts at psychotherapy with delinquents can be attributed to the fact that "although the pathology exists in the parents, the symptoms appear in the child." Elkind utilizes the concept of "parental exploitation" in accounting for middle-class delinquency and feels that with lower-class delinquents there is often exploitation by society as well as by parents.

The dramatic transition from middle- to lower-class delinquency is revealed most vividly in the paper by Susan M. Fisher. This disquieting description of the way society allows lower-class delinquent black children to be treated will be revolting to many readers. This form of institutional treatment seems to ensure that troubled youngsters will learn to behave more like pathological adults.

In the final paper, Irwin G. Sarason again mentions the failure of traditional "talking therapy" to modify undesirable behavior of juvenile delinquents and describes an experimental treatment project that represents an outgrowth of social learning theory (Bandura & Walters, 1959, 1963). Sarason gropes with the problem of determining what kinds of personal characteristics make for good role models for delinquents. Rather surprisingly, he found that using former delinquents as cottage parents did not work out well since these reformed adults often harbored negative attitudes toward delinquent youth.

Use of modeling and observational learning as a primary treatment approach with delinquents seems to hold considerable promise, although there are many unsolved problems with this approach. If society's true concern were to guide deviant children onto a path leading to psychologically healthy adulthood, it would not allow them to be caged in settings more jungle-like than those they must cope with when they return to the streets of the city.

References

Bandura, A., & Walters, R. H. *Adolescent aggression.* New York: Ronald Press, 1959.

Bandura, A., & Walters, R. H. *Social learning and personality development.* New York: Holt, Rinehart & Winston, 1963.

Conger, J. J., Miller, W. C., & Walsmith, C. R. Antecedents of delinquency: Personality, social class, and intelligence. In P. H. Mussen, J. J. Conger, & J. Kagan (Eds.), *Readings in child development and personality.* New York: Harper & Row, 1965.

Cortes, J. B., & Gatti, G. M. *Delinquency and crime: A biopsychosocial approach.* New York: Seminar Press, 1972.

Craig, M. M., & Glick, S. J. Ten years experience with the Glueck social prediction table. *Crime and Delinquency,* 1963, **9,** 249–261.

Glueck, S., & Glueck, E. *Unraveling juvenile delinquency.* New York: The Commonwealth Fund, 1950.

Glueck, S., & Glueck, E. *Delinquents in the making.* New York: Harper & Row, 1952.

Glueck, S., & Glueck, E. *Physique and delinquency.* New York: Harper & Row, 1956.

Glueck, S., & Glueck, E. *Predicting delinquency and crime.* Cambridge, Mass.: Harvard University Press, 1959.

Kvaraceus, W. C., & Miller, W. B. *Delinquent behavior: Culture and the individual.* Washington, D. C.: National Education Association, 1959.

Massimo, J. L., & Shore, M. F. The effectiveness of a comprehensive vocationally oriented psychotherapeutic program for adolescent delinquent boys. *American Journal of Orthopsychiatry,* 1963, **33,** 634–642.

Massimo, J. L., & Shore, M. F. Comprehensive vocationally oriented psychotherapy: A new treatment technique for lower-class adolescent delinquent boys. *Psychiatry,* 1967, **30,** 229–236.

Offer, D., Sabshin, M., & Marcus, D. Clinical evaluations of normal adolescents. *American Journal of Psychiatry,* 1965, **121,** 864–872.

Porterfield, A. L. Delinquency and its outcome in court and college. *American Journal of Sociology*, 1943, **59**, 199–208.

Quay, H. C. Patterns of aggression, withdrawal, and immaturity. In H. C. Quay & J. S. Werry (Eds.), *Psychological disorders of childhood*. New York: Wiley, 1972.

Sheldon, W. H. *Varieties of delinquent youth: An introduction to constitutional psychiatry*. New York: Harper, 1949.

Slack, C. W. Experimenter-subject psychotherapy: A new method of introducing intensive office treatment for unreachable cases. *Mental Hygiene*, 1960, **64**, 238–265.

Weiner, I. B. *Psychological disturbance in adolescence*. New York: Wiley, 1970.

12. Middle-Class Delinquency

David Elkind

The research literature on juvenile delinquency is already vast and continues to grow at an increasing pace (1). By and large, however, this research tends to deal with lower-class children living in slum areas of large cities. Much less is known about the young people from suburban, middle-class homes who also get into trouble with the law.

Some writers (2, 3) have suggested that delinquent youngsters from "respectable homes" are acting out the parents' repressed antisocial impulses and are subtly encouraged by the parents in this regard. Although this explanation probably holds true in a certain number of cases, my own experience (as consulting psychologist to a suburban juvenile court) suggests that the vicarious satisfaction of needs is but one of many forms of parental exploitation that can lead to delinquent behavior on the part of children. In what follows I shall elaborate on some of the forms of parental exploitation and some of the possible adolescent reactions to such exploitation.

Before proceeding, however, it is necessary to distinguish among three quite distinct groups of middle-class delinquents. There are, first of all, those adolescents whose delinquency is a direct manifestation of a long-standing emotional disturbance and for whom the remedy is usually psychiatric rather than probationary. Secondly, there are those young people who come before the court almost by accident—quite often for pulling some prank that turned out to be more serious than they had anticipated—and who are seldom, if ever, adjudicated for a second time. By far the largest group, however, are those adolescents who get into trouble more or less regularly and who have a series of past charges filed against them. Although these young people do not appear to have serious internalized conflicts, they are usually in quite open conflict with their parents.

It is with the etiology of delinquent behavior in this third group of young people that the present paper is primarily concerned.

The Contract

The concept of parental exploitation makes sense only if there is an implicit contract between parents and their offspring. In middle-class families such a contract does exist. For their part, the parents agree to provide for the physical and emotional well-being of their children, who, in return, agree

From *Mental Hygiene*, 1967, **51**, 80–84. Copyright 1967 by the National Association for Mental Health. Reproduced by permission.

to abide by the norms of middle-class society. Although minor infractions of this contract on the part of both parents and children are to be found in most middle-class families, they tend to be temporary. For the most part, the contract is honored on both sides.

This appears not to be true in the families of the delinquent children under discussion. If one inquires deeply enough into the family relationships of these children, one finds that the contract has been broken by one or both parents *over a prolonged period of time*. More particularly, that part of the contract is broken which ensures that the parent will take responsibility for the emotional well-being of his child. What one finds in these cases is that the parent not only puts his own needs before those of the child, but, more significantly, attempts to use the child as an instrument in the satisfaction of those needs. It is because the parent violates the contract with his child while demanding that the child hold to his end of the bargain that such violations are legitimately called "parental exploitation."

Forms of Parental Exploitation

Although particular instances of parental exploitation are almost infinite in their variety, they can nonetheless be grouped under a few reasonably comprehensive headings. We have already noted that the *vicarious satisfaction of parental needs* is one frequent form of exploitation.

This form of exploitation is illustrated by a case in which a sexually frustrated mother encouraged her daughter to act out sexually. When the daughter returned from a date, the mother would demand a kiss-by-kiss description of the affair and end by calling the girl a tramp. When I saw the girl, who was being adjudicated for sexual vagrancy, she told me, "I have the name so I might as well play the role." When she left my office, her mother, who had been waiting outside, teasingly asked her how far she had gotten with the "cute psychologist."

A somewhat different form of parental exploitation might be called *ego bolstering*. In this category fall those parents who demand academic or athletic achievement far beyond what the young person is able, or has the capacity, to produce. This form of exploitation has an element of vicarious satisfaction in it, but the dominant affect seems to be the need to bolster flagging parental self-esteem. Although it is normal to want to take pride in one's child's achievements, it becomes pathologic when the parents' own needs to bask in reflected glory take precedence over the emotional welfare of the child.

A somewhat different variety of this form of exploitation is illustrated by the father who encouraged his 17-year-old son to drink, frequent prostitutes, and generally "raise hell." This particular father was awakened late one night by the police who had caught his son in a raid on a so-called "massage" parlor. The father's reaction was, "Why aren't you guys out catching crooks?" This same father would boast to his co-workers that his son was "all boy" and a "chip off the old block."

Still another form of parental exploitation occurs when parents use their youngsters as *slave labor*. In one instance, a father who owned a motel demanded that his son do all the lawn work and help to clean up the rooms and make the beds. To top it off, he insisted that the boy take the lids off all the cans in the trash barrels and then flatten the cans so that the volume of trash, and hence the cost of disposal, would be lessened. The boy barely had time to do his homework, much less to visit with his friends. Mothers who get their teenage daughters to do more of the housework and the baby-sitting than is reasonable or equitable provide another example of slave labor exploitation.

A fourth form of parental exploitation is frequently encountered in broken homes in which the mother, who usually retains custody of the children, is relatively young and attractive. In one case a mother took a lover, much younger than herself, into her home over the protestations of her teenage daughter, who had to cope with the curiosity of friends and the indignation of neighbors. Another young divorcee had a baby out of wedlock whom she kept in the home without any explanation to her teenage children. Still another mother, who had lost her husband under tragic circumstances, took to drinking away her afternoons with a younger man, to whom she gave large sums of money. She could not understand why her teenage son ran off to Mexico.

In all such cases, the mothers demand not only that their children accept the situation, but that they condone it. By demanding that their children accept and condone their behavior, these mothers hope to use their children to *assuage their own consciences*.

One of the saddest forms of parental exploitation is engaged in by parents who are very much in the public eye, particularly school principals, clergy-men (of whatever faith), and judges. If a parent in one of these professions sees his child's behavior primarily in terms of what it means to his career, he may demand a degree of conformity to middle-class mores that is quite unreasonable from the young person's point of view. When young people of this kind get into trouble, it is not because the parents are too strict, but rather because the parents are using their children to *proclaim their own moral rectitude*. As in all cases of parental exploitation, the dominant effect in such children is not so much the feeling of being restricted as it is the feeling of being *used*.

Reactions to Parental Exploitation

When a worker is exploited he has at least four courses of action open to him. He can either quit, go out on strike, sabotage the plant, or passively submit to the exploitation.

Parallel types of reaction are found in middle-class delinquents. Some young people literally quit the scene. They may quit school and become truant, quit the home and become runaways, or quit the family psychologi-cally and become incorrigible. Other adolescents go on strike. They continue to go to school, but refuse to perform; they stay in the home, but refuse to do their fair share of the chores; they stay out late, and they go with a group of whom the parents don't approve. In short, they defy parental authority generally. More serious reactions are observed in young people who wish to sabotage their parents. These kids get pregnant, steal cars, vandalize schools, get drunk, sniff glue, or take drugs. Such reactions cost the parents plenty in worry, time, money, and bad publicity. The saddest reaction of all is that of the youngsters who passively submit to parental exploitation in the hope of winning or regaining parental love.

Despite the variety of these reactions, they all have one feature in common: parental exploitation is essentially private and is seldom recognized by anyone outside the home. Whereas the worker often has a union to voice his grievances and to stand up for his rights, there are no unions for children. Consequently, the delinquent behavior of adolescents who are being exploited by their parents often serves as a kind of "cry for help." Put differently, delinquent behavior often has as one of its components the desire to make exploitation public, to let the world know what is happening behind the drawn drapes and closed doors. The sad thing about such cries for help is that they are as injurious to the young person as they are to the parents.

Treatment

To say that middle-class delinquency is difficult to treat psychotherapeutically is a gross understatement. The major reason for this is the fact that, *although the pathology exists in the parents, the symptoms appear in the children*. Since it is the children who are in trouble, the parents find it hard, except on a superficial basis, to accept their responsibility in the matter. Blind to their own violation of the parent-child contract, they insist that the young person live up to his side of the bargain. For his part, the young person feels that he has been used and abused and generally will not take responsibility for his actions.

With both parents and children blaming each other for the difficulty, there is little motivation for change on either side. Usually, however, the children are more tractable than the parents on this score. In many cases all that one can do is either remove the young person from the home, or help him to understand and deal with the exploitation in a more effective and less self-injurious way.

Summary and Implications

In the foregoing discussion, I have argued that middle-class delinquency is essentially a reaction to parental exploitation and have tried to enumerate some of the forms of exploitation as well as some of the reactions to it. Such a position clearly places the burden of blame for middle-class delinquency upon the parents. To some extent, this is perhaps unjust, since children may encourage exploitation on their own behalf and may well exploit their parents in return. In many cases the exploitation is as likely to be circular as it is to be unidirectional. And yet, my impression is that in the majority of cases the parents are much more to blame than are their children.

It should be said, too, that I don't offer the notion of parental exploitation as a complete explanation of middle-class delinquency. It is probably true that many of these young people have ego and superego defects of long standing. It is also true that we don't know why one form of exploitation will lead to a particular kind of delinquency and not another. In some cases, the connections seem direct and clear-cut, whereas in others they remain obscure. Unknown, too, is how prolonged the exploitation must be and how much of it is needed to incite an adolescent to delinquent acting-out. Such threshold values are probably a joint function of the child's personality and the quality of parental exploitation.

In short, a detailed understanding of any particular case of middle-class delinquency will have to involve a psychodynamic evaluation of the personalities of both parent and child. On the other hand (or so it seems to me), a psychodynamic evaluation of the parent-child interaction, although providing an explanation in a particular case, may well miss the common theme that seems to run through all cases of middle-class delinquency, namely, parental exploitation. Taken together, however, the concept of parental exploitation and psychodynamic evaluations may well provide a general, as well as a specific, explanation for middle-class delinquency.

The value of such a general explanation of delinquency as parental exploitation is shown in the way it helps to make plausible why certain familial conditions are regularly associated with delinquent behavior. Broken homes, for example, have routinely contributed more than their fair share to the delinquent population (4–7). It seems reasonable to assume that in broken homes one is more likely to find unmet parental needs than would be the case in intact families. Under these conditions, the temptation to put one's own needs ahead of those of the child and to use the child as an instrument in the satisfaction of those needs would probably be greatly enhanced. In short, the concept of parental exploitation might allow one to predict, or at least hypothesize, the kinds of family constellations that would be most likely to produce delinquent behavior.

Before closing, I want to take up one more point that has been raised by those who attribute middle-class delinquency to the antisocial impulses of parents that are vicariously satisfied through the child. It has already been noted that the vicarious satisfaction of parental needs is indeed one form of parental exploitation. Where I disagree with this position is in the implication that middle-class delinquency is antisocial, regardless of whether or not this is true of the parental need. If antisocial means the intent to harm or injure society in general, then I do not believe middle-class delinquency is antisocial. I do believe it is antifamilial. Looked at from the point of view of the adolescent, and not necessarily from the point of view of society, delinquent behavior may be the most psychologically adaptive action a young person can take in the face of parental exploitation. Delinquent behavior not only calls attention to his plight, but also may remove him from the home on temporary or permanent basis.

Although I have limited the application of the concept of exploitation to the question of middle-class delinquency, it is possible that all delinquency is, at least in part, a reaction to exploitation and that society, as well as parents, can be culpable in this regard.

References

1. Quay, H. C. (ed.): Juvenile Delinquency. Princeton, Van Nostrand, 1965.
2. Giffin, M. E., Johnson, A. M., and Litin, E. M.: American Journal of Orthopsychiatry, **24**:668, 1954.
3. Johnson, A. M., and Burke, E. C.: Proceedings of the Staff Meetings of the Mayo Clinic, **30**:557, 1955.
4. Burt, C.: The Young Delinquent. New York, Appleton, 1929.
5. Glueck, S., and Glueck, E. T.: Unraveling Juvenile Delinquency. New York, Commonwealth Fund, 1950.
6. Monahan, T. P.: Social Forces, **35**:250, 1957.
7. Nye, F. I.: Family Relationships and Delinquent Behavior. New York, Wiley, 1958.

13. Life in a Children's Detention Center: Strategies of Survival

Susan M. Fisher

The children come out of vans, handcuffed to policemen. Their belongings are taken, except a comb. They wait in the lobby from ten minutes to half a day. No one looks at them. From the start, no one wants to know them. They are there awaiting trial. Some for ten days, some for three hundred, they never know when they will go to court, when they will see their probation officer, when they will be visited. If convicted, the time spent waiting does not count in their sentence; time in the detention center is not related to time before or time that will come. A twelve-year-old waits from October to June to be screened. He has been forgotten. The children are issued clothes, stripped, and searched for drugs. Sometimes drugs are in balloons, swallowed, to be vomited up later. No rules are explained to them. They are put onto the units without introductions. Girls are separated. The boys are grouped by age, except the armed offenders, and a special unit for homosexuals, transvestites, and the rare white boy. Segregation by race, poverty, education, capacity to adapt, has occurred already. One counselor watches thirty children in space meant for fifteen. Eight hours. Brick

From *American Journal of Orthopsychiatry*, 1972, **42,** 368–374. Copyright © 1972 the American Orthopsychiatric Association, Inc. Reproduced by permission.

walls, naked light bulbs, loud music; no solitude is permitted voluntarily. They must stay together in the main room of the unit, yet for any alleged infraction—smoking outside the allotted smoking period, cursing back to a counselor—or for no specific violation at all, they can be put into isolation. Officially all isolation detentions are to be reported; reports are often not made, and any child can be locked up within the eight hours of a shift, and no one will know. And with other such institutions it shares: one hundred degrees in summer, smells of urine and unwashed bodies. Twenty-three beds in a sleeping room; some isolation rooms have only a toilet bowl, and the counselor can turn off the water supply. To fight roaches, the rooms are heavily sprayed. Physical abuse with no redress; the word of a child is never accepted against that of a staff member.

These children are innocent before the law. Some are accused of major crimes—assaults, armed robbery, rape, murder. Others are not held for crimes at all but for being unmanageable and intractable in homes and schools where rebellion may be a measure of vigorous health; such children are designated "beyond control." Some are detained because mental hospitals refuse them and they are caught in a circuit between detention center, foster home, and hospital. They have the same needs for "rules of the game" as any incarcerated person, the same needs to create an internal social structure in which to participate, but it is hard to establish one when the formal roles and relationships of the institution are undefined, illusive, even contradictory. They are innocent but treated as guilty. Counselors are to maintain safety, watch, and protect them but often abuse and threaten them. Held within a legal system designed to insulate them from depersonalized adult bureaucracies, they have no civil rights and are isolated from the world of their origins. The atmosphere within the detention center is chaotic for the children and the staff. The chaos mirrors the inner state of the children and the social existence they came from.

The children are almost all black, between seven and eighteen. White children are not so quickly picked up for similar offenses. Frequently, black parents are not called from the station house and their children are detained before the parents know where they are, whereas white parents are usually located and the children released into their custody.

Some common perceptions of the world unite these children before they reach the detention center. They have learned to view social authorities as persecutory and punishing, coming at them with prejudged expectations of their responses and performances—guilty, stubborn, irresponsible, unlovable. They have been faceless objects to be manipulated, as others are to them; and manipulation is effected through behavior, not language. The establishment figures of their world—teachers, police, welfare workers, storekeepers, bus drivers—are to them arbitrary and rejecting; while their sources of food and shelter, the intimate associates to count on, are precarious. Psychiatrists might call these children paranoid, except that their perceptions are accurate most of the time; and the model for dealing with outer danger and uncertainty perpetuates a style of projection of internal distress.

On the units they are passive. They lie on the floor, near or on each other, sometimes playing games. Occasionally they riot, fight, or gang bang.

Sudden swings from immobility to violence are part of accepted and expected behavior, for staff and children alike. They pass in lines from unit to school to meals to recreation. Unexplained shifts in schedule for work, school, and play occur almost daily; rules vary according to the counselor on duty.

One's fate is sealed on arrival day. Each new boy is physically challenged. If he doesn't defend himself, he will be beaten up or threatened sexually. If he fights but loses he will still be accepted. He must not back off or cry. Group homosexual assaults are common among the older boys. Younger boys are simply taken sexually; sometimes they offer themselves. A shrewd newcomer can ally himself with tougher kids by being a good "cracker," a style of speech to be discussed later. The genuinely innocent kid—the eight- or nine-year old who is not street-wise and is physically weak—gets it in every way and learns fast.

Throughout the system, anger is vented on weaker members, and weakness is defined in physical struggles. A tough counselor can alter the threats of violence on a unit by being the strong man himself. Often a less punitive counselor will ally himself with the toughest boy to maintain order and survive. A rare counselor interrupts this pecking order by engaging children in group activities and loyalties and presenting different values of strength. Such counselors, though respected by the children, usually do not last long.

Once a child has entered the unit, what are his strategies for survival? The only method with positive rewards is to con the system. This means being deliberately friendly with counselors and administrators, thereby getting jobs in the kitchen, the offices, school, and laundry. This gives extra privileges—more food, smoking, new contacts, and, most important, movement off the unit. All conning activities are safe as long as they are perceived by the other kids as tongue-in-cheek, as long as a child is not thought a "patsy" or a "ratter."

The second major tack to survive, by far the most prevalent, is to disappear into the woodwork, to be utterly passive, faceless, non-existent. Even bizarre behavior is not seen. I learned from one therapy group of a sixteen-year-old boy drinking his own urine, burning his forehead with cigarettes, and calling himself "black Jesus." He was not noticed by the staff. From another, I met a group member who used different names each time he came to the detention center without anyone ever recognizing it was the same child.

Only rarely will a child beat down the system. These are big kids who are good "crackers" and physically overbearing. They are the brightest boys, who supersede whatever alliance a counselor makes with other tough kids and become a kind of spokesman. They are feared by the staff because of their cunning, their power to disrupt. The hostility toward them is intense but they are left alone. The system often expels them and, for some, the penalty is high. Sammy was a master at this, and intimidated the staff to its limit. Having traveled between hospital and detention center, he was released to his home, where he was stabbed to death by his father.

Closely tied to survival is the informer system. The administration corrals, bribes, and frightens certain children into informing on their peers. The rules are strict. If discovered, informing is tolerated by the other children if suffering would have been the penalty for silence—if you would have gotten more time, or been severely punished. But one can never inform to gain something. The penalty for this is physical abuse, rape, or ostracism.

An important aspect of survival is called "cracking." It is a mocking, jeering, joking use of language that establishes with words the same pecking order as physical strength does initially. You crack *on* someone, you don't crack *with* him. "Ass-kissers," boys who con about going straight when they get out, are particular targets. This is vicious humor and in therapy groups it is important to cut through it but not threaten its effectiveness on the units. It is the major non-physical cohesive force that allies them. Cracking represents an implied ability to fight and to withstand and dish out verbal abuse. You put people down, put feelings down, always mocking tenderness and sentiment. Feelings are hidden. Language is not a neutral vehicle for contact or communication. When not cracking, the boys sit silently on the floor. It is the only conversation.

When is there tenderness? When is there protection? Only under extreme circumstances. Most of the time, extreme physical helplessness is protected. A severe stutterer on a very tough unit cannot be teased. I learned of a boy in isolation for twenty-four hours in severe drug withdrawal. The administration had refused to send him and several others to the hospital, accusing them of malingering; some were, but some weren't. He lay with his head on a roll of toilet paper, his face in his vomitus, shaking under blankets. Outside the door, keeping check, was a boy from the unit who had watched him throughout the day, keeping him warm.

Psychological helplessness is not so protected, and the disturbed are good subjects for cracking. Out of fear, the extremely bizarre are left alone; sometimes boys will point out to a mental health consultant sick kids, ignored by the staff. Vince had been in isolation for six days and had not been visited except for food put in his room. He was locked up to finish an isolation punishment meted out a year before in a previous period at the detention center, unfinished because he had gone to court and been released. When I saw him, he was incoherent, babbling, drooling, terrified; his ravings soon became comprehensible to me. He wanted a particular doctor every day—a man who had been kind to him four years before. He had held the gun during an armed robbery because he wanted "those guys" to like him and he couldn't say no. He was afraid to go back to the unit because he would be raped.

The primary defense mechanisms operating on every level in the detention center are projection, denial, and dissociation. One's internal wretchedness, when experienced at all, is "because of them." Children are tormented by counselors, counselors are threatened by administrators, administrators are endangered by "downtown," and "downtown" is harassed by the legislators. Too often, they are right; the concrete realities of these people's lives makes interruption and examination of these defenses almost impossible. Few people within the detention center distinguish external and internal sources of misery or notice any personal difficulty in tolerating painful feelings.

Who are the counselors and administrators, and how do they function? Like the children, they have no options. Their supervisors and senior administrators offer them no intimacy, no range of techniques to handle problems; only authoritarian strength or deflection of responsibility to a vague "other." As the counselors fail the children, so the senior administrators permit no identifications or sharing, acknowledge no conflictual feelings. Like the children, counselors receive no positive rewards, only negative reinforcement. If they fly through a window to prevent an escape, that is expected behavior. If they are five minutes late, it is written into their record. They are frequently spied upon and lied to.

Like the children, they wait—for promotions, commendations, course certificates that don't ever come or are delayed without explanation. They too have no privacy. Personnel files lie open, rumors abound and threaten everyone. Counselors rarely protect each other, and children are pawns in staff rivalries. Three boys were left naked in one isolation room in a struggle over which counselor would get them clothes.

The relationship between counselors and children is a deadly game, and the main rule is "beat them or they'll beat you." A drug user is caught by a counselor. In the morning statistical report, without intended irony, is printed, "Congratulations, Mr. X. You are the biggest drug catcher of them all." Counselors try to outguess and outfox the children, as in a ruthless sport. Understanding, empathizing, helping is emasculating. Fundamentally, the children must never be seen as like themselves; they cannot imagine their own children in such a setting.

Respectful intimacy is non-existent in the detention center and the counselors use the children in different ways. Like objects of pornography, they are erotically used. Some stimulate the kids by teasing them and egging them on. One counselor has the boys talk about homosexual exploits into a tape recorder. Some female counselors are visibly titillated by illegitimate pregnancies and stories of prostitution. Occasionally, a counselor rapes a child, with or without consent. One senses that the children are discharging the forbidden aggressive and sexual impulses of the staff, who reestablish their self-image, distance, and self-control by massively suppressing the children.

Most counselors cannot tolerate any physical and verbal show of aggression in the children, and some hit and even beat them at the first sign. Once, a counselor called a psychologist for himself because he was putting a child into isolation for no apparent reason, yet he knew he was going to hit him unless he got rid of him. That amount of self-observation is rare. Encouraging and watching violence is irresistible for some, and their fascination is not acknowledged. A female counselor stood and impassively watched a girl bite out a piece of another girl's cheek and told me later, "Nice girls don't fight."

Always there is the reality of actual danger working with severe overcrowding. This too is used, and counselors often flirt with danger, provoking avoidable situations that excite them, and provide an opportunity to watch, experience unacceptable behavior, and then divorce themselves from it entirely. When overcrowding occasionally diminishes, there is no change in staff behavior.

The counselors use language as the children do—bitter cracking with each other; they rarely have shared, matter-of-fact exchanges. With their senior authorities, they retreat into sullen silence. Meetings between them reveal similarities with the children on the units. Counselors are impassive, talked at, immobile, and then break into fits of temper, screaming, physically threatening, banging chairs. These outbursts by counselors are dealt with by their bosses as tangentially and immaterially as the fires and riots of the children. I once dared a senior administrator to risk telling the counselors at such a meeting that he was sometimes depressed working there. They fell into an astonished calm.

Occasionally more flexible persons are hired. Senior administrators don't want to hear their complaints and suggestions, and will harass them until they quit. Often such men cannot tolerate the frustration and depression. A powerful clique of authoritarian counselors makes life miserable for a more flexible person, and very few remain. The detention center is a place to get out of—for everyone who can. What remains is a group of people who feed on the chaos within the center to avoid facing their own doubts and fears, and issues of their own competence. Tactics to improve working conditions are never gripped and applied vigorously; they hide behind the system's inadequacies and extrude more effective people. What is rewarded is security, passivity, immobility, no overt conflict. And the staff lives with a sense of impending destruction—each television interview, meeting, call from a judge is potentially the loss of safety, job, promotion, status, perhaps reflecting deep projected guilts.

Although of different backgrounds, staff, like the children, are locked within constricted character structures with little internal mobility. Almost all black, with some higher education, the staff struggles to maintain a middle-class identity in jobs that have little social status. Significantly, a large number come from the rural South, farms or small towns, where angry outbursts were often forcibly suppressed, and the need for control was related to the dangers of white society "out there." Rarely, a counselor will admit his outrage at seeing these urban boys doing what they never could; sometimes senior administrators, who spend far less time with the children, connect their dislike of the new music, new haircuts, new freedoms to the compromises they made to "make it" in a white bureaucracy. Their hatred of the children, which is felt after a few hours in the detention center, is a necessary piece of the delicate equilibrium required to maintain their self-esteem.

Cracking, the only language effective on every hierarchical level of the detention center, is also a metaphor for the cracks, the split, the dissociation that mark this institution. Everywhere one meets the illusion of infinite distance and difference. These children are a different species, not human. Top administrators are unreachable, unknowable bosses. Distance between castes is experienced as a non-crossable space. Yet each level is partially identified with and living through the other, dependent on the other; the illusion of infinite separation masks an unconscious fusion between the groups based on mutual projection—a partial symbiosis. Fusion versus infinity—on every level the same image is reflected, like facing mirrors.

No one trusts here, and everyone is hungry. In therapy groups, in consultations with senior administrators, in talks with counselors, the imagery is oral. Beneath the hatred, the backbiting, the projections, the chaos, lie enormous reservoirs of depression. Ultimately, the maintenance of the chaos may itself be defending against the hopelessness and lack of mobility in their lives, which get perpetuated throughout the institution.

At the core of several decisions by the United States Supreme Court has been its recognition that the juvenile court system, established to protect the special interests of children before the law, has violated not only their civil rights under the Constitution, but has perpetrated those very abuses of human growth the special systems were created to avoid.

This detention center represents the failure of all structures in urban society—family life, schools, courts, welfare systems, organized medicine, hospitals. It is a final common pathway to wretchedness. Occasionally a scandal in the newspaper, an outraged lawyer, an interested humanitarian judge makes a ripple. The surface smooths rapidly over again, because, locked away in a distant part of town, society forgets the children it does not want or need.

14. Verbal Learning, Modeling, and Juvenile Delinquency

Irwin G. Sarason

What possible connection might there be between the pristine beauty of the memory drum and the rough and tumble world of juvenile delinquency? I shall attempt to show that these seemingly different worlds can be bridged, and that this is possible in terms of concepts related to modeling and observational learning. In the process of doing this, I shall describe an ongoing investigation of psychological variables which bear upon the problem of the prevention and control of juvenile delinquency. The subjects of the investigation are institutionalized delinquents. The basic hypothesis underlying the investigation is that systematic exposure to meaningful identification models can have a discernible and salutary influence in modifying the behavior of the acting-out teenager.

Excerpted from *American Psychologist,* 1968, **23,** 254–266. Copyright 1968 by the American Psychological Association and reproduced by permission.

The significance of this topic is obvious. Few social problems rival juvenile delinquency as a source of concern and urgency. The general public has called stridently—at times, even with terror—for the development of procedures for the control of crime and delinquency and for the prevention of recidivism. Professional workers often become dismayed at the apparent failure of extant and traditional cognitively oriented "talking therapy" to modify the undesirable behavior of juvenile and adult criminals.

The research which I shall describe is an outgrowth of social learning theory and research dealing with the process of observational learning. Sociological and clinical evidence relating to the behavior of crime and delinquency have also influenced its development. My present work with delinquents is a cognitively complex product and sibling (believe it or not!) of another, and more venerable, ongoing research interest in the relationship of anxiety and the observation of models to learning and performance. . . .

One contribution of these verbal learning experiments is the impetus that they provide for the investigation of modeling effects in a variety of performance and learning situations. Observing others in a novel situation may serve to increase task familiarity and to reduce the apprehension of an individual when he enters that situation. In addition, observing others may provide the observer with helpful cues for his own behavior. It would seem necessary, now, to begin to explore intensively the nature of observational cues and the effects of observational experiences on cognitive processes. One practical possibility is that manipulation of the composition of learning and social groups could have salutary effects on members' behavior. For example, underachieving college students might be given the opportunity to reside in dormitory units alongside more competent and successful students. Or, socially disadvantaged children might be given the opportunity to attend school with more fortunate children. What sorts of vicarious benefits might accrue to the underachiever or disadvantaged pupil in such a situation? Might observation by students of filmed models be an effective means of education? Might it be an especially effective means for certain students, such as those characterized by high test anxiety? The value of further experimentation on the modeling process in intellectual performance resides in the possibility of uncovering variables which have potent effects on learning and on achievement. This experimentation is relevant both to the development of the theory of observational learning and to the enhancement of educational opportunities. . . .

The Delinquency Leap

Let us turn at this point to the seemingly only abstract relationship between verbal learning studies of relatively well-put-together college students and the behavior of acting-out youth. I shall not inflict upon you the complex and, no doubt, at least in part, poorly wired cognitive circuitry which made this connection. In fact, in candor, I shall admit that as the verbal learning research proceeded I simply became increasingly interested in the question: Might observational opportunities prove to be a useful behavior-modification vehicle with persons who display behavior problems?

The behavior of juvenile delinquents is clearly a serious social problem. It seemed an appropriate focus for approaching the question of behavior modification, for a number of reasons. The major one is that a good bit of juvenile delinquency need not be viewed in terms of a mental illness conception. Rather, it can be seen as a reflection of inadequate learning experiences. The delinquent is someone who has fallen out of the mainstream of his culture; he is someone who is deficient in socially acceptable and adaptive behavior. His deviant behavior may be viewed as part of a rebellion against societal norms and as a failure to have introjected socially useful ways of responding. This failure, it seemed to me, comes about as a result of inadequate opportunities to observe, display, and, subsequently, receive reinforcement for socially useful behavior. This interpretation is consistent with empirical evidence, social learning theory, sociological theories such as those dealing with differential association, and clinical observations.

These considerations, together with the social importance of the problem of juvenile delinquency, contributed to development of the research which I shall now describe. I should point out that one determinant of the decision to study delinquents was that two groups of delinquents could be compared: those which are characterized by moderate to strong degrees of anxiety and those where anxiety is relatively absent (for example, as in many cases of character disorders). Thus, the research on delinquency really was not just a product of poorly wired cognitive circuitry. It is being carried out in order to find out the generality of the verbal learning research which I have described. Are anxious juvenile delinquents more responsive to observational opportunities than those who are low in anxiety?

The specific foci of our investigation were the vocational and educational plans of juvenile offenders, their motivations, interests, attitudes towards work, and their meager repertory of socially appropriate behavior. Our hypothesis is that systematic exposure to identification models who exhibit relevant socially appropriate behavior can have a salutary and positive influence in changing the behavior of the juvenile offender.

The project began in the fall of 1966. It was an obviously necessary first step to establish a good working relationship with the personnel at the locus of our research, the Cascadia Juvenile Reception-Diagnostic Center, located in Tacoma, Washington. Meetings were held with supervisory and staff members of the administration, psychology, education, recreation, and social service departments, and with the personnel of the cottages in which the research was to be conducted. Concurrently, time was spent learning the details of the diagnostic process, educational programs, and schedules to which delinquents at Cascadia are subjected during their stay at the institution and in determining the extent to which portions of the institution's diagnostic data and information could be utilized for research purposes. Within a relatively short period of time it became clear that both cooperation with and support of the project characterized every level of Cascadia's personnel.

Cascadia's cottages, in each of which 20–25 children reside, are staffed by a Supervising Group Life Counselor, an Assistant Counselor, and four staff counselors. These six persons staff the cottage in shifts round the clock. The children at Cascadia represent a 100% sample of children committed to the Department of Institutions by the juvenile courts of Washington. Approximately 1,700 cases per year are seen at Cascadia.

The models were clinical psychology graduate students (I shall have more to say about this fact later on). An early activity of the project was the development of the project's research assistants' skills in role playing and working with groups. Meetings, discussions, and practice sessions were devoted to maximizing the assistants' effectiveness as models, with emphasis on techniques appropriate for a population of adolescents.

At the outset of the research it was felt that three requirements would have to be met in order to attain our objectives. These requirements were:

1. Modeling opportunities afforded adolescent delinquents would have to be provided under controlled conditions.

2. Relevant comparison and control conditions would have to be investigated.

3. Objective behavioral indices would have to be developed in order to determine the efficacy of our experimental procedures.

The work of the first year was concerned with meeting these requirements. This initial period was also used for pilot work dealing with several specific questions, including these:

1. What types of observational opportunities would be interesting and ego involving for juvenile delinquents?

2. How should models behave toward the subjects in order to maximize the effects of observational opportunities?

3. What sorts of control groups are needed?

4. What specific types of dependent variables should be obtained in order to assess the effects of modeling opportunities?

It soon became clear to us that the more objective and uncomplicated the modeling situation is, the greater its applicability to various kinds of situations and the more useful and practical it will be to others as a rehabilitation aid. We concluded that two ingredients were needed for modeling opportunities to be effective: (a) an objectively describable modeling situation and (b) good rapport between models and subjects—the models must be liked by the subjects and must be objects with whom boys would want to identify.

Early preliminary studies led us to the conclusion that, while the models should interact informally with subjects in Cascadia's cottages, modeling sessions should be clearly labeled and easily discriminable situations. We have spent much time working on these situations and training our research assistants to be effective models and empathic, reinforcing individuals.

Preliminary work with several dozen subjects resulted in the development of a series of 15 modeling sessions to which Cascadia's delinquent boys were exposed. All of these sessions were explained to them as opportunities to develop more effective ways of coping with problems that are important and common for people like themselves. A practical problem-solving atmosphere was created during each session. This initial orientation was given to the boys:

First, let's all introduce ourselves, starting with me. I'm Mr. _____ and this is Mr. _____ (boys introduce themselves). We are working with small groups of boys here at Cascadia. We are doing something new to show you some different ways of handling common situations and problems that will happen in your lives. The situations we'll work with and emphasize are often particularly important for fellows like yourselves. We say this because just the fact that you're going through an institution will have important effects on your lives, and we want to work with you to teach you better ways of handling some of these effects. In other words, we want to work together with you to teach you new ways to handle problem situations. These are situations which we feel will be of importance to you in the future. They are things that probably all of you will run into from time to time and we think that you can benefit from learning and practicing different ways to act in these situations.

The way we want to do this isn't by lecturing or advising you. Having people watch others doing things and then discussing what has been done is a very important way and a useful way to learn. It is easy to learn how to do something just by observing someone else doing it first. Often times, just explaining something to someone isn't nearly as effective as actually doing it first while the other person watches. For example, it is easier to learn to swim, or repair a car, if you have a chance to watch someone else doing it first.

We think that small groups, working together, can learn a lot about appropriate ways of doing things just by playing different roles and watching others play roles. By role, we mean the particular part a person acts or plays in a particular situation—kind of like the parts actors play in a movie scene, only this will be more realistic. These roles will be based on actual situations that many young people have trouble with, like how to control your anger, or resist being pressured into doing destructive things by friends. Other roles are directly related to fellows like yourselves who have been in an institution. These are situations such as your review board, or the ways you can best use the special skills of your parole counselor to help you after you leave here. Things like this are things that not everyone can do well. We want to emphasize better ways of doing these things and coping with similar problems which will be important in the future for most of you. Everyone in the group will both play the roles for themselves and watch others playing the same roles. This is like acting, only it is realistic because it involves situations in which you might really find yourselves. We feel that the situations are realistic because they are based on the real experiences of a lot of fellows who have gone through Cascadia.

There are seven of us here at Cascadia who are working in these small groups. We are not on the Cascadia staff. We are here because we are interested in working with fellows like yourselves and in helping you improve your skills in how you approach the situations I've just described. Since we are not on the Cascadia staff, we do not have anything to do with the decisions made concerning you or where you will go after leaving here. We do not share any of our information with the regular staff. Everything this group does or talks about is kept strictly confidential and isn't available to or used by the staff in any way at all.

This group is one of several we have been working with here on _____ Cottage. Each group meets three times a week for about 40 minutes at a time. This same group will meet together each week during the time you are all here at Cascadia, but different ones of us will be with this group on different days. We will be playing different roles in different situations on each day. This is how we will do it. First, we will describe the situation to you. Then we will play out the roles that are involved. We want you to watch us and then take turns in pairs, playing the same roles yourselves. We will also discuss how everyone does and what is important about the particular roles or situations and how they may be related to your lives. We will want you to stick closely to the roles as we play them but also add your own personal touch to your role. As you will see, it is important that we all get involved in this as much as we can. The more you put yourself into the role you play, the more realistic it will be to you and to the rest of the group. We see these scenes as examples of real situations that you will all find yourselves in sometime, and it is important to play them as realistically as possible. We will outline each scene as we go along.

Also, each meeting will be tape-recorded. We use these tape-recordings for our own records of how each group proceeds. These tapes are identified by code numbers and no one's name actually appears in the tape. The tapes are confidential too, and will be used only by us. As we said, none of this information is used by the regular staff.

Before going any further, we want to give you an example of what we're talking about. Mr. _____ and I will play two roles which involve a scene that has really gone on right here on your cottage. This scene is based on information we got from a cottage counselor and other boys who have been on this cottage. This situation involves a common cottage problem and we will show you some things that can be done about it.

Each session had a particular theme, e.g., applying for a job, resisting temptations by peers to engage in antisocial acts, taking a problem to a teacher or parole counselor, foregoing immediate gratifications in order to lay the groundwork for more significant gratifications in the future. In each situation, an emphasis was placed on the generality of the appropriate behaviors being modeled in order to emphasize their potential usefulness. An example of one of these situations is the job interview scene, in which roles are played by an interviewer and a job applicant. The dialogue emphasizes the kinds of questions an interviewer might ask and the various positive, coping responses an interviewee is expected to make. Also, such factors as proper appearance, mannerisms, honesty, and interest are stressed.

Job Interview Scene

Introduction: Having a job can be very important. It is a way that we can get money for things we want to buy. It is a way we can feel important because we are able to earn something for ourselves through our own efforts. For this same reason, a job can make us feel more independent. Getting a job may not always be easy. This is especially true of jobs that pay more money and of full-time jobs. A job may be important to guys like you who have been in an institution because it gives you a way of showing other people that you can be trusted, that you can do things on your own, that you are more than just a punk kid. However, because you've been in trouble, you may have more trouble than most people getting a job. In the scene today you'll have a chance to practice applying for a job and being interviewed by the man you want to work for. Being interviewed makes most people tense and anxious because interviewers often ask questions which are hard to answer. After each of you has been interviewed, we'll talk about the way it felt and about what to do about the special problems that parolees may face in getting jobs.

Scene Ia

A boy who is on parole from Cascadia is applying for a job at a small factory in his home town. He is 18 and has not finished high school but hopes to do so by going to school at night. Obviously, the boy has a record. This will come up during the interview. Pay careful attention to how he handles this problem. This is a two part scene; first, we'll act out the job interview, then a part about another way of convincing an employer that you want a job.

(Mr. Howell is seated at his desk when George knocks on the door.)

Howell: "Hello. Have a seat. I'm Mr. Howell, and your name?"

(Mr. Howell rises—shakes hands.)

George: "George Smith."

Howell: "Have a seat, George."

(Both sit down.)

"Oh yes, I have your application right here. There are a few questions I'd like to ask you. I see that you have had some jobs; tell me about them."

George: "They were just for the summer because I've been going to school. I've worked on some small construction jobs and in a food processing plant."

Howell: "Did you ever have any trouble at work, or ever get fired?"

George: "No trouble, except getting used to the work the first couple of weeks. I did quit one job—I didn't like it."

Howell: "I see that you have only finished half your senior year in high school. You don't intend to graduate?"

George: (showing some anxiety) "Yes, I do. I intend to go to night school while I'm working. It may take me a year or so, but I intend to get my diploma."

Howell: "How did you get a year behind?"

George: "I've been out of school for awhile because I've been in some trouble. Nothing really serious."

Howell: I'd like to know just what kind of trouble you've had, serious or not."

George: "Well, I was sent to Cascadia for six weeks but I'm out on parole now. I just got out a couple of weeks ago. One of the reasons I want a job is to help keep me out of trouble."

Howell: "What kind of trouble were you involved in?"

George: "A friend and I stole some car parts and parts off an engine. I guess we were pretty wild. I'm not running around like that any more though."

Howell: "You sound like you think you can stay out of trouble now. Why do you think so?"

George: "In those six weeks at Cascadia I thought about myself and my future a whole lot, and realized it was time to get serious about life and stop goofing off. I know I haven't been out very long yet, but my parole counselor is helping me with the problems that come up. I'm trying to stay away from the guys that I got into trouble with. I really think that if I could get a job and be more on my own it would help a lot."

Howell: "Yes, I think you're probably right—but, I'm afraid we don't have any openings right now. I'll put your application on file though and let you know if anything turns up. I have several other applications too, so don't be too optimistic."

George: "All right. Thank you."

(George stands and starts to leave as he says this line.)

Scene Ib

Introduction: It is now two weeks later. George has called back several times to see if an opening has occurred. He now stops by to check again.

(George knocks on Mr. Howell's door.)

Howell: "Come in."

George: (enters room while speaking) "I stopped by to see whether you had an opening yet."

Howell: "You certainly don't want me to forget you do you?"

George: "No sir, I don't. I really want a job, I think its the best thing for me to do now."

Howell: "You know, I believe you. I wasn't so sure at first. It's pretty easy for a guy who has been in trouble to say that he's going to change and then do nothing about it. But the way you've been coming here and checking with me so often, I think you're really serious about it."

George: "Yes, sir, I am. I started night school this week. I think I'll be able to get my diploma in a year. So, if I had a job now I'd be all set."

Howell: "Well, I've got some good news for you, George. I have an opening for a man in the warehouse and I think you can handle the job if you want it."

George: "Yes, very much. When do you want me to start?"

Howell: "Tomorrow morning at 7:30."

George: "O.K."

Howell: "I'll take you out there now and introduce you to Mr. Jones, who will be your supervisor."

Scene Ic

Introduction: Same as Scene Ib.

(George knocks on Mr. Howell's door.)

Howell: "Come in."

George: "I stopped by to see whether you had an opening yet."

(enters room while speaking)

Howell: "You sure are persistent. Have you tried other places?"

George: "Sure, I'm checking back on them too. Getting a good job isn't easy."

Howell: (uncomfortably) "Ah, well, look. We're not going to have a place for you here. I wouldn't want you to waste your time coming back again. We can't use you."

George: (rises to go) "Well ... (pause) ... O.K. Thanks for your trouble. Look, what's up? I know that your company is hiring other fellows like me right now."

Howell: "Er ... that's true. Uh, I'm afraid that we have a company policy not to hire anyone with a record."

George: "How come? That doesn't sound fair to me."

Howell: "Well, er, ahem ... that's just the company's policy. I'm sorry, but my hands are tied. There's nothing I can do about it."

George: "Well, I would have appreciated knowing that right away."

Howell: "I'm really sorry. I can see you're trying ... I hope you get a job."

George: "Well, do you know of a place that could use me? Since you're in personnel, maybe you've heard something."

Each subject played George's role. At the end of the session, these discussion points were emphasized:

1. Importance of presenting oneself well. Getting a job is "selling yourself" too. In both scenes the boy takes the initiative instead of waiting around passively for things to happen.

2. How to deal with the fact that you have a record. Here, the boy had to admit to having a record because of the time in school gap. If he had lied, the interviewer would have caught this and formed the impression of dishonesty. Discuss the possibility of cases when telling about a record is unnecessary. Situational factors are very important.

3. It is understandable to feel anxious when being interviewed, because getting the job is important.

4. Persistence is a trait employers like. In this case, it is an important reason why the kid got the job.

Each session was attended by six persons. Two models (advanced graduate students in clinical psychology, especially interested in the field of delinquency) and four boys between the ages of 15½ and 18 years. A session began by one of the models setting the stage. He defined the topic for the session and the scene which everyone present would role play. Following this introduction, the two models would act out the scene which had previously been carefully planned. For example, one model might play a parole counselor and the other might play the role of the delinquent parolee. One pair of subjects would then act out the same scene. Following this, soft drinks would be served, during which time a discussion of the various aspects and the strengths and weaknesses of the scene as acted out by the subjects would take place. After this, the other subjects would act out the same scene.

Our procedures were arrived at after a number of preliminary runs. They gave every indication of being interesting to the boys, who seemed to accept the modeling situations as they were presented to them: learning opportunities designed to enhance their ability to cope with situations that, for them, are problem areas.

We did our first pilot study in the winter of 1967. The general aims of this investigation were threefold: (a) to compare the relative effectiveness of a modeling approach and a more traditional role-playing approach as behavior-modification techniques with a suitable control (no treatment) group, (b) to assess the adequacy and efficiency of our dependent behavioral and attitudinal measures and rating scales which we had assembled, and (c) to assess the feasibility of the research design and procedures employed prior to initiation of a major experimental effort.

As I have mentioned, in one of our groups the subjects were exposed to the modeling sessions described above. Another group, the control group, received neither the modeling experience nor any other kind of special treatment. The role-playing group was a comparison group similar to the modeling group except that the same roles were only verbally described to the boys, who then spontaneously enacted them. That is, the subjects were not given the opportunity to act out the several scenes.

In the spring of 1967 we did an additional study which was similar to the first one except that in the spring the subjects were exposed to lengthier modeling sequences and more detailed group discussions than those employed in the winter procedure. No role playing was used in the spring study. The spring scenes were revised in a number of respects, and a greater emphasis was placed on the personal meaning of the group meetings to the subjects. Also, in the spring study, at the conclusion of the experimental sequence, the boys made up and acted out one scene in the group meeting.

In both studies, we looked at a number of dependent variables. Some of our measures were obtained prior to beginning the modeling and role-playing sequences. Some measures were obtained both before and after, and some measures were obtained only after the subjects had gone through the modeling and role-playing sequences. Our measures consisted of subjects' self-reports and data from the Cascadia staff. Two self-ratings were forms of the semantic differential and Wahler's Self-Description Inventory. The semantic differential consisted of concepts and words such as "me as I am," "me as I would like to be," "man," "work." These were rated on a 7-point scale along 11 bipolar dimensions. The Self-Description Inventory contained an assortment of positive and negative self-descriptive items, for example, "has a good sense of humor," "am often depressed or unhappy." These statements are evaluated in terms of the mean score of all favorable items endorsed versus the mean score of unfavorable items endorsed.

Cottage staff supplied two kinds of pre- and post-ratings. One was a Behavior Rating Scale which all staff filled out on each boy. The scale consisted of 25 items describing different types of behavior, for example, table manners, lying, self-control. Each item was checked on a 9-point scale from high to low. The second rating, the Weekly Behavior Summary, included seven categories of behavior, for example, peer relationships, staff relationships, and work detail performance. Ratings were made for each boy after his initial 10 days on the cottage, and again just prior to his discharge from Cascadia. The two main post measures were taken from Cascadia Review Board decisions. These were the diagnosis of the boy and the Review Board placement decisions, that is, where the boy was to be sent from Cascadia. A breakdown of diagnostic categories was made on the basis of neurotic versus character disorder and combinations of these categories. Placement ratings were assigned numerical scores on the basis of rank ordering of possible placements along the dimension of most to least favorable for boys of the type seen at Cascadia.

The following have been our major findings. There has been a consistent tendency for experimental boys to show less discrepancy between "me as I would like to be" and "me as I am now," than control subjects. One of the most suggestive findings is that boys who have received the modeling condition became more personally *dissatisfied* with themselves as their stay at Cascadia proceeded. Control subjects, on the other hand, became more *satisfied* with themselves as their stay in Cascadia proceeded. At this point the meaning of these results is not immediately obvious. But one strong possibility is that untreated delinquents in an institution are initially anxious because of the strangeness of being in the institutional environment for the first time. As they adapt and "rest up," their anxiety level goes down and they, therefore, become more self-satisfied. If this is true, it may be that the experimental procedures we have been employing have been successful in stirring up the treated boys at Cascadia. If so, this has important theoretical implications, since the process of observational learning may be much more complex than simply observing someone else making a response and then attempting to replicate that response. Ignored thus far in research on observational learning has been what might be called cognitive modeling or the cognitive aspect of the modeling process. Our results concerning self-satisfaction suggest that lessened defensiveness and greater willingness to admit to having problems and difficulties have characterized the responses of the experimental, but not the control, boys.

In general, the findings for our two pilot studies showed that boys who were members of our experimental groups showed more change in their behavior and attitudes than did matched control groups of boys who did not participate. The results were strongest and most positive in the case of the modeling groups, and second in order of potency was the role-playing condition. We obtained numerous kinds of ratings by cottage personnel of the behavior of our subjects. Overall, the experimental subjects were rated as showing more positive behavior change than control subjects. It should be noted that our groups had been matched for: (a) age, (b) intelligence level, and (c) severity and chronicity of delinquency. In addition, our data permit us to compare boys varying along the anxiety-sociopathy dimension. In view of our verbal learning research this dimension is of great interest to us. Preliminary analyses have suggested that boys who are characterized by high degrees of anxiety and neuroticism respond most favorably to observational opportunities. . . . Thus far, our studies of the behavior of juvenile delinquents seem consistent with the verbal learning findings.

One interesting difference between the winter and spring studies was that some of our results were much stronger for the winter study than for the spring one. This was true even though we felt at the time that most of our conditions were far superior in the spring study. In looking at our procedures we noted an important difference between the winter and spring studies. In the winter there were virtually no discussions following the modeling sessions, whereas discussion did follow the role-playing sessions. In the spring there were rather extensive discussion periods after the modeling sessions. One possibility which has occurred to us is that there may be something like a Zeigarnik effect at work; that is, when discussion follows either the modeling or the role-playing activity, subjects may achieve a degree of closure by virtue of the discussion. On the other hand, in the winter study no opportunity for closure was provided. It is possible that the winter study's seemingly "less smooth" procedure may, in fact, be better in that when questions are left unanswered adolescents tend to continue to come to grips with them after the experimental session is over.

We have been challenged and encouraged by the results of our pilot work and have just begun an experiment which will probably take 10 to 12 months to complete. It involves better defined conditions, larger *N*s, and more reliable dependent measures than we had for our pilot studies. Also, we have formulated procedures for following up the Cascadia boys a year after they leave that institution. These dependent measures will include a number of specific indices of vocational and educational adjustment. Will the various groups differ in the level of jobs which they got? How many of them will be repeat offenders? How many of them will finish high school?

Not surprisingly, some of the procedures which we are now employing are different from those of our pilot studies. There are two which I should briefly mention. One is that we are using a comparison group different from the role-playing group which I have described. This change grew out of a need to achieve more fully the original aim of the research. This was to develop a behavior-modification procedure which would be both simple and direct. Since psychotherapy is a frequent technique employed with delinquents, we decided to use, for comparison purposes, a procedure more similar to psychotherapy than was that of role playing. This procedure will consist of guided group discussion meetings. Subjects in guided discussion groups of our experiment will have the same number of sessions as the modeling groups will have. In addition, the content of each session will be similar. That is, while the modeling group will act out a job interview scene, the guided discussion groups will discuss the problems posed by and solutions to the problems of job interviews. What follows suggests the orientation given to boys in the guided discussion groups. They are the guidelines which the group leaders follow in introducing the guided discussion sessions to the boys.

First, let's all introduce ourselves, starting with me. I'm Mr. _____ and this is Mr. _____ (boys introduce themselves). We are working with small groups of boys here at Cascadia. During the times we meet together, we will be talking about common situations and problems that happen in your lives. The situations we'll work with are often particularly important for fellows like yourselves. We say this because just the fact that you're going through an institution will have important effects on your lives, and we want to work with you by discussing some of these effects. In other words, we want to work together with you in talking about problem situations. These are situations which we feel will be of importance to you in the future. They are things that probably all of you will run into from time to time, and we think you can benefit from talking and thinking about them.

The way we want to do this isn't by lecturing or advising you. Your talking about these situations is an important way to learn. Often we don't take time to think about things that get us into trouble, or about situations that make us feel bad. It's kind of disturbing to think about it in the first place, and it's also hard to pull out words to describe what's going on. In the group you will find that you have experiences in common and you can help each other think through what happens.

We think that groups working together can help each member of the group learn a lot about what makes him tick . . . just by talking frankly about the topic. The topics will be real situations that many young people have trouble with: controlling your anger, or being pressured into doing destructive things by friends. Sometimes we will talk about the situations you fellows have to cope with as persons who have been in an institution. There are situations such as your Review Board, or the experiences you have had with your probation officer and anticipate having with your parole counselor when you get out of here. Subjects like this are often not carefully talked about and we think that the time we spend together talking about them will be important in the future for most of you. We use four rules in these groups: (1) One person talks at a time; (2) everyone contributes to the discussion; (3) what goes on here won't be taken outside the group—it will be confidential and not used by staff; and (4) no ranking—constructive criticism and comments are good, but ranking doesn't help anyone.

There are seven of us here at Cascadia who are working in these small groups. We are not on the Cascadia staff. We are here because we are interested in working with fellows like yourselves and in helping you understand yourselves and your experiences better. We want to emphasize that we are not connected with the Cascadia staff. Since we are not on the staff, we do not have anything to do with the decisions made concerning you or where you will go after leaving here. We do not share any of our information with the regular staff. Everything this group does or talks about is kept strictly confidential and isn't available to or used by the staff in any way at all.

This group is one of several we have been working with on _____ cottage. Each group meets four times a week for about 40 minutes at a time. This same group will meet together each week during the time you are all here at Cascadia, but different ones of us will be with this group on different days. We will meet on _____, _____, _____, and _____. We will be talking about different situations on each day. This is how we will do it: First, we will describe the situation to you. Then we will turn the hour over to you except for the comments and questions we will add to the discussion from time to time. You can share with each other any experiences you have had, describe your feelings about what has happened, also question and make comments to each other. There is no certain way the discussion must go . . . it is pretty much up to what you think will be useful.

Also, each meeting will be tape-recorded. We use these tape-recordings for our own records of how each group proceeds. These tapes are identified by code numbers and no one's name actually appears on the tape. The tapes are confidential, too, and will be used only by us here. As we said, none of this information is used by the regular staff.

Before going on any further, we want to give you an example of what we're talking about. Mr. _____ will describe a situation here on your cottage, etc. . . .

The following are our guidelines for the guided discussion group, analogue of the Job Interview Scene. The guidelines are those employed by the group leaders.

Having a job can be very important. It is a way to get money for things we need, but it is also a way to earn something for ourselves through our own efforts and it makes us feel more independent. Getting a job isn't easy. Today we want to talk about some of the things involved in getting jobs. Also, since you fellows have been in trouble with the law, you may have some extra problems getting jobs that other young fellows wouldn't have. We can talk about that too. Let's start today by finding out what sorts of jobs you fellows have had (ask each person in the group to describe the kinds of jobs he has had in the past).

A very important part of getting a job is, of course, the job interview. There are lots of ways to handle a job interview, so let's talk about that for awhile.

The leader then asks the boys what sorts of interviews they have had, if any, and what kinds of questions were asked and how they handled these questions. He asks others to comment on each boy's discussion. He begins a discussion about what kinds of things are important in an interview, for example, how should one look, what does it mean when an interviewer says, "We'll keep your application and call you." He raises the question of applying for more than one job at a time. There is a discussion of how each boy deals with the question of his record, whether or not he admits it, and, if not, why.

Besides employing the guided group discussions, the other new element in our major experiment is the introduction of closed-circuit television as a means of increasing the numbers of exposures subjects will have to obser-vational opportunities. I mentioned earlier that our modeling sessions seemed to be successful in stirring up the boys. This suggested that, while the modeling sessions seemed to contribute to a desirable step forward for them, they needed more observational trials in order to strengthen their pro-social repertoires. Therefore, we are increasing the number of modeling sessions, and, in addition, we are televising them and playing them back to the boys. This will give them an opportunity, not only to observe others (models and peers), but also to observe themselves. Since the use of television is part of the experimental design, it will be used with half of the modeling and half of the guided discussion groups, which will enable us to assess its effectiveness as a behavior-modification technique. Another of our interests in video taping the modeling sessions is ultimately to carry out a study to determine the relative effectiveness of live modeling sessions and video-taped sessions.

There is one problem which we shall not study directly in our present experiment. We hope to study it in the future. That problem concerns the personal characteristics of the models. Our models are primarily middle class psychologists in training. They have some very positive characteristics: more than a little psychological *savoir faire*, and a deep interest in helping mixed-up people. We have seriously considered the possibility that the best models would be those who are more peerlike for delinquent boys. Within the institutional setting in which we now working the use of peer models administratively and practically is not possible. It is interesting, however, that the Cascadia staff itself has made an effort in the recent past to use former delinquents as cottage personnel. This was done on the assumption that "Cascadia graduates" who had righted themselves might more easily establish rapport with delinquent boys than cottage personnel with other characteristics. The outcome of this effort was quite negative, because people who had been in Cascadia and who had managed to overcome the tendency towards delinquency often harbored quite negative attitudes toward delinquent boys. This seems analogous to the oft-observed situation in which people who have grown up in quite poverty-stricken environments may become quite unsympathetic and often antagonistic to their poor brethren when they reach the level of the *nouveau riche*. We hope soon to enter the planning stage of a study, to be carried out in the community, that would systematically explore characteristics of models as variables in achieving behavior modification among delinquents.

To summarize briefly, we have come to two conclusions. First, observational opportunities seem to be potentially powerful behavior-modification influences, and, second, it is important to have a proper respect for the complexities of the process of observational learning. Modeling is a potentially valuable behavior-modification vehicle, but there is much empirical and theoretical ground to be broken in understanding, developing, and validating its various ramifications.

Chapter Six

Childhood Psychosis

Of the numerous perplexities in the psychiatric literature, there is no greater confusion and lack of agreement than in the area of childhood psychosis. Chapter Six will attempt to clarify this baffling area.

Historical Overview

More than 100 years ago, the noted British psychiatrist Maudsley wrote about "insanity of early life" and opened the topic of childhood psychosis to psychiatric study. In 1906, De Sanctis in Italy studied psychotic symptoms in mentally retarded children and was concerned about similarities and differences in the disorders of mental deficiency and dementia praecox. In 1908, soon after this pioneering investigation, an Austrian educator named Heller described a rare childhood disorder occurring in the third or fourth year of life following normal development. This affliction, known as Heller's disease, was characterized by increasing malaise, lack of interest in surroundings, loss of speech and, finally, complete regression in behavior.

Around 1911, Kraeplin's term "dementia praecox" (that is, early intellectual deterioration) was being superseded by Bleuler's term schizophrenia (split mind or personality). Clinicians and investigators were already having considerable trouble agreeing about diagnostic labels or causative (etiological) factors. Most of the theorizing and clinical study was devoted to adult psychotics, but similar problems were encountered by those attempting to understand severe psychopathology in children; some theorists emphasized constitutional factors (heredity, disease, brain damage, biochemical imbalances), and others viewed them as functional disorders (caused by life experiences).

Potter (1933) reported the first systematic study of schizophrenic children who showed retraction of interest in their environment and behavior change ranging from agitated excitement to catatonic stupor. Physical and neurological examinations revealed no evidence of constitutional factors in these children, and neither did their family backgrounds appear to be especially conducive to development of psychopathology.

Bradley (1941) wrote the first book devoted to childhood schizophrenia describing the following characteristics: seclusiveness, daydreaming, bizarre behavior, lack of personal interests, sensitivity to criticism, and physical inactivity. While Potter had mentioned the sudden onset of this type of disorder following seemingly normal development, Bradley reported that parents tended to note these abnormalities during the first two years of life. Another early worker in this field, Despert (1938), also reported that these symptomatic behaviors usually appeared with acute onset following normal development. However, Despert and Sherwin (1958) subsequently described three types of onset of schizophrenia: (1) insidious (slow building), (2) acute (previously normal), and (3) insidious with acute onset (precipitated by some specific event).

Another influential child psychiatrist during the past quarter century has been Bender (1947), who takes a very strong position favoring constitutional etiological explanations of childhood schizophrenia. She maintains that the developmental inadequacies evidenced in varied areas of functioning in these children are attributable to organic defects.

Mahler (1952) introduced the concept of "symbiotic child psychosis," emphasizing the pathological relationship between mother and child. From this viewpoint, the primary disorder is of a psychodynamic nature (interaction between parent and child) rather than attributable to organic malfunctioning. According to this theory, the child's ego does not become differentiated from the mother's. The mother's own psychopathology is believed to play an important role in preventing the child from acquiring independence.

Another theoretical position advanced some years ago by Rank (1949) introduced the concept of the "atypical child" and further emphasized the role of maternal psychopathology. According to this view, the major difficulty is "ego fragmentation" as a result of seriously disturbed relations between mother and child. This position is largely influenced by orthodox psychoanalytic theory.

Probably the most important contribution to this field in recent times was Kanner's (1943) description of the syndrome of "early infantile autism." Major characteristics found in the autistic children in Kanner's original studies were: inability to relate to people and situations, failure to use language appropriately, obsessive maintenance of "sameness" in the environment, and certain areas of exceptionally high cognitive potential. This disorder, which Kanner considered to be very rare, is believed to be present from birth. Kanner viewed infantile autism as a subcategory within the broader classification of childhood schizophrenia.

Differential Diagnosis

Diagnostic possibilities are not exhausted by the categories mentioned above. In addition to differentiating among childhood schizophrenia, infantile autism, symbiotic psychosis, and atypical development, there are additional closely related diagnostic categories such as mental deficiency and chronic brain syndrome. Thus, when clinicians are presented with a child who shows these gross behavioral abnormalities, they must decide whether the child is brain damaged, retarded, or psychotic.

Rather than attempting to differentiate among varieties of psychosis, many workers use the broad term "childhood psychosis" to encompass all types that have been described. On the other hand, some workers believe that the most pressing problem in this field is refining diagnostic categories and developing a more homogeneous group of subtypes. Rimland has strongly advocated differentiating between childhood schizophrenia and infantile autism and has published a diagnostic behavior checklist designed to provide scores for schizophrenia and for autism. As a result of parents' answers to questions on this inventory, the child receives an objective score revealing whether he is predominantly schizophrenic or autistic.

Rimland (1964) has discussed several criteria that differentiate between these two forms of childhood psychopathology. Following are some of the important features of infantile autism: (1) present from birth, (2) physically healthy child, (3) normal electroencephalograms (EEG), (4) stiff and unresponsive to adults, (5) aloneness, (6) perseveration of sameness, (7) unoriented, aloof, detached, (8) language disturbance, (9) no hallucinations or delusions, (10) good motor skill, (11) idiot-savant performance, (12) not conditionable, (13) first-born children, (14) normal siblings, (15) low family incidence of psychosis, (16) intact families (low divorce rate), and (17) bright, highly educated parents.

On the other hand, Rimland describes very different characteristics of schizophrenic children, including: (1) normal early development, (2) physically frail, sickly child, (3) abnormal EEG, (4) dependency on adults (tendency toward physical molding), (5) disoriented, confused, in conflict, (6) language development may be abnormal, (7) hallucinations and delusions, (8) poor motor skill, (9) no special abilities, (10) easily conditionable, (11) high family incidence of psychosis, and (12) unstable home background.

Goldfarb (1961) makes a further differentiation within the category of childhood schizophrenia, dichotomizing it into children with detectable organic impairment and those without known organic deficit. Detailed investigations revealed very different performance and behavior in these two subgroups of psychotic children, as well as differences in home backgrounds and responsiveness to psychiatric treatment.

Menolascino (1965) has been concerned with problems involved in differentiating among psychotic, brain-damaged, and mentally retarded children. He distinguishes the three disorders of (1) early infantile autism, (2) chronic brain syndrome with psychotic reactions, and (3) mental retardation with psychotic reactions. Sarason and Doris (1969) also discuss the many difficulties encountered in diagnosing infantile autism, especially in differentiating it from retardation; they refer to this issue as the "continuing controversy."

In view of these diagnostic ambiguities and disagreements, it is not surprising that accurate figures concerning the incidence of childhood psychosis are not easily obtained. Regardless of the specific diagnostic categories used, however, a reliable finding is that boys outnumber girls by a ratio of four to one. On the basis of an epidemiological study, Lotter (1966) reports that pathological autism was found in 4.5 per 10,000 children between the ages of 8 to 10 years. Based on studies in England, Hermelin and O'Conner (1970) reported a rate of 4 cases per 10,000 children. Working with clinic samples (that is, among children seen in psychiatric facilities), Kessler (1966) reports a finding of 2.7 percent psychotic children, and Bender (1955) found a surprisingly high incidence of childhood schizophrenia of 8 percent in a group of 7000 child patients seen over a 20-year period. Kanner (1958) reports a much lower incidence of infantile autism, finding only about 150 cases among 20,000 children (less than 1 percent) seen at the Johns Hopkins clinic over a 19-year period.

In general, then, the incidence in the general population of children is probably not very high. But as Sarason and Gladwin (1958) have emphasized, the study of childhood psychosis and attempts to understand further the syndrome known as infantile autism have theoretical and practical implications well beyond what might be expected from working with such relatively small numbers of cases. As psychiatrists and behavioral scientists unravel the baffling problems pertaining to causes, prevention, and effective treatment of these severely disturbed children, they are likely to gain knowledge that will make major contributions to increased understanding of normal child behavior and development.

Etiology

Closely related to problems of diagnosis are differing views on causes of psychotic disorders in childhood. On the one hand, some theorists believe that psychogenic factors are primary, while other equally qualified experts maintain that the causative factors are biogenic. According to the psychodynamic position, the psychotic child has undergone traumatic experiences in relations with the mother during the earliest stages of life; consequently, he turns away from the world, thus evidencing the strange behaviors indicative of autism. From this perspective, childhood psychosis results from pathological interpersonal relations, usually originating in the oral stage of psychosexual development and worsening throughout the later developmental stages.

Most theorists who assume this position favoring sociopsychological causation are psychoanalytically oriented. They tend to see the mother's personality as playing a crucial role in psychologically damaging the child. Often the mother is described as cold, detached, aloof, and rejecting. In fact, the literature contains descriptions of "refrigerator mothers" who have no warmth or love to give to the child. Another unflattering term applied to these mothers is "schizophrenogenic," suggesting quite emphatically that the mother's personality traits, attitudes, and child-rearing behaviors cause the child to become psychotic. Kanner has remarked about the intellectual, compulsive, career-oriented parents seen so frequently in his work with autistic children. And Bettelheim (1967) is an outstanding example of one who adheres to the psychodynamic interpretation of infantile autism.

Probably the most influential proponent of the biogenic viewpoint is Rimland (1964), who maintains that autistic children suffer from neurological deficits that are present from birth. He has marshalled a vast amount of supporting data for this position and presents a convincing case against the psychogenic position. The evidence for his theory of neurobiological causation, however, is still somewhat speculative. Rimland hypothesizes that autistic children may suffer from impairment of the reticular formation in the brain, which makes it difficult for them to connect incoming sensory information with memories from past experience. That is, sensory input from the environment does not become associated with previously learned material that normally would be stored in the child's brain; much of the seemingly bizarre behavior of autistic children can be understood in terms of this neurological malfunction.

According to Rimland, this physical defect occurs during the process of childbirth and is in no way attributable to psychological characteristics in the parents. He has gone to great lengths to lessen the feelings of guilt and inadequacy that parents of psychotic children often show. From this perspective, the parents' personalities are not implicated any more than if they had conceived a mongoloid child, cerebral palsied child, or some other form of physically damaged offspring. Rimland agrees that the parents of autistic children tend to be highly intelligent, well-educated, and hard-working, but he interprets this in a positive light, emphasizing their competence at work and their ability to raise other normal children at home.

Goldfarb (1961) found a wide range of personalities among the parents of schizophrenic children he has studied. As mentioned earlier, he differentiated two subgroups, one with organic impairment and the other physically normal. Findings from the parents of these psychotic children revealed greater psychopathology in parents of the non-organic children, and relatively normal psychological adjustment in parents of the children with known organic deficits. These findings suggest two different etiologies, with one subtype more likely resulting from negative psychological experiences and the other subtype showing psychotic behaviors caused mainly by neurobiological factors.

Based on years of careful study in this area, Rutter (1968) believes that language and perceptual abnormalities lead to the autistic behaviors. He maintains that cognitive deficits, probably with a neurological basis, make it difficult for the child to function normally and cause the behaviors symptomatic of autism. According to this view, the social withdrawal and tendency toward isolation result from the child's inability to comprehend spoken language. Other behavioral abnormalities in the autistic syndrome are also believed attributable to the confusion resulting from the child's inability to understand fully sounds and other perceptual stimuli from the environment.

Hermelin and O'Conner (1970) also believe that the basis of autistic disorder is a cognitive defect. According to these theorists, sensory aspects of the nervous system function adequately, but the children suffer from an expressive deficit. In other words, the sensory input is normal but the encoding and expressive aspects are defective. Based on their experiments, Hermelin and O'Conner report that autistic children have good immediate memory, but are not influenced by meaning. They hear properly, but do not understand the meaning, and therefore tend to withdraw and act strangely. Often the parents are unable to handle the seemingly bizarre behavior, and the child withdraws even more.

DesLaurier and Carlson (1969) use a neurological model to explain autism. They envision two arousal systems in the central nervous system, one associated with the reticular activating system and primarily concerned with attention, and the other associated with the limbic-mid-brain system and concerned with reward. It has been hypothesized that these two arousal systems work in an integrated way to produce learning and memory. When the organism is exposed to a stimulus, the first system is activated and energizes responses. After the responses are made, system two is activated, inhibiting system one and enabling connections between responses and rewards to be consolidated. Basic neurological research conducted with laboratory animals has provided evidence supporting this theoretical account.

At the human level, DesLaurier and Carlson propose that in autistic children, system one is in a continual state of ascendancy over system two, thus the child is unable to make associations between responses and rewards and, consequently, is unable to learn. At this point, this explanation is largely hypothetical, and it will require much further research with humans to provide the needed empirical confirmation. However, DesLaurier and Carlson (1969) are able to use this neurological theory to account for several conspicuous characteristics of autistic behavior.

There are other organic theories of childhood psychosis but, as of now, none have been either proved or disproved. In this regard, Kugelmass (1970) presents views similar to Rutter's, referring to disorganization of the central nervous system in autistic children. According to Kugelmass, the child cannot transfer auditory and visual patterns into meaningful experiences. He reports that brain-damaged children behave in a fashion similar to those suffering from infantile autism. As mentioned above, Bender also believes that childhood schizophrenia results from disordered integration in the central nervous system. She describes a "maturational lag" (Bender, 1961) that is evidenced throughout varied facets of the physical and neurological development of schizophrenic children. From this viewpoint, the proper treatment of these disorders is medical, using procedures such as electric shock therapy (Bender, 1955), heavy dosages of medication (Fish, 1960), or even surgical operations on the brain (Freeman & Watts, 1947).

In keeping with an organic emphasis, according to Bender (1947), the parents' emotional problems do not "cause" the child's psychotic development but rather they result from having to cope with the psychotic child. In further defense of parents, Schopler and Loftin (1969) presented results from psychological studies showing that parents of psychotic children do not have thought disorders nor are they emotionally maladjusted. These experiments reveal that it is only in regard to the psychotic child that the parents show any difficulty in thinking unemotionally. Thus, the parents are not pathological in thought or behavior but are troubled by the psychotic child in the family.

So concerned is Schopler about what he considers to be unfair blaming of parents that he presented a paper before the American Psychological Association, "Parents of Psychotic Children as Scapegoats." In this presentation, he stated:

> Over the past several decades the most prevalent views of autism and childhood psychosis have considered parents to be the primary cause of the child's disturbance. Psychoanalytic theory has been used to identify interpersonal trauma, rejecting mothers, and destructive parental motives as producing the child's emotional withdrawal and ego disorganization. During the last few years, however, there has been growing evidence that autistic and psychotic children suffer from neurological, biochemical, or other organic impairments which predispose them to psychotic development. This new knowledge suggests that regardless of what other adjustment problems they may have, parents also react with emotional and intellectual confusion to their problem child (Schopler, 1969).

Schopler considers various reasons why parents have been regarded as primary agents in their child's psychosis; he attempts to understand these reasons in terms of the age-old mechanisms of scapegoating. He points out ways in which members of the mental health professions can take out their own personal hostilities and biases on the parents of severely disturbed children. He also indicates how ambiguity and lack of knowledge in this field can serve to frustrate and threaten the security of professionals, thus encouraging them to project their aggression onto others. Moreover, the parents' confusion, perplexity, and guilt feelings make them ready victims for scapegoating. In the attempt to remedy this unhealthy situation, Schopler enumerates some methods for combating scapegoating. Among them is the suggested use of parents as therapists in treatment of their own psychotic children.

Treatment and Prognosis

Therapeutic approaches to treatment of childhood psychosis can be classified as psychodynamic therapy, behavior therapy, or developmental therapy. Psychodynamic therapies have used varying approaches, but all are aimed at correcting the traumatic emotional experiences that are believed to underlie the child's psychotic adjustment. Some dynamically oriented therapists believe it is necessary to enter into and fully accept the child's world in order to reduce gradually the child's fear of personal contact (see Despert, 1947; Rank, 1955). Some therapists advocate that the therapist be very active and directive in his manner of entering the child's world, while others recommend a more cautious approach. Some stress the importance of the therapist having bodily contact with the child (Eickhoff, 1952), and Mahler (1952) recommends that the therapist assist the symbiotic child to face reality but do so at an unhurried pace.

In general, the intent of psychotherapy is to remove the autistic barrier that the child has erected against what, according to psychodynamic theory, he perceives as a hostile and terrifying world. To accomplish this goal, Bettelheim (1967) and some other therapists believe that it is essential to remove the autistic child from his home environment. Most of the cases described by Bettelheim—and the impressive therapeutic results he has reported—have come from children undergoing residential treatment. In these institutional settings, it is usually felt that the parents have had a damaging effect on the child and, therefore, it is beneficial to keep them apart until psychodynamic changes have occurred in parents and child. Most psychodynamic approaches try to have the parents seen for psychotherapy or psychiatric casework as well as having the child treated by these techniques. Thus, this approach usually attempts to involve the parents as much as possible in the therapy but often while also keeping the parents and child apart.

Schopler and Reichler (1971) advocate a very different approach. In fact, they maintain that psychodynamic theory and psychoanalytically oriented therapy are actually harmful and detrimental to both the children and their parents. This sentiment has been voiced even more strongly by Rimland (1964), who on occasion has used the term "pernicious" in referring to the effect that psychoanalytic thinking has had on these unfortunate families. As a more effective treatment technique, Schopler and Reichler (1971) recommend developmental therapy, with parents functioning as primary developmental agents for their own psychotic children.

Another form of therapy that has had a marked impact on this field in recent years is behavior therapy. (This technique is described and documented in Chapter Ten, on behavior therapy.) Leff (1968) has published a comprehensive review indicating the considerable utility and success enjoyed by this approach to modifying the behavior of psychotic children. Also, as we will see in Chapter Ten, Ney, Palvesky, and Markely (1971) have recently shown behavior therapy to be more effective than play therapy in treating a group of schizophrenic children.

A major publication pertinent to treatment and prognosis is the Rutter, Greenfield, and Lockyer (1967) five- to fifteen-year follow-up study of psychotic children. In general, these children, who were adolescents or young adults at the time of the follow-up assessment, were not faring very well. Of 63 former child patients, 10 had developed fits in adolescence, most continued to show developmental abnormalities, and few were gainfully employed. On the basis of this research and review of several other follow-up studies, Rutter (1966) concluded that crucial prognostic factors are adequacy of speech and level of intellectual functioning. If the child does not show meaningful speech by age 5 and/or if his IQ on a standard intelligence test is not above 50, the prognosis is particularly poor. Very few children with these kinds of deficits at a young age are able to ever function anywhere near a normal level in later years.

Thus, the prognosis is quite discouraging regardless of the particular therapeutic approach applied with these severely disturbed youngsters. Davids (1972) and others have suggested that the best predictors of therapeutic outcomes are the kinds of behaviors the child shows before treatment. In other words, there appears to be little relationship between specific aspects of the therapy process and the outcome found at the follow-up assessment. Those psychotic children who were able to speak and to play appropriately at the time of initiating treatment are usually found years later to be the ones who have evidenced some degree of long-range successful outcome.

A unique and particularly revealing follow-up study was recently published by Kanner (1971), reporting on the adult status of the children who formed the basis for his original study in 1943. This paper was published in a newly founded scientific journal devoted exclusively to theory and research concerned with infantile autism and childhood schizophrenia. Of the original group of eleven autistic children, only two were found to be functioning as normal adults, and the remainder had continued to live as non-contributing members of society or as inmates of institutions for the retarded or the mentally ill. In describing the dismal outcomes found in those who had been institutionalized Kanner stated, "One cannot help but gain the impression that state hospital admission was tantamount to a life sentence, ... a total retreat to near-nothingness." On the other hand, the few cases who had made an adequate adjustment in later life were those who had been placed with foster parents, working as tenant farmers, in their early years.

The Issues

Kanner is obviously disappointed with the amount of progress that has been made in this area, stating, "There has been a hodge-podge of theories, hypotheses, and speculations, and there have been many valiant and well-motivated attempts at alleviation awaiting eventual evaluation." He hopes that the years ahead will witness considerable advances, citing as positive factors the tendency toward interdisciplinary collaboration, biochemical explorations, genetic investigations, and including parents in therapeutic efforts. On this latter point, Kanner urges that parents be viewed " ... not as etiological culprits, nor merely as recipients of drug prescriptions and of thou-shalt and thou-shalt-not rules, but as actively contributing co-therapists."

In the first paper presented in this chapter, I discuss Bruno Bettelheim's psychodynamic view of infantile autism, in which parents are believed to play a fundamental role in causing this childhood disorder. In the second paper, Bernard Rimland takes a very different position, maintaining that infantile autism results from biological malfunctioning. In the last paper, Eric Schopler and Robert J. Reichler describe a treatment program in which parents participate actively as co-therapists for their own psychotic children. From the numerous unresolved issues mentioned in this introduction and in these papers, it should be abundantly evident that 30 years after Kanner's original study we still have a tremendously long way to go before attaining any significant degree of understanding and mastery of these problems.

References

Bender, L. Childhood schizophrenia: Clinical study of 100 schizophrenic children. *American Journal of Orthopsychiatry*, 1947, **17**, 40–56.

Bender, L. The development of a schizophrenic child treated with electric convulsions at three years of age. In G. Caplan (Ed.), *Emotional problems of early childhood*. New York: Basic Books, 1955.

Bender, L. Twenty years of clinical research in schizophrenic children with special reference to those under six years of age. In G. Caplan (Ed.), *Emotional problems of early childhood*. New York: Basic Books, 1955.

Bender, L. The brain and child behavior. *Archives of Child Psychiatry*, 1961, **4**, 531–548.

Bettelheim, B. *The empty fortress*. New York: The Free Press, 1967.

Bradley, C. *Schizophrenia in childhood*. New York: Macmillan, 1941.

Davids, A. *Abnormal children and youth: Therapy and research*. New York: Wiley, 1972.

DesLaurier, A., & Carlson, C. *Your child is asleep*. Homewood, Ill.: Dorsey Press, 1969.

Despert, J. L. Schizophrenia in children. *Psychiatric Quarterly*, 1938, **12**, 366–371.

Despert, J. L. Psychotherapy in child schizophrenia. *American Journal of Psychiatry*, 1947, **104**, 36–43.

Despert, J. L., & Sherwin, A. C. Further examination of diagnostic criteria in schizophrenic illness and psychoses in infancy and early childhood. *American Journal of Psychiatry*, 1958, **114**, 784–790.

Eickhoff, I. F. W. The etiology of schizophrenia in childhood. *Journal of Mental Science*, 1952, **98**, 229–243.

Fish, B. Drug therapy in child psychiatry. *Comprehensive Psychiatry*, 1960, **1**, 55–61, 212–227.

Freeman, W. J., & Watts, J. W. Schizophrenia in childhood: Its modification by prefrontal lobotomy. *Digest of Neurology and Psychiatry*, 1947, **15**, 202–219.

Goldfarb, W. *Childhood schizophrenia*. Cambridge, Mass.: Harvard University Press, 1961.

Hermelin, B., & O'Conner, N. *Psychological experiments with autistic children*. Oxford, England: Pergamon Press, 1970.

Kanner, L. Autistic disturbances of affective contact. *Nervous Child*, 1943, **2**, 217–250.

Kanner, L. The specificity of early infantile autism. *Zeitschrift für Kinderpsychiatrie*, 1958, **25**, 108–113.

Kanner, L. Follow-up study of eleven autistic children originally reported in 1943. *Journal of Autism and Childhood Schizophrenia*, 1971, **1**, 119–145.

Kessler, J. W. *Psychopathology of childhood*. Englewood Cliffs, N.J.: Prentice-Hall, 1966.

Kugelmass, I. N. *The autistic child*. Springfield, Ill.: Charles C Thomas, 1970.

Leff, R. Behavior modification and the psychoses of childhood. *Psychological Bulletin*, 1968, **69**, 396–409.

Lotter, V. Epidemiology of autistic conditions in young children: I. Prevalence. *Social Psychiatry*, 1966, **1**, 124–137.

Mahler, M. S. On childhood psychoses and schizophrenia: Autistic and symbiotic psychoses. In *The Psychoanalytic Study of the Child*. Vol. 7. New York: International Universities Press, 1952.

Menolascino, F. J. Autistic reactions in early childhood: Differential diagnostic considerations. *Journal of Child Psychology and Psychiatry*, 1965, **6**, 203–218.

Ney, P. G., Palvesky, A. E., & Markely, J. Relative effectiveness of operant conditioning and play therapy in childhood schizophrenia. *Journal of Autism and Childhood Schizophrenia*, 1971, **1**, 337–349.

Potter, H. W. Schizophrenia in children. *American Journal of Psychiatry,* 1933, **89,** 1253–1269.

Rank, B. Adaptation of the psychoanalytic technique for the treatment of young children with atypical development. *American Journal of Orthopsychiatry,* 1949, **19,** 130–139.

Rank, B. Intensive study and treatment of preschool children who show marked personality deviations, or "atypical development," and their parents. In G. Caplan (Ed.), *Emotional problems of early childhood.* New York: Basic Books, 1955.

Rimland, B. *Infantile autism.* New York: Appleton-Century-Crofts, 1964.

Rutter, M. Prognosis: Psychotic children in adolescence and early life. In J. K. Wing (Ed.), *Early childhood autism: Clinical, educational, and social aspects.* London: Pergamon Press, 1966.

Rutter, M. Concepts of autism: A review of research. *Journal of Child Psychology and Psychiatry,* 1968, **9,** 1–25.

Rutter, M., Greenfield, D., & Lockyer, L. A five- to fifteen-year follow-up study of infantile psychosis. *British Journal of Psychiatry,* 1967, **113,** 1169–1200.

Sarason, S. B., & Doris, J. *Psychological problems in mental deficiency.* New York: Harper & Row, 1969.

Sarason, S. B., & Gladwin, T. Psychological and cultural problems in mental subnormals: A review of research. *Genetic Psychology Monographs,* 1958, **57,** 3–290.

Schopler, E. Parents of psychotic children as scapegoats. Presented at meeting of the American Psychological Association, Washington, D. C., September 1969.

Schopler, E., & Loftin, J. Thought disorders in parents of psychotic children. *Archives of General Psychiatry,* 1969, **20,** 174–181.

Schopler, E., & Reichler, R. J. Parents as co-therapists in the treatment of psychotic children. *Journal of Autism and Child Schizophrenia,* 1971, **1,** 87–102.

15. On Bettelheim's View of Infantile Autism

Anthony Davids

One of the most influential figures in the field of childhood psychosis over the past several years has been Bruno Bettelheim. This psychologist and educator is director of the Orthogenic School in Chicago. In this residential treatment setting, he conducts intensive psychotherapy with psychotic children. His publications have been numerous and include key reference works on residential treatment of severely disturbed children (Bettelheim, 1955, 1967).

Most of his views on infantile autism have been presented in *The Empty Fortress* (1967) and in an interview conducted by Hall (1972). Material presented in these two sources serves as the basis for this paper.

Essentially, Bettelheim maintains that infantile autism has a psychological origin and is caused mainly by negative interactions between mother and child during early stages of the child's life. He believes that during the first few years there are critical periods in development in which various experiences have particularly marked effects on the growing organism. During these developmental stages, according to Bettelheim, unhappy experiences and hostile interactions with the mother cause the child to withdraw from the world around him. That is, the child in response to these mother-child relations develops a psychotic withdrawal reaction to his social environment. Bettelheim has described a case known as "Joey, A 'Mechanical Boy,' " which vividly demonstrates how psychotic children are prone to become preoccupied with mechanical objects and to avoid interactions with human beings.

In the interview with Hall, in response to the question, "Exactly how does the autistic child differ from the schizophrenic child?" Bettelheim replied "Autism is only an extreme form of childhood schizophrenia. While the schizophrenic child withdraws from the world, the autistic child fails ever to enter it." According to Bettelheim, schizophrenic children are convinced that they are threatened with total destruction, and thus they are afraid to enter into human interactions. In this connection, Bettelheim states that "Both the schizophrenic child and the concentration camp prisoner live in an extreme situation, a condition without hope."

Bettelheim feels that through intensive psychological treatment, schizophrenic children can be cured of their severe psychopathology. In his conversation with Hall, Bettelheim described a boy who came to him as a clear case of childhood schizophrenia, who years later became a successful college student and eventually a professor at a major university. Thus, Bettelheim feels that schizophrenia is curable, but only through intensive psychotherapy with kind, accepting, understanding adults who are able to provide a setting in which the child's entire psychosocial development can be restructured.

In describing the failures reported by the other clinicians and investigations in this field, Bettelheim feels that they do not work sufficiently long with their children. He describes the work by the psychiatrist Lauretta Bender, who treats schizophrenic children at the Bellevue Hospital in New York, and feels that her relatively brief, organically oriented approaches to treatment are bound to be ineffective. According to Bettelheim, it takes two or more years before psychotic children start to move out of their psychosis. If they are sent back to the same environment, there is no chance they will ever recover. In discussing forms of physical therapy practiced by some psychiatrists, Bettelheim states, "I have never seen shock treatment given before puberty do anything but damage." Neither has he seen any beneficial effects of drugs despite others' claims of their effectiveness with psychotic children. Bettelheim feels that if you administer drugs to these children they can probably be managed more easily at home, but that this is vastly different from trying to effect any lasting cures. In this regard, Bettelheim stated in his interview, "I have never seen a case subjected to prolonged drug treatment that became a full human being. If someone ever finds a drug that will cure schizophrenia, I will be delighted. Until that time, I wish they'd go back into their labs and work quietly."

When asked by Hall how many of the "hopeless" children he treated had been "cured," Bettelheim replied that with those who were allowed to remain at his treatment center for long periods, his success rate had been 85 percent. Note that this degree of success has been reported by *no other workers* who have devoted their energies to the treatment of psychotic children. In fact, many treatment centers have reported dismal rates of improvement, and these findings of failure with approaches like conventional psychotherapy have generated much of the interest and enthusiasm about other approaches, such as physical treatments and behavioral therapy.

Let us now turn from the Bettelheim interview to some of the important views presented in Bettelheim's book, *The Empty Fortress* (1967). One chapter, on the etiology and treatment of childhood autism, has provided most of the material discussed here.

According to Bettelheim, while Kanner (1943) in the beginning implied that infantile autism had an innate organic basis, he also stressed the peculiar nature of the parents of these children. Thus, while hereditary factors were implicated in Kanner's original writings on this topic, these papers also suggested the possibility that the parents were different from ordinary parents and might well play an important role in their children's psychopathology. Bettelheim cites a symposium in which Eisenberg and Kanner (1956) referred to "the emotional refrigeration" produced by the cold, intellectual, rejecting parents of autistic children. Bettelheim, however, feels the implication that parents can have a pathological effect on these children does not fit with the notion that autistic children are unresponsive to humans.

In other words, Bettelheim feels that these children are very responsive to emotional and psychological factors in the parents and that their symptomology is a result of withdrawing from these unhappy social interactions.

In discussing the origins of autism, Bettelheim reviews evidence presented by proponents of biogenic causation and finds considerable fault with their interpretations and conclusions. Bettelheim cannot accept the notion that autistic children are different from the beginning of their existence. In this regard he states, "Despite the most careful scanning of the literature and study of the many cases that have come to our attention at the Orthogenic School, we found no tangible evidence that autism was recognized at birth or right afterwards. . . . Autism has essentially to do with everything that happens from birth on. . . . It will tend to become most apparent during the second year of life when more complicated contact with the world would normally take place [1967, pp. 392–393]."

Bettelheim also reviews evidence from animal studies and from studies of infants reared in institutions and other deprived backgrounds showing the seriously damaging effects that traumatic experiences during early stages of life can have on the organism's development and later functioning. He feels that autistic children may have had a heightened sensitivity and responsiveness to stimuli from their environment during their earliest periods of development and thus react even more strongly to traumatic experiences. After reviewing these studies, Bettelheim states that stories about autistic children being unresponsive from birth do not necessarily suggest an innate disturbance. Rather, it may be a very early negative reaction to the mother triggered during the first weeks of life. In concluding his views on the origins of autism, Bettelheim states " . . . there is reason to question the inborn nature of autism until such time as it is actually observed in newborn infants before mothering can have made a difference; or until such time as organicity is established not on the basis of speculation but of objective neurological findings or other incontrovertible evidence." Bettelheim states that if infantile autism should ever become curable through pharmacology or any other organic treatment of the central nervous system, he would cease his efforts to cure it on a psychological basis, but not before.

With these strong feelings in regard to the psychological etiology of infantile autism, Bettelheim quite naturally advocates a psychoanalytically oriented approach to understanding and treatment of these seriously disturbed children. In discussing treatability, Bettelheim states that wherever infantile autism is viewed as an inborn impairment, the resultant attitude toward treatment will be defeatist. However, among those who trace the causes of autism to environmental influence, outlooks will be more optimistic because of the belief that what environment has caused, environment may also be able to correct. He feels that the pessimism shown by many workers in this field is unwarranted and ascribes this to the fact that most treatment efforts have not been sufficiently intensive nor sustained for a long enough period. To Bettelheim's way of thinking, adequate therapy with psychotic children is bound to require a very long period, usually in the confines of a residential treatment center. He discusses a follow-up study conducted by Eisenberg (1956) in which a "fair" or "good" outcome was found in only 30 percent of the group of 63 children. Since, however, most of these autistic children were seen on an outpatient basis once or twice a week, and usually for a period not exceeding two years, Bettelheim feels that the treatment was inadequate to provide a fair test of the treatability of psychotic children.

According to Bettelheim, Kanner has vacillated in his opinions about the effectiveness of psychotherapy. Kanner has occasionally reported that psychotherapy seems to be of little avail in effecting cures with psychotic children; at other times he has mentioned certain successes in treating psychotic children psychotherapeutically. Rimland, however, shares none of these doubts, having stated categorically that "no form of psychiatric treatment has been known to alter the course of autism [Bettelheim, 1967, p. 407]." Bettelheim strongly disagrees with Rimland, citing some of his own successful cases as supporting evidence. He seems convinced that therapeutic success can be obtained with these children, especially if they are treated at a relatively young age, are removed from their home environment, and the mother is treated separately.

On this issue of treating the mother and child separately, Bettelheim is quite adamant. He maintains that much of the child's difficulty is attributable to disturbed interpersonal relations with the mother; therefore, to expect the mother to participate actively in his therapy is a definitely misplaced emphasis. In this regard, Bettelheim states, "And as if to crown the irony, some treatment methods rely on efforts to understand and help the schizophrenic child through the very person who (it is assumed) kept him from developing normally in the first place—his mother."

Bettelheim takes issue with the approach advocated by Mahler (1952), who has emphasized the symbiotic nature of childhood psychosis. Mahler sees the relationship as being of paramount importance and, as a major tool of treatment, attempts to reconstruct the mother-child relationship by treating them simultaneously. Bettelheim feels this is very wrong, stating "Just because it is so extraordinarily important for the infant's initial well-being and later healthy development to have a good mother, it is erroneously assumed that any mother-child relationship is so valuable that it must be salvaged, even when it is damaging to the child." Bettelheim further states that if we listen to what those schizophrenic children who can talk tell us, we will find out the kind of treatment they truly need and will discover that it is only through study and treatment of the child, not his mother, that he can be helped.

While strongly advocating psychoanalytically oriented treatment of psychotic children in residential treatment, Bettelheim is very critical of attempts to treat infantile autism through operant conditioning. In discussing this form of behavior therapy, which attempts to modify behavior through the application of positive and negative reinforcements, Bettelheim maintains that "autistic children are being reduced to the level of Pavlovian dogs."

In further discussing the issue of conditioning disturbed children, Bettelheim agrees that this approach can temporarily break down a child's defenses against facing the frustrations of reality and thus stir him into action, but that these behaviors are strictly conditioned responses in keeping with the experimenter's desires. Even in the area of speech training with mute autistic children, Bettelheim feels that the only responses conditioned are imitative and represent non-meaningful use of language. He emphasizes further that speech, in the sense of human communication, cannot be forced out of people but can be acquired only through satisfying personal relationships. Forcing children into echolalia by shouting, bribing, or spanking them leads only to greater dehumanization. Bettelheim feels that operant conditioning is meant to achieve certain results with autistic children, but without concern for the permanent injury that may also result from application of these techniques. He states that these unfortunate children are treated as objects and are forced to face a painful reality regardless of the consequences to them.

Bettelheim discusses other forms of treatment of mental patients that he finds particularly abhorrent, such as the use of shock treatments and application of physical punishments. He feels there are many reasons for the application of these treatments. One is that they produce results by making patients fearful and stripping them of whatever humanity they might have had. Another is that these aggressive manipulations serve to satisfy the desire to punish recalcitrant patients. Bettelheim likens operant conditioning to the use of lobotomy—a neurosurgical operation destroying parts of the brain. He feels that both operant conditioning and lobotomy serve to change a functional disorder that could have been cured into an organic disorder for which there is no adequate treatment. Bettelheim obviously feels that it would be much better to leave autistic children free to live in whatever way they choose rather than training them to live what he calls a "conditioned response existence" merely because it makes things more convenient for those who are responsible for their care.

In summarizing his views on psychogenic versus biogenic causation of infantile autism, Bettelheim states that none of those who propose a neurological or biological theory of causation have shown significant improvement in children treated by methods derived from their theories. However, he adds that the majority of clearly autistic children who were treated at the Orthogenic School for several years were eventually returned to society. Thus, it is obvious that Bettelheim disagrees with many of the other views in this area and is quite optimistic about the therapeutic potential in autistic children. On the basis of his years of clinical experience, he feels confident that given sufficient time and with the child removed from the mother's negative influence, he can effect positive changes to an extent that will in many cases later enable the child to live as a member of ordinary society.

In considering the parental background in these cases, Bettelheim reports that his data do not confirm some of the reports in the literature. Neither do they confirm previous reports on the sex ratio and birth order of autistic children. While Rimland (1964) has summarized a good bit of evidence designed to indicate that autistic children tend to come from highly intelligent parents, Bettelheim does not believe that this is in fact true. His review of the literature and findings from many cases he has studied over the years lead him to believe that high intelligence is not a usual characteristic in parents of autistic children. In this regard, Bettelheim states that findings from the Orthogenic School fail to support the assertions of Kanner, Rimland, and others regarding the parents' superior intelligence. In attempting to account for the discrepancies between his data and those of Kanner and others, Bettelheim mentions possible differences among groups of the population who seek out and have access to psychiatric treatment. He maintains, as have other sociologically oriented writers, that there is overwhelming evidence that well-educated middle and upper classes seek psychiatric service, while the uneducated lower classes do not. It has also been pointed out that autistic children from lower classes in past years may well have been relegated to institutions for the retarded, while comparable children from better educated upper-class parents were brought to the attention of psychiatrists and were treated in psychiatric institutions. These factors could serve to bias the findings, leading erroneously to the conclusion that parents of autistic children tend to be highly intelligent.

Bender is convinced that autism results from an inborn neurological impairment, but she also feels that there is no relationship to superior parental intellect. According to Bender (1959), who has worked with the unselective services of large cities and state public facilities, "as many autistic children come from a background of defective or mediocre intellectual attainment, with all kinds of family, social, and personality constellations, as come from families of cold and over-controlled intellectuals described by Kanner." Thus, as Bettelheim points out, while Bender and Rimland are both proponents of the organic etiology of autism, they differ quite markedly in their opinions about the intellect of parents of autistic children.

Another issue on which Bettelheim disagrees with statements made by Kanner and Rimland is the sex ratio among autistic children. It has been reported that the ratio is about four boys to every girl, with first-born males predominating. In the original studies by Eisenberg and Kanner (1956), in a sample of 100 cases there were 80 males and 20 females. However, Bettelheim states that his findings do not show the same degree of dominance of male first-borns as has been reported by others. Bettelheim's sample reveals a dominance of boys over girls and of first-born over later-born children, but to a much lesser degree than that suggested by reports in the published literature.

On one point, however, Bettelheim's findings agree with those described previously by Kanner and Rimland. They have mentioned the large percentage of Jewish children among reported cases of infantile autism, and Bettelheim found that 21 of the 46 children he had studied intensively had one or two Jewish parents. However, Bettelheim points out that this may be again attributable to the kinds of parents who are able to send their chilren to the Orthogenic School and who consult psychiatrists about their disturbed children. In support of this point, Bettelheim mentions that not only is there a preponderance of Jewish children at the Orthogenic School, but also the number of Jewish delinquents seen there is disproportionate to the expectations based on random distribution of ethnic background. Thus, Bettelheim presents additional evidence that the proportion of Jewish children among autistic cases is much higher than would be expected by chance. But, in this regard, he recommends that until large random samples of the population are studied and provide evidence of the overall incidence of infantile autism, it would be much better to disregard claims pertaining to the ethnic origin of such children and their parents' superior intelligence and professional achievements.

Bettelheim concludes his discussion on the etiology and treatment of autistic children with the statement that a study of all three-year-old children in one of our metropolitan areas would probably reveal that infantile autism is more frequent than is generally assumed and more evenly distributed among all groups of the population. He admits, however, that this is merely a guess and stresses the need for much further research and increased factual information beyond what is currently available.

These, then, are some of the major issues in the writings of Bruno Bettelheim, who has certainly been one of the most influential theorists in this area of childhood psychopathology. While he has had a major influence on the formulation of ideas that have been adopted by professionals in the recent past, at present there is much dissatisfaction and disagreement with Bettelheim's viewpoint. Rimland criticized the views Bettelheim expressed in the Hall interview (1972). Rimland said, "It would be a pity if ... readers were left with the impression that Bruno Bettelheim's views on infantile autism and childhood schizophrenia represent more than the opinions of a member of the rapidly dying cult of psychoanalysis. Bettelheim's statements on the cause and treatment of mental illness in children are not only *unsupported* by any objective researcher—the scores of research studies published on these topics in the past two decades directly *contradict* Bettelheim's fatuous assertions. His great claims for his treatment methods have never been supported by any objective study, and are regarded by those of us active in research on these problems as having no merit whatsoever ... [Rimland, 1972, p. 660]." This is certainly a very negative evaluation offered by a man who is now regarded as one of the foremost authorities in the field of infantile autism.

In his capacity as Director of the Institute for Child Behavior Research, Rimland publishes a newsletter that is sent to parents of autistic children and to professionals who work with these disturbed children in varied treatment settings. In the May 1972 issue of the newsletter, Rimland included a comprehensive list of published books pertaining to autism and related problems. For each book, Rimland presented a brief evaluative statement. In the case of Bettelheim's *The Empty Fortress,* Rimland made the following comment: "Very imaginative, inaccurate, writing. Referred to by Leo Kanner as *The Empty Book!*"

Thus, while there may be much of value in the Bettelheim interview and in his comprehensive book, critics find serious fault with Bettelheim's contributions to the literature on infantile autism. At this stage, there certainly are no final answers, but it does seem that the weight of current evidence is not in favor of theories of psychogenic causation or psychoanalytically oriented therapy. The biogenecists have much to say and should be listened to, and the mounting evidence suggests also that operant conditioning and behavior therapy must be given serious consideration as more fruitful approaches to treating autistic children than the techniques used in the past.

References

Bender, L.   Autism in children with mental deficiency. *American Journal of Mental Deficiency,* 1959, **64,** 81–86

Bettelheim, B.   *Love is not enough: The treatment of emotionally disturbed children.* New York: Free Press, 1955.

Bettelheim, B.   *The empty fortress: Infantile autism and the birth of the self.* New York: Free Press, 1967.

Eisenberg, L.   The autistic child in adolescence. *American Journal of Psychiatry,* 1956, **112,** 607–612.

Eisenberg, L., & Kanner, L.   Early infantile autism, 1943–1955. *American Journal of Orthopsychiatry,* 1956, **26,** 556–566.

Hall, M. H.   A conversation with Bruno Bettelheim. In *Readings in Psychology Today.* (2nd ed.) Del Mar, Calif.: CRM Books, 1972.

Kanner, L.   Autistic disturbances of affective contact. *Nervous Child.* 1943, **2,** 217–250.

Mahler, M.   On childhood psychosis and schizophrenia: Autistic and symbiotic infantile psychoses. In *The Psychoanalytic Study of the Child.* Vol. 7. New York: International Universities Press, 1952.

Rimland, B.   *Infantile autism.* New York: Appleton-Century-Crofts, 1964.

Rimland, B.   A conversation with Bruno Bettelheim. In *Readings in Psychology Today.* (2nd ed.) Del Mar, Calif.: CRM Books, 1972.

16. The Etiology of Infantile Autism: The Problem of Biological versus Psychological Causation

Bernard Rimland

In the previous chapter we have presented what appears to the present writer to be incontestable support for Kanner's finding of unusual personality-intelligence configurations in the parents of children with early infantile autism. Many who have written on the problem of autism regard this finding as evidence for psychogenic etiology of the disease. This appears to be a plausible hypothesis and so should be subjected to critical evaluation to determine if it merits acceptance. Unfortunately, plausibility rather than consistency with evidence seems to be the criterion for many of the writers on early infantile autism. Consequently the hypothesis has been accepted without evaluation, and the literature on autism contains many papers in which it is asserted rather than suggested that psychogenic factors play a major part in the etiology of the disease. Indeed, a substantial proportion

From *Infantile Autism: The Syndrome and Its Implications for a Neural Theory of Behavior,* by Bernard Rimland. Copyright © 1964. Reprinted by permission of Appleton-Century-Crofts, Educational Division, Meredith Corporation.

of these papers carry no indication that biological factors may play even a minor part in the disease.

This chapter will be devoted to a detailed consideration of the problem of the etiology of infantile autism. The present writer disagrees with Eisenberg and Kanner's assertion that "Arguments that counterpose 'hereditary' versus 'environmental' as antithetical terms are fundamentally in error. Operationally defined, they are interpenetrating concepts" (1956, p. 563). That heredity and environment are "interpenetrating" cannot be denied. But the conclusion that their interpenetration precludes analysis does not follow. Complex problems require that we *increase,* not diminish our analytical efforts, if we are to have hope of solving the problems confronting us (Burt, 1958; Cattell, 1960).

There are several reasons for drawing close attention to the consideration of etiology in infantile autism. These are, in order of increasing generality:

1. The welfare of individual autistic children and their families hinges closely upon the problem of specific etiology, as van Krevelen has amply demonstrated (e.g., 1958, 1960). If the disease is psychogenic, the causative factors need to be identified. On the other hand, if autism is determined solely by organic factors, there is no need for the parents of these children to suffer the shame, guilt, inconvenience, financial expense and marital discord which so often accompany the assumption of psychogenic etiology. (For examples of this, see May, 1958; Peck, Rabinowitz and Cramer, 1949. Oppenheim, 1961, and Stuart, 1960, are also germane.)

2. So long as the practitioners who actually deal with autistic children feel satisfied that the disease is largely or entirely psychogenic, biologically trained research workers will feel disinclined to concentrate their efforts on the problem. It should be added at his point, in all frankness, that while the purpose of the review which follows was to investigate the specific etiology of early infantile autism, the issue is a broad one and a good deal of the material covered relates closely to the problem of causation of childhood behavioral disorders in general. The results of this work were surprising to the present writer and discordant with his previous beliefs. They may also be so to the reader. It is largely because of the large discrepancy between research findings and the remainder of the published literature that such detailed consideration is given the problem of etiology in this chapter.

Failing to find any adequate formulations of many of the inexplicit assumptions on both sides of the issue, the writer has attempted to articulate these, in his belief that a good part of the unique function of the psychologist is to try to articulate what seems ineffable.[1] No doubt much of this formulation will be challenged, and additional points will need to be added to those listed. We can do no better on this issue than to refer to Bacon's assertion that truth is more likely to emerge from error than from confusion.

3. There is yet another reason, one of considerable theoretical importance to psychology and psychiatry, for giving careful and reasoned attention

---

[1]There are certain arguments, however, which defy our attempt to reformulate them in any testable way: "I believe that the child who shows autistic behavior has been traumatized in the early months of life since he symbolizes to the mother so definitely the hated sibling" (Ribble, in discussion of Despert, 1951, p. 350).

to the etiology of early infantile autism. Sufficient evidence pointing toward a very unique and specific personality-intellectual configuration in the parents of children having early infantile autism has been adduced to permit little doubt of the accuracy of Kanner's original observations on this point. If it should turn out that early infantile autism is biologically—not psychologically—determined, then the only logical way of accounting for the parents' unusual personalities and intelligence is biologically. This would mean that basic personality structure may, in at least some cases, be far more closely tied to the biological makeup of the individual than has heretofore been realized. Unless autism can be shown to be largely psychogenic in origin, or the evidence presented by Kanner and others concerning the parents can be disqualified, the conventional view that heredity must invariably act only in general and unspecific ways as a determinant of human behavior must be reconsidered.

This point appears to have escaped most writers in the field. Kanner, while he has not emphasized the implications of his finding, does refer to "the astounding fact" that his "search for autistic children of unsophisticated parents" had remained unsuccessful (1949, p. 421) and the "remarkable" absence of mental disorders in the children's parents and relatives.

Fuller & Thompson (1960) explain in their book *Behavior Genetics* that they hold Eysenck's work on the introvert-extrovert factor to be of great importance because, "Here is a clearcut case of a basic variable of temperament, relating to both personality and learning ability, that is strongly dependent on genetic factors. More work along these lines will undoubtedly be of great value" (p. 241). Because the study of infantile autism may lead to even more striking findings, it seems essential that close and thorough examination of the etiology of infantile autism be undertaken.

A. The Arguments for Psychogenesis of Infantile Autism

The case for psychogenesis of autism would appear to rest on the following arguments and assumptions:

1. No consistent physical or neurological abnormalities have been found in autistic children which could account for their condition.
2. Many autistic children have been raised by parents apparently deficient in emotional responsiveness, which could have pathogenic effects on the child.
3. Certain children raised in hospitals or orphanages where maternal contact was sparse have been reported to show an undue frequency of emotional difficulties.
4. The behaviors of the child—his indifference or aggressiveness, his refusal to speak (or "elective mutism"), his apparent withdrawal from the outside world —are interpreted as signs of "punishment" or "retaliation" against the parents.
5. Certain incidents in the life of the autistic child appear to be pathogenic and permit the disorder to be traced to them.
6. Psychotherapy or otherwise placing the child in a kind and understanding environment has beneficial effects.
7. The high incidence of first-born and only children suggests that parental attitudes may be causative. . . .

B. The Case for Biological Causation

Unlike the hypothesis that autism is psychogenically determined, there are a number of points of information which support the hypothesis that autism may result from a rare recessive trait, or be otherwise determined by biological factors. Kanner, in his various publications (especially with Eisenberg, 1956), has cited the first five points listed below as evidence against the psychogenic view. The remaining points have been identified by the present writer or others who have concerned themselves with this problem.

1. Some clearly autistic children are born of parents who do not fit the autistic parent personality pattern.
2. Parents who do fit the description of the supposedly pathogenic parent almost invariably have normal, non-autistic children.
3. With very few exceptions, the siblings of autistic children are normal.
4. Autistic children are behaviorally unusual "from the moment of birth."
5. There is a consistent ratio of three or four boys to one girl.
6. Virtually all cases of twins reported in the literature have been identical, with both twins afflicted.
7. Autism can occur or be closely simulated in children with known organic brain damage.
8. The symptomatology is highly unique and specific.
9. There is a absence of gradations of infantile autism which would create "blends" from normal to severely afflicted. . . .

C. Psychogenesis as an Inadequate and Pernicious Hypothesis

Perhaps it should be made explicit at this point that the writer does not presume to have shown that autism is biologically determined and that the psycho-social environment plays no part in its etiology. What the writer *does* assert is that a careful review of the evidence has revealed no support for the psychogenic point of view. The evidence is instead highly consistent with expectation based on organic pathology.

Our finding with regard to autism coincides with the more general view formulated by the participants of a recent conference on the causes of mental disorder (Milbank Memorial Fund, 1961):

> There seems to be no clearly demonstrated instance of either a cultural or social factor being known to be a predisposing factor in mental illness. . . . The absence of clear-cut evidence does not show that the hypothesis is incorrect but only that it has not been demonstrated even once (p. 379).

Neither Creak and Ini (1960), who intensively studied 100 sets of parents of psychotic children, nor Peck, Rabinowitz, and Cramer (1949), who studied 50 sets of parents, were able to find evidence of a psychogenic nature. What they did find was a good deal of suffering brought on by the child's behavior and a good deal of intense (and we might add unnecessary) feelings of guilt.

It is probably too early to suggest that psychogenesis as a *hypothesis* no longer be considered. ("Hypothesis" is used advisedly, because there appears to be too little evidence to support use of the term "theory.") No avenue for learning all that we can about the etiology of mental disorder should be unexplored. The detailed explication in this chapter of the arguments concerning the etiology of autism was in part intended to facilitate, and perhaps even to provoke, some long-overdue, rational and articulate consideration of the problem, even at the expense of jointly provoking a measure of articulate and inarticulate wrath.

It is not questioned that distinction should be maintained between a disproven and an unproven hypothesis, but neither should there be a failure to distinguish between an unproven and an uninvestigated hypothesis. The psychogenic hypothesis is by no means uninvestigated.

Whatever may be the merit in being patient with psychogenesis as a hypothesis, there is much less in being patient with it as an assumed force-in-fact. The all too common practice of blatantly assuming that psychogenic etiology *can* exist or *does* exist in any individual case or in any given class of disorders is not only unwarranted but actively pernicious.

It is perhaps permissible for writers such as Weiland & Rudnik (1961) to "postulate" that "the expectation of murderous attack or of symbiotic engulfment by a psychogenic mother results in a failure to progress beyond autism and in panicky attempts to escape from symbiosis into autism..." (p. 552), especially when they add (in a footnote) "We do not believe this has been demonstrated conclusively..." It is something else again when the implications of this view are translated into action, and psychogenic causation is assumed to be a reality rather than merely a hypothetical possibility.

Ross (1959) presents an interesting and instructive case history of an autistic girl whose mother had been held to be responsible for her child's plight because the mother's affection was considered "intellectualized and objectified." Only when the child died did the fact of extensive brain damage become evident. Intensive neurological examination had failed to reveal the difficulty before the child's death, which interrupted intensive psychotherapy. It was fortunate for the mother that the brain damage was of a sort that present-day techniques could disclose, else she would to this day be held responsible for her daughter's death.

Consider the case of "Jonny" (Rothenberg, 1960). After stating that Jonny, at 1½ pounds, was one of the smallest premature babies ever born in the United States to survive, and after noting that 3½ months spent in an incubator under high oxygen tension and heat lamps had turned the infant's hair orange and his skin chocolate brown, the author attributed his later severe behavior disturbance to lack of mothering while being incubated. "Cure" was said to be greatly facilitated by suddenly confronting Jonny with a model of the incubator—a personification of the mother who supplies only material needs and no nourishment of the ego. The possibility that organic brain damage might have resulted from such adverse physical conditions was apparently not seriously considered, yet it had been known for some time that a high concentration of oxygen is able to cause destruction of nerve tissue in infants.

Bettelheim (1959a) interpreted the psychosis of "Joey, the Mechanical Boy" as a reaction to his mother's hostility when the evidence was also quite consistent with hereditary determination, since the mother appeared to be severely mentally disturbed herself. (See also the reply by May to this article.) In this case, as in Rothenberg's, the appeal of the psychogenic concept appeared to preclude consideration of concealed organic defect. Somehow the adherents of the psychogenic hypothesis tend to overlook the possibility that the complex and little understood cerebrum could be structurally or chemically impaired.

In another case Bettelheim (1959b) found emotional isolation to have caused the psychosis of a girl who had been conceived, born, and raised by her Jewish parents in World War II in a small hole beneath a farm building in Poland. The hole was too cramped to permit an adult to stretch out. German soldiers were nearby (sometimes firing shots into the building) so that the mother had to smother the infant's cries. Not considered by Bettelheim was research showing the adverse effects on the offspring's emotionality of prenatal stress in the mother (e.g., Thompson, 1957), nor of sensory deprivation in the child.

It should not be thought, however, that workers in this field are universal in accepting environmental determination. Some writers have been frank in rejecting the psychogenic hypothesis. Keeler (1957), for example, has said, "I certainly do not adhere to the opinion put forth by some that infantile autism stems from a very specific type of pathological parent-child (especially mother-child) relationship." Anthony (1958) notes, "I do not think that traumata which sometimes seem to precipitate a psychosis in childhood are anything greater than normal developmental hazards (sibling birth, etc.). It is the predisposition that makes them vulnerable." Chapman (1960) also believes the role of the psycho-social environment has been overestimated: " ... the degree of interpersonal pathology between parents and child rarely seems sufficient to explain the catastrophic interpersonal disorder of the child." Goldstein (1959), in his very illuminating discussion of autism, has pointed out clearly the gratuitousness of assuming psychogenesis as an etiologic factor in the disease.

In discussing the obvious prejudice against the hereditary viewpoint, Noland Lewis (1954) points out, "It would seem that most of the prejudice against genetic inheritance stems from a feeling in the realm of wish fulfillment, based on the idea that acceptance of genetic factors would create an attitude of therapeutic hopelessness." Williams (1956) cites this point among others in his attempt to penetrate the prejudice against heredity. He notes that hopelessness is by no means justified by the evidence, and cites the ready correction of the effects of diabetes, phenylketonuria and hypothyroidism as examples.

It should not be necessary to ask for recognition of the role played by genetic factors among persons trained in scientific thinking, but Williams has seen the need to do so:

> We therefore make a plea for an unprejudiced facing of the facts of heredity. We urge that such facts be accepted with as great readiness as any others. This plea seems necessary in view of the attitude which we have repeatedly noted, namely, that of willingness to arrive at "environmentalistic" conclusions on the basis of slender evidence while rejecting points of view which would emphasize the role of heredity, even though the weight of the evidence, viewed without prejudice, appears overwhelming (p. 16).

When dark-haired and dark-eyed parents produce a dark-complexioned child, we all are quick to agree, "Mendel was right!" But when introverted parents produce a child who similarly shows little interest in socialization, the refrain inexplicably changes to "Aha, Freud was right!"

In arguing for more critical use of the diagnosis of autism, Kanner says:

> The misuse of the diagnosis of autism has played havoc with the comfort and finances of many parents of retarded children, who were made to feel that their attitudes and practices were primarily responsible for their offspring's problems, were made to submit themselves and the child to lengthy, expensive, and futile therapy, and were pauperized and miserable to the time the true state of affairs was brought to light (1958, p. 111).

Kanner's appeal for the protection of the parents of children misdiagnosed as autistic is certainly to be commended, but what of the parents of *accurately* diagnosed cases? In view of the present status of research on the efficacy of psychotherapy, and of the fact that the evidence for psychogenic etiology of autism is not, to use Kanner's term, "unequivocal" (1958), it would seem that the parents of properly diagnosed autistic children might also be deferred from being made "pauperized and miserable," for the time being.

In a court of law it is impermissible to convict a person solely on evidence consistent with the hypothesis that he is guilty—the evidence must also be inconsistent with the hypothesis that he is innocent. This simple point of justice has been neglected, consistently, by those who deal with families having children afflicted with autism, and the damage and torment this practice has wrought upon parents whose lives and hopes have already been shattered by their child's illness is not easy to imagine nor pleasant to contemplate. To add a heavy burden of shame and guilt to the distress of people whose hopes, social life, finances, well-being and feelings of worth have been all but destroyed seems heartless and inconsiderate in the extreme. Yet it is done, as May (1958), Oppenheim (1961), Stuart (1960), and van Krevelen (1960) amply illustrate.

In view of these pernicious implications and the absence of scientific evidence, the wide acceptance of the psychogenic view is difficult to understand. A partial explanation for the prevalence of this view may be found in Kanner's unguarded admission that he is perplexed by the fact that the great majority of the parents of autistic children have been able to rear non-autistic children, while other parents who fit the parental typology perfectly, raised children who responded aggressively rather than by withdrawal: "... the existence of these exceptions is puzzling.... It is not easy to account for this difference of reaction" (1949, p. 426). The same "puzzling" inconsistency is clearly present in other childhood mental disorders, such as mongolism, Tay-Sachs disease, and phenylketonuria, and is readily explained in terms of recessive inheritance.

Despert provides another example of a child psychiatrist who does not apply what she must certainly know of genetics to her thoughts on etiology:

> It is sometimes argued that these mothers had other children who were normal or relatively normal, but it must be remembered that a mother, biogenetically identical for all her children, may nevertheless psychogenetically differ widely from one child to the other (1951, p. 345).

"Biogenetically identical"—100 years after Mendel!

Perhaps we are painting too dark a picture. There are signs of a growing recognition that the failure to find support for psychogenesis may possibly lie in the inadequacy of the concept rather than in a lack of resourcefulness among its investigators. Despert, whose 1951 view was quoted immediately above and who in 1947 wrote of cases in which neurological disorders had been "ruled out" by examination, has written in 1958 that the possibility of finding constitutional factors in infantile autism was particularly strong (Despert & Sherwin, 1958). Ekstein, Bryant, and Friedman (1958) show a willingness to question "our prejudiced, one-sided consideration of etiological factors" (p. 653); and Bettelheim, for years a leader of the psychogenic school, was recently willing to "reserve judgment" about what causes autism, although he is still "pretty sure" that psychogenic factors "contribute" (1959b, p. 463).

Szurek, who started in 1946 "to test the hypothesis that the etiology of psychotic disorders of childhood are entirely psychogenic" (Boatman & Szurek, 1960; p. 389) takes a much weaker stand today in stating that certain "facts" "... seem to lend weight to the possibility that psychogenic factors are at least important" (p. 430). (The reader may wish to see these "facts.")

To the present writer these indications of a retreat from the psychogenic hypothesis, like Bowlby's previously cited disavowal of the maternal deprivation hypothesis, represent a timely and welcome willingness to let conviction be subordinated to evidence. The history of science proves this to be the first step toward progress.

References

Anthony, J. An experimental approach to the psychopathology of childhood: Autism. *British Journal of Medical Psychology,* 1958, **31,** 211–225.

Bettelheim, B. Joey: A "mechanical boy." *Scientific American,* 1959, **200,** 116-217. (a)

Bettelheim, B. Feral children and autistic children. *American Journal of Sociology,* 1959, **64,** 455–467. (b)

Boatman, M. J., & Szurek, S. A. A clinical study of childhood schizophrenia. In D. D. Jackson (Ed.), *The etiology of schizophrenia*. New York: Basic Books, 1960.

Burt, C. The inheritance of mental ability. *American Psychologist,* 1958, **13,** 1–15.

Cattell, R. B. The multiple abstract variance analysis equations and solutions: For nature-nurture research on continuous variables. *Psychological Review,* 1960, **67,** 353–372.

Chapman, A. H. Early infantile autism: A review. *Journal of Diseases of Children,* 1960, **99,** 783–786.

Creak, M., & Ini, S. Families of psychotic children. *Journal of Child Psychology and Psychiatry,* 1960, **1,** 156–175.

Despert, J. L. Psychotherapy in child schizophrenia. *American Journal of Psychiatry,* 1947, **104,** 36–43.

Despert, J. L. Some considerations relating to the genesis of autistic behavior in children. *American Journal of Orthopsychiatry,* 1951, **21,** 335–350.

Despert, J. L., & Sherwin, A. C. Further examination of diagnostic criteria in schizophrenic illness and psychoses of infancy and early childhood. *American Journal of Psychiatry,* 1958, **114,** 784–790.

Eisenberg, L., & Kanner, L. Early infantile autism, 1943–1955. *American Journal of Orthopsychiatry,* 1956, **26,** 556–566.

Ekstein, R., Bryant, K., & Friedman, S. W. Childhood schizophrenia and allied conditions. In L. Bellak & P. K. Benedict (Eds.), *Schizophrenia.* New York: Logos Press, 1958.

Fuller, J. L., & Thompson, W. R. *Behavior genetics.* New York: Wiley, 1960.

Goldstein, K. Abnormal mental conditions in infancy. *Journal of Nervous and Mental Disease,* 1959, **128,** 538–557.

Kanner, L. Problems of nosology and psychodynamics of early infantile autism. *American Journal of Orthopsychiatry,* 1949, **19,** 416–426.

Kanner, L. The specificity of early infantile autism. *Zeitschrift für Kinderpsychiatrie,* 1958, **25,** 108–113.

Keeler, W. R. In discussion. *Psychiatric Reports of American Psychiatric Associations,* 1957, **7,** 66–68.

van Krevelen, D. A. Zür problematik des autismus. *Praxis Kinderpsychiatrie,* 1958, **7,** 87–93.

van Krevelen, D. A. Autismus infantum. *Acta Paedopsychiatrie,* 1960, **27,** (3), 97–107.

Lewis, N. D. C. In discussion. *Proceedings of the Association for Research on Nervous and Mental Disease,* Baltimore: Williams and Wilkins, 1954.

May, J. M. *A physician looks at psychiatry.* New York: John Day, 1958.

Millbank Memorial Fund. *The causes of mental disorders.* New York: Author, 1961.

Oppenheim, R. C. They said our child was hopeless. *Saturday Evening Post,* June 17, 1961, 56–58.

Peck, H. B., Rabinovitch, R. D., & Cramer, J. B. A treatment program for parents of schizophrenic children. *American Journal of Orthopsychiatry,* 1949, **19,** 592–598.

Ross, I. S. An autistic child. *Pediatric Conferences,* 1959, **2,** 1–13.

Rothenberg, M. The rebirth of Jonny. *Harper's Magazine,* February 1960, 57–66.

Stuart, N. G. Scream in the night. *Ladies Home Journal,* September 1960, 163–172.

Thompson, W. R. Influence of prenatal maternal anxiety on emotionality in young rats. *Science,* 1957, **125,** 698–699.

Weiland, I. H., & Rudnik, R. Considerations of the development and treatment of autistic childhood psychosis. *Psychoanalytic Study of the Child,* 1961, **16,** 549–563.

17. Parents as Cotherapists in the Treatment of Psychotic Children.

Eric Schopler
Robert J. Reichler

Severely disturbed children have been exposed to a remarkable array of therapies in the past three decades, including custodial isolation, electroconvulsive shock, drug therapies, psychoanalytic therapy, operant conditioning, electronic typewriters, and megadose vitamin therapy. This variety attests to a mounting experimental interest in helping those children and understanding their disorders, as well as to the lack of professional consensus. Developmental therapy, discussed in this report, is a method in which parents function as the primary developmental agents for their own severely disturbed child. The goals are to prevent the elaboration of psychosis, to increase adaptation between the child and his family, and to promote recovery where possible.

Since we do not yet have sufficient knowledge of specific causes for childhood psychosis, it may be helpful to explain the theoretical framework and the focal propositions that guide such a program. It is assumed that the directions of a child's development are based on the interactions with his parents. By and large, the normal child's behavior is shaped around parental expectations; the child in turn has an effect on the parent's behavior. The human infant is born with a biologically determined set of reflexes and responses that appear in regular sequence, relatively unaffected by learned experience. Some of these responses are basic to social development. Some infants, for example, smile a great deal, whereas others smile less. The infant's smile increases his mother's involvement. Infants who smile frequently tend to be fatter than infrequent smilers (Freedman, 1966). For an autistic infant with impaired social responses, the mother is negatively reinforced for her mothering efforts. The interaction cycle is directed more by the biological limitations than it is for the normal child.

The presence of such constitutional adaptational rigidities was alluded to in Kanner's original discovery of autism, which has subsequently been elaborated and clarified in the review of Eisenberg (1967) and Rutter (1970). From these reviews a consensus about the nature of childhood psychosis appears to be evolving. Several factors are important to developmental therapy: (1) the causes are multiply determined, (2) in individual cases the

From *Journal of Autism and Childhood Schizophrenia,* 1971, **1,** 87–102. Copyright 1971 by Scripta Publishing Corporation. Reproduced by permission.

primary causes are usually unknown, and (3) it is most likely that the primary causes involve some form of brain abnormality resulting in language impairment and other symptoms, depending on the child's age, severity of disability, and time of onset.

Learned experience has had less effect on preschool children than on older children, increasing the likelihood that for the younger child, adaptational difficulties involve biological processes. Our own studies (Schopler, 1965, 1966; Schopler & Reichler, 1970) agree with those of others (Ornitz & Ritvo, 1968; Rutter, 1968) in suggesting that the primary defect in childhood psychosis involves impairment in communication and understanding with manifestations in both cognitive and perceptual processes.

New knowledge about the personalities of parents of psychotic children has been perhaps even more prominent in the evolution of developmental therapy than what is known of their children. Until very recently parents were generally looked upon as the primary causative agents. However, little of the care lavished on classifying and describing the children was spent on understanding the parents. Based largely on psychogenic theories, they were bestowed with such homey epithets as "refrigerator parents," "smothering mothers," "cold," "intellectual," "rejecting," and "schizophrenogenic." Since the clinical history of childhood psychosis is relatively brief, it is possible that the psychogenic theory, placing the etiologic emphasis on parental feeling and thought, was an attempt at substituting theory for lack of information (Schopler, 1969). To date the psychogenic theory has generated virtually no specific research which may help explain the nature of childhood psychosis. Its persistent application has evoked scientific and parental indignation against such unsubstantiated bias. Besides inhibiting research, the theory may also be implicated in social-political processes that appear to go against the best interests of the children. Parents of retarded children, whose child-rearing practices have rarely been considered as a primary cause of retardation, have long been effectively organized toward promoting educational resources for their children. Parents of autistic children, on the other hand, did not form a national organization until Rimland spoke out in 1964 against the psychogenic emphasis and then became the founder of the now growing National Society for Autistic Children.

Clinical observations of parents have ascribed to them emotional and intellectual deviations far more frequently than these characteristics have been demonstrated through controlled research. Pitfield and Oppenheim (1964) found that some of the stereotyped characteristics did not apply to their sample of 100 mothers of psychotic children. Meyers and Goldfarb (1961), on the other hand, found mothers imposing their perplexities on their schizophrenic offspring. Parents' aberrant thinking has been repeatedly linked to the thought structure found in their schizophrenic offspring. Such "schizophrenogenic" thinking has been reliably measured in several studies (Singer & Wynne, 1965; Lovibond, 1954; Lidz, 1958; Wild, 1965; and Rosman, 1964) using the Goldstein Scherer Object Sorting Test. In each of these studies parents showed more disordered thinking than did control groups. The primary interpretation of the findings placed the emphasis on parental thought disorder as generating similar impairment in their child.

These studies have recently been extended (Schopler & Loftin, 1969a, b) with parents of psychotic children. The results showed that they were impaired in their thinking when tested in association with their psychotic child in the context of psychodynamic evaluation. When another group was tested in the context of an interview asking them how they were able to raise successfully their normal children with a problem child in the family, they showed no more impaired thinking than a control group of parents of retarded children. It has become increasingly clear that parents of psychotic children are disorganized in reaction to their disorganized, psychotic child.

Some of the current trends concerning the nature of the psychotic child and his parents are discussed in greater detail elsewhere (Schopler & Reichler, 1971). The following propositions were derived as the framework for developmental therapy: (1) the causes of autism are as yet unknown, (2) the classification must therefore, for the time being, remain broad but descriptively explicit, (3) the most likely causes are those involving biochemical and neurological brain abnormalities, (4) these result in perceptual inconstancies involving speech and communication impairment, and (5) parents' personalities fall within the "normal range," differing from the general population only in that they react with perplexity and confusion to their unresponsive children.

Some theories of autism are locked tightly to the prescribed therapy for their verification. Thus, Bettelheim's therapy involves separating the child indefinitely from his parents, replacing them with warm, accepting parent surrogates. This parentectomy therapy and the psychogenic theory are often presented as evidence of one for the other. A similar relationship exists between the position taken by many learning theorists and their operant conditioning procedures. The therapy assumes that behavior can be shaped if the right reinforcement contingencies can be found. Ferster (1961) proposed that autistic behavior is caused by parental inability to provide a proper reinforcement history for the child. Such circular reasoning is not the link between developmental therapy and the propositions formulated above.

Program Structure

Following a pilot study in 1966, using parents of psychotic children as cotherapists, a 5-year project was begun. Since it is only in its second year, some of the outcome data reported here are incomplete and based on clinical observations. The structure for the program, however, has been established. Three main admissions criteria are used:

   1. The child must have diagnosis of autism or psychosis based on the Creak (1961, 1964) criteria.

2. He must live at home in an intact family, with parents who are willing and able to participate in the Child Research Project.
3. He must be functioning on a pre-school level.

Families are referred from all parts of the state within commuting distance from the Project. Decisions for admission are made after a 2-hour diagnostic evaluation which, like all subsequent sessions with the child, is conducted in a one-way observation room. Prior to this, all previous work-ups have been reviewed. Both parents accompany the child for this session.

Diagnosis of Psychosis or Autism

An objective rating system has been developed for measuring the degree of psychosis found in each child referred with a suspicion of autism or childhood psychosis. The child is rated on observations made during a semistandardized interaction. The ratings are based on the criteria worked out by Creak's (1961) working party and elaborated by Rutter (1970). These criteria, offering only a broad descriptive classification, have the advantage of avoiding premature closure and impediments for the subsequent identification of more discrete subgroups as more specific knowledge becomes available. Rutter has suggested that the term childhood psychosis be used to designate the broad range of severe disorders in which autistic characteristics are prominent. It is in this sense that the term childhood psychosis is used to select children for the Project. Ratings of the young psychotic child may be grouped in two levels of importance for differentiation from other conditions.

Specific Response Patterns

Relatedness. The absence of age-appropriate relatedness can often be distinguished between a lack of attachment to people or a lack of attachment to objects or places. Perhaps because people are themselves more complex and changing from day to day, lack of social responsiveness is more frequent. The child is aloof, or excessively clinging, avoids eye-contact and does not imitate verbal or non-verbal signals. He is impaired in communication and understanding, both of which are basic to age-appropriate human relatedness.

Speech impairment. Equally important, though developmentally subsequent to the relatedness impairment, is the absence, delay, or peculiarity of speech development. The child may speak slowly, late, and with poor ability to communicate. Sometimes he plays with sounds, words and phrases unintelligibly. He echoes certain words repeatedly, often the one heard most recently. This also results in pronoun reversal.

Sensory peculiarities. These children show various expressions of unusual sensory processes. Nearly all appear deaf or have been suspected of deafness. The child tends to be inattentive especially to auditory and visual stimuli. He may also show special sensitivity to selective sounds or have panicky reactions to certain visual stimuli. He may persist in excessive examination of things around him by touch and taste. He may feel textures and tap on surfaces like a child who is born blind. He may appear indifferent to pain, unable to sense, locate, or respond to pain-producing stimuli.

Other Characteristics

The second level of psychotic signs includes peculiar motility patterns, such as rocking, spinning, toe walking, and hand flapping. The child manifests abnormal activity levels, appearing either hyperactive or hypoactive. He may have a preoccupation with the repetitive use of the same toy or object. Intellectual functioning is on a retarded level, but hints of normal or superior potential in some areas are common. Excessive and often unpredictable mood changes occur with severe temper tantrums and self-destructive behavior. The assessments of these behavior items during the diagnostic session can be made with satisfactory reliability between different raters.

Parent-Child Interaction

Both parents are also observed in an interaction with their child. They are asked to bring along some of the toys or objects he is currently most interested in and then to get him as involved with them in organized activity as they can, and to get him to help them return the materials to their container. This enables the staff to get an initial measure of the kinds of difficulties parents are having in interacting with their child. It also gives the parents an idea of how they will be expected to work with their child should they be admitted to the Project.[1]

Staff Background

All staff members function both as therapists and parent consultants, though not usually with the same family. This dual role enables them best to maintain a balanced perspective on parent-child interaction. Their past training and experience may have been in the discipline of education, psychiatry, psychology, or social work. They are selected for their interest and skill in teaching autistic children and their parents rather than for their professional identity. Experience with such children, enthusiasm, and willingness to learn have so far proven to be the best qualifications.

Parent Participation

Parents attend twice weekly for 45-minute sessions, with mothers and fathers usually alternating. During these visits parents may observe the

---

[1]When a family is admitted, an agreement of collaboration between them and the staff is made for a specific period of time.

therapist's demonstration, discuss problems in other areas of their home life with the parent consultant, or demonstrate their home program with the child. Occasionally other family members, such as siblings, are also involved in working with the child.

Therapy Demonstration

Parents observe through a one-way screen with their consultant, who focuses their attention on relevant aspects of the demonstration and answers questions parents may raise. This observation has several important advantages:

1. It avoids the mystique and unfounded authority of the therapist who reports to parents from only private observations of the child.
2. It guards the parents against recommendations which are more easily made than carried out.
3. It provides stimulation stemming from constructive competition between parents and therapist and also affords a realistic opportunity for parents to use the therapist for modeling behavior.
4. Direct demonstrations have a more immediate impact than verbal interpretation. They are more easily understood, especially by unsophisticated parents, than are eloquent verbal explanations.
5. When parents are allowed to see the therapist's struggles, frustrations, and occasional mistakes, they become less self-critical and are better able to resume responsibility for the bond with their own child.

The demonstrations play a key role in encouraging parents to use as guidelines their knowledge of successful experience in normal child rearing, but to apply this knowledge in the special way required by their autistic child. To do this, the parents have to develop a degree of self-consciousness inappropriate to normal child rearing. Indeed, they need to become experts on their own autistic child. Therapist demonstrations contribute to this in two general ways: They offer the therapist as a model for general attitudes and approaches, and they demonstrate specific teaching methods.

The therapist confers with the parent consultant prior to the demonstration and they agree on the session's focus. For example, parents often have unusual difficulties in controlling the child's behavior and they have adopted an air of resignation in accepting anything the child does. The therapist will show how to get the child seated at the table, how to give him a swat on the behind to clarify communication, and how to maintain a meaningful interaction when the child withdraws. Specific interventions are evolved appropriate to the child's development. These can be grouped conveniently in four main areas of function with examples of typical interventions in each.

Human Relatedness

The children are impaired in their responsiveness to adults, including both social attachment and differentiated awareness. Since subsequent development, especially imitation for communication, is dependent on such responsiveness, improvement is especially useful during initial phases. This involves the adult's nonspecific impingement on the child and striving for clarity in both positive and negative responses. The child is not allowed to do anything—move about the room or use any object without the mediation of the adult, similar to the common-sense suggestions of Des Lauriers and Carlson (1969). Gradually, as the child takes the adult into account, increasing degrees of frustration are imposed, such as demanding some action or task before satisfying the child's wishes. Self-stimulation and withdrawal by the child are met with immediate and direct intervention by the adult. With a child at a higher level of development, the therapist may be more passive and allow the child to initiate contact by responding immediately and positively. After breaking through a child's severe withdrawal, some object or food may be used as a means of exchange.

Competence Motivation

The appropriateness of materials used is important. The aims include helping the child to develop pleasure and interest in increasingly organized exploration and use of toys and educational materials. Increase in the child's sustained and spontaneous interest with materials when he is by himself appears to be one of the more efficient ways of promoting competence motivation. Initially, however, it is fostered externally and increased by improved relatedness to the therapist. As the child becomes more responsive to external motivation and his perceptual-cognitive organization increases, he is allowed to follow his own interests more freely. Exploration is then encouraged by association with meaningful use of materials. One child's perceptual skills may develop, enabling him to explore new materials spontaneously. For example, he may learn how to put a new puzzle together on his own. While such success is self-rewarding, the child also is encouraged to explore new materials. For another child human relatedness may be undeveloped, while his motivation to meaningful exploration of materials is increasing quite rapidly. His motivation to organize materials may be used to improve responsiveness by making such materials contingent on responding to the adult. The main aim, however, is to enable the child to develop spontaneous, organized activity and play, reinforced by his own success. Methods such as these are specified for each child on a continuous basis and translated into specific tasks in a home program.

Cognitive Functions

The primary concern here is the child's development of both receptive and expressive communication skills. These involve recognizing and naming subjects, discriminating colors and shapes, learning concepts, action verbs, and their meaningful application. When special education is not productive, operant conditioning procedures are often effective.

A child without speech may first need to learn non-verbal imitations. He will be required to look at the adult's mouth while a desired object is named before it is given to the child. At higher levels of development, a sound already produced by the child may be encouraged and identified with an object. At still higher levels, concepts are encouraged through the use of modalities with immediacy for the child. "Up and down" can be taught initially by swinging the child up and down accompanied by the appropriate word. Eventually the word is required from the child before he is picked up. One child, for instance, would be held upside down until he asked to be picked "up." These concepts are then generalized through other activities.

Perceptual Motor Function

Exercises are developed for improving the child's awareness and coordinated use of his body. This may include practice with coordination between his eyes and hands, exercises for developing pincer grasp and other functions such as jumping, climbing, and balancing. Some children at very low levels of development initially need passive manipulation of their limbs to learn to use them. For example, one child never brought his hands together. In another, pincer grasp might be developed by manipulating materials that could not be grasped in any other way. For some children, experience with a graded series of puzzles or cups fosters increased perceptual discrimination, which often interacts with cognitive development as language is added. Development is uneven and sometimes unpredictable. One young child, after learning to discriminate geometric shapes, developed an interest in letters. Although this interest did not follow the normal developmental sequence, he was helped to learn the alphabet. This increased his overall organization of his perceptual world and supported language development as well.

Home Program

Concurrent with their observations of sessions, parents are also given home programs, which are revised at regular intervals. These describe objectives, methods and materials for working with the child in daily sessions. The content of the home program is based on the therapist's assessment of the child and the parents' experience at home. Both parents are expected to share in these home sessions, though mothers usually work more frequently with their children than do fathers.

At regular intervals, parents demonstrate the home program with their child while therapist and consultant observe. Parents bring along the materials they had made or purchased for home use. They are aware of being observed and occasionally filmed. Although many of them are at first nervous about performing behind a one-way screen, the nervousness disappears after they have observed the therapist for a while. In fact, sooner or later most parents request additional demonstration sessions to show new developments of which they are especially proud. Not only do spontaneous demonstrations of new progress boost the parental ego, these sessions also maintain some motivating competition for understanding and improving the interaction with the child.

Generally the parents' daily home program sessions are more easily organized into an enjoyable and successful interaction than are problems in other areas of home life. To work out solutions to these problems the parent meets with his consultant in an office other than the observation room. The problems discussed often involve issues not practical or feasible for handling during demonstration sessions, such as sleeping, eating, and difficulties with toilet training.

> One child did not go to bed until eleven o'clock. He sat in the living room rocking himself for a half hour every night, and then slept in his parents' bed every night. This had been going on for several years. The parent consultant helped the parents to divide this bedtime problem into several units. First the rocking chair was moved into the child's bedroom as was a radio he liked listening to. After he became accustomed to this change he was consistently moved from the parents' to his own bed. A difficult struggle ensued, requiring parents to move the child 15 times to his own bed during the first few nights. Within three weeks, however, he was sleeping in his own bed.

Parents are required to complete daily logs. On this form each section of the home program is rated for changes in the child's responses. Once each week both parents complete the second part of the log, rating the child's progress in the other areas of home life. These logs form an important part in tracking changes and development in the child over time.

Research Participation

Parents have been involved directly in research relating to therapy. During the first year of the Project's operation, parents expressed considerable confusion about the meaning of "structure." How to differentiate between rigidity, clear structure, and lack of structure? Some of the parents had read about or had their children involved in relatively unstructured, nondirective, or psychoanalytic play therapy. Although these traditional therapies have certain ground rules of time, place, and safety, they have contributed to the belief that a disturbed child's difficulties can be improved if he is allowed free expression with a minimum of impingement of frustrating expectations from adults. This attitude played into the parents' own perplexity in dealing with the child and hence it became relatively easy for them to accept uncritically any of the child's autistic behavior.

Other parents had been exposed to operant conditioning therapy involving more rigid structures. A certain target behavior to be modified is explicitly identified by the therapist and specific reinforcement contingencies are established. The child is conditioned in a direction independent of his own preference or developmental organization. Even in this highly organized situation, factors outside the therapist's control affect his carefully designed structure. Such effects are rarely measured or reported; nevertheless they obviously exist.

Without dichotomizing therapeutic structure as present or absent, the parents were involved in a systematic study investigating the effects of degree in structure on the child's functioning. Both parents and therapist were asked to alternate the structure in working with their child at two-week intervals for an eight-week period. The interactions were rated by a time-sampling method. Results detailed elsewhere (Schopler & Reichler, 1971), showed that the children were able to function more appropriately during structured than during unstructured sessions on all variables rated. The degree of disorganization varied among children. There was less disorganizing effect in the unstructured condition for children functioning at higher levels of development. Conversely, children at lower levels reacted to the change in conditions with more disorganization.

These findings and their implications for education and therapy were consistent with our clinical observations. The autistic child responds best to relatively high structure. Accordingly, relatively unstructured play therapy is not an appropriate treatment. On the other hand, a rigidly applied technique, such as operant conditioning, may not offer the best help for an autistic child if the rates and levels of the child's development are disregarded. The optimal learning situation for autistic children, as for others, is one which has more external structure for acquiring new learning patterns, and relative freedom from structure for practicing those patterns which have been mastered and internalized. The parents' direct participation in this study contributed to their interest and sensitivity to more accurate appraisal of their child's functioning level. They used this information for becoming more active in finding and using appropriate methods of intervention.

Outcome Trends

Although developmental therapy with parent-child interaction was begun 4 years ago, only during the past 2 years has the program included at least 10 children. There has not been sufficient time to complete longitudinal evaluation. Even in this beginning phase, however, we have some clear indication for the success of this process for both parent and child.

Of the 10 families in the Project during the first 18 months, the following social class distribution occurred: using the Hollingshead Index (1957), three families are in social class I, three fall into class II, two into class III, and two into class IV. This trend is consistent with the distribution reported by Rutter and Lockyer (1967). Four of the 10 families are Negro, 6 are Caucasian. The direct demonstrations were especially effective at the lower educational level where verbal facility is limited. Although less verbal, these parents were capable observers and were effective in putting their observations to good use.

Parent involvement has been greater than anticipated. Attendance has been quite regular although parents have to drive from 1 to 4 hours for each visit. Daily logs documenting the home program sessions have been maintained with high regularity. Mothers were more frequently involved in working with their children than were fathers, though both participated. Often, at the very beginning of the parents' participation, fathers were able to understand the child with more objectivity and to control the interaction more effectively than mothers. Mothers were often more confused, hopeless, and exhausted; spending most of their time with the child, they were more continuously affected adversely by his unresponsiveness. Nevertheless, improvement in the child was more noticeable when mothers became more involved with the home program than when fathers attempted such dominant involvement. However, parents' capacity to shift primary involvement to each other made for greater adaptability in the child's behalf.

Recently a comparison was made between the ratings on the child's activities during sessions with his therapist and ratings on the demonstration sessions of parents. These time-sampled ratings were made on the child's attention, affect, relatedness, verbal behavior, and nonpsychotic behavior. The ratings for seven children who had been in the program for at least 6 months were averaged for a 4-month period. In spite of individual variation, there was a trend for parents to obtain higher ratings on these five variables more frequently than did the therapist during the same period. This is perhaps not surprising considering that parents spent much more time with their child than the therapist and worked with him in daily home program sessions. However, it also confirms our observation that parents often pull ahead of the therapist in their effectiveness in implementing therapy demonstrations. Nevertheless, parents continue to seek support for maintaining their efforts.

Many parents, especially mothers, have developed a degree of objectivity, investment, and skill found only in top-notch teachers. Indeed, 3 out of 10 of the mothers in our program have become actively involved in teaching and 3 more have expressed a lively interest in this direction.

In the Child Research Project, therapists and parent consultants have come from the fields of psychiatry, psychology, social work, and education. Their successful fulfillment of their roles seems less related to their professional training than it does to their enthusiasm and motivation to work with autistic children and their knowledge of normal child development. In the field of mental health, there is a reluctant but increasing acceptance that paraprofessional and relatively untrained workers are conducting important therapeutic interventions. This is usually justified with the explanation that the increase in demand for service accompanied by a shortage of trained personnel makes such use of subprofessionals necessary. Our experience suggests that it is not only expedient to use parents to supplement the shortage in manpower, but that they are also frequently the most effective developmental agents for their children.

In addition to working directly with their own children, the parents in our program have recently organized their own state chapter of the National Society for Autistic Children. They have been dedicated and effective in working toward the establishment of special education programs for their children in the public schools. Through meetings with legislators, educators, and professionals, they have succeeded in setting up two demonstration programs for special education of autistic children. Parents have extended their capacity to bring more meaningful organization into their children's lives, into the broader social implications of the disorder.

Several trends for change in the children can be identified after this relatively brief period of time. For some, a recovery from autism to relatively normal function can be predicted.

One of our children had no communicative speech, did not relate, and had an IQ of 57. During the 3-year period of therapy, he learned to function sufficiently to attend a regular public school and not to be distinguished from other children in his grade. This youngster's IQ went to 101, advancing 44 points. He developed a personality that made him appealing to both teachers and peers. The only traces of his early difficulty can be detected in perceptual-motor awkwardness showing up in poor handwriting. It is quite likely that the traces of this impairment will become sufficiently camouflaged with further development to be unnoticeable.

For another child the psychotic symptoms, screaming, self-destructive behavior, and lack of relatedness, are no longer a problem. Even after the psychosis was no longer an issue, this child continued to function on a retarded level with an IQ of 56. It was possible to place her without any difficulty in a special class for retarded children in a public school, where previously she had been excluded.

A third child showed extremely slow progress during the period of therapy. His IQ remained about 39. There was some improvement in relatedness, and he was able to learn a few words. However, advances in his development were not firm and tended to disappear without continuous practice. Eventually, he showed symptoms that made it possible to report a diagnosis of tuberous sclerosis. Even before this diagnosis could be made medically, the staff and parents recognized that his rate of development was profoundly slow and unstable and suspected an active biological process. But even in this case involving progressive brain disease, some degree of improvement could be measured.

These trends in the children are consistent with those reported by Gittelman and Birch (1967) and Rutter (1968), linking prognosis with IQ. IQ's of less than 50 suggest a poor prognosis for normal development. IQ's over 50 indicate a greater variability in prognosis. Depending on the severity of the underlying impairment and the consistency of appropriate education, the child may reach optimal or normal levels of development.

In all our families, the parents' realistic appraisal of the child contributed to making their best energies available to him while either maintaining or improving the adjustment among all family members. Apparently, the recognition of the child's disabilities helps to improve the family equilibrium. Attention to the coping abilities of families faced with a difficult problem releases resources, energies, and abilities. These resources are often dissipated in other therapeutic enterprises in which parental adjustment difficulties are the primary emphasis. It is time to recognize the autistic child's parent as the integral agent to the solution of his child's problems rather than as having caused them.

References

Creak, M. Schizophrenic syndrome in childhood: Progress report of a working party. *Cerebral Palsy Bulletin*, 1961, **3**, 501–504.

Creak, M. Schizophrenic syndrome in childhood: Further progress report of a working party, *Developmental Medicine and Child Neurology*, 1964, **4**, 530–535.

Des Lauriers, A. M., & Carlson, C. F. *Your child is asleep—early infantile autism.* Homewood, Ill.: Dorsey Press, 1969.

Eisenberg, L. Psychotic disorders in childhood. In L. D. Eron (Ed.), *Classification of Behavior Disorders.* Chicago, Ill.: Aldine Press, 1967.

Ferster, C. B. Positive reinforcement and behavioral deficits of autistic children. *Child Development,* 1961, **32,** 437–456.

Freedman, D. G. The effects of kinesthetic stimulation on weight gain and on smiling in premature infants. Paper presented at the annual meeting of the *American Orthopsychiatric Association,* San Francisco, 1966.

Gittelman, M. & Birch, H. G. Childhood schizophrenia: Intellect, neurological status, prenatal risk, prognosis, and family pathology. *Archives of General Psychiatry,* 1967, **17,** 16–25.

Hollingshead, A. *Two factor index of social position.* New Haven, Conn.: privately published, 1957.

Lidz, T. Intrafamilial environment of the schizophrenic patient: VI. The transmission of irrationality. *Archives of Neurology and Psychiatry,* 1958, **79,** 305–316.

Lovibond, S. The object sorting test and conceptual thinking in schizophrenia, *Australian Journal of Psychiatry,* 1954, **5,** 52–70.

Meyers, D. I., & Goldfarb, W. Studies of perplexity in mothers of schizophrenic children. *American Journal of Orthopsychiatry,* 1961, **31,** 551–564.

Ornitz, E. M. & Ritvo, E. R. Perceptual inconstancy in early infantile autism. *Archives of General Psychiatry,* 1968, **18,** 79–98.

Pitfield, M., & Oppenheim, A. Child rearing attitudes of mothers of psychotic children. *Journal of Child Psychology and Psychiatry and Allied Disciplines,* 1964, **1,** 51–57.

Rosman, B. Thought disorders in the parents of schizophrenic patients: A further study utilizing the object sorting test. *Journal of Psychiatric Research,* 1964, *2,* 211–221.

Rutter, M. Concepts of autism: A review of research. *Journal of Child Psychology and Psychiatry,* 1968, **9,** 1–25.

Rutter, M. The description and classification of infantile autism. Proceedings of the Indiana University Colloquium on Infantile Autism. Springfield, Ill.: Charles C Thomas, 1970.

Rutter, M., & Lockyer, L. A five to fifteen year follow-up study of infantile psychosis. *British Journal of Psychiatry,* 1967, **113,** 1169–1182.

Schopler, E. Early infantile autism and receptor processes. *Archives of General Psychiatry,* 1965, **13,** 327–335.

Schopler, E. Visual versus tactual receptor preferences in normal and schizophrenic children. *Journal of Abnormal Psychology,* 1966, **71,** 108–114.

Schopler, E. Parents of psychotic children as scapegoats. Paper presented at Symposium of the American Psychological Association, Washington, D.C., September, 1969.

Schopler, E., & Loftin, J. Thought disorders in parents of psychotic children a function of test anxiety. *Archives of General Psychiatry,* 1969, **20,** 174–181. (a)

Schopler, E., & Loftin, J. Thinking disorders in parents of young psychotic children. *Journal of Abnormal Psychology,* 1969, **74,** 281–287. (b)

Schopler, E., & Reichler, R. J. Psychobiological referents for the treatment of autism. Proceedings of the Indiana University Colloquium on Infantile Autism. Springfield, Ill.: Charles C Thomas, 1970.

Schopler, E., & Reichler, R. J. Developmental therapy by parents with their own autistic child. Paper presented at Symposium under the auspices of CIBA and the Institute for Research into Mental Retardation, London, June, 1970. A version of this paper will appear in M. Rutter (Ed.), *Infantile autism: Concepts, characteristics and treatment.* London: Churchill (in press), 1971.

Singer, M., & Wynne, L. Thought disorder and family relations of schizophrenics. *Archives of General Psychiatry,* 1965, **12,** 201–212.

Wild, C. Disturbed styles of thinking: Implications of disturbed styles of thinking manifested on the object sorting test by the parents of schizophrenic patients, *Archives of General Psychiatry,* 1965, **13,** 464–470.

Chapter Seven

Mental Retardation and Learning Disorders

These two categories of childhood abnormality are far from identical; in a conventional textbook, they are usually treated in separate chapters. With the selective nature of this book's coverage, and since these two areas share many common problems and issues, it seems more efficient to consider them together.

Definitions and Prevalence of Learning Problems

Most mentally retarded children have difficulties in learning, and many children with learning problems show some degree of intellectual deficit. However, the learning disorder category includes a much broader range of disability than mental subnormality, including several other types of so-called exceptional children, which denotes children suffering from disorders such as emotional disturbance, brain damage, physical handicaps, and sensory defects.

In a paper devoted to problems of classifying and educating children with learning disabilities, McDonald (1968) described the lack of agreement in use of terms, making it practically impossible to define clearly the population of children included in this category. Of 35 experts who were questioned about their experiences in working with such children, McDonald obtained 22 different synonyms for "learning disorder," including "disability," "difficulty," "problem," "dysfunction," "deviation," "impairment," "imbalance," and so forth. McDonald quoted William Cruickshank, one of the world's leading authorities in this area: "I can well imagine that you are having some difficulty with the vocabulary relating to the general problem of children with learning disorders. We have recently identified 43 terms used in the current literature, all referring to practically the same group of children. Learning disabilities was one of these terms [McDonald, 1968, p. 373]."

Some experts in this field specifically exclude mentally retarded children from their accepted definition of learning disability, but others maintain that mildly retarded children should be the proper concern of those who specialize in working with learning disabilities. The following quotation from Samuel Kirk, a renowned leader in the education of exceptional children, provides both a definition of "learning disability" and a clear statement of its relationship to mental retardation:

> A learning disability refers to a specific retardation or disorder in one or more of the processes of speech, language, perception, behavior, reading, spelling, writing, or arithmetic. The word "specific" is very important in this definition since it implies that the child has a definite retardation in one or more areas but that the retardation is at variance with certain assets. . . . This point of view does not imply that a mentally retarded child, diagnosed as such by ordinary mental tests, cannot also have a learning disability. If he has discrepancies among abilities, or if he has special abilities and marked disabilities, he could be classified as a child with a learning disability rather than overall mental retardation [Kirk, 1968, p. 398].

In spite of inconsistent terminology, there is unanimous agreement that learning disabilities are extremely prevalent in contemporary society. Myklebust and Johnson (1962) have stated that "at least five percent of school children have some type of psychoneurological learning disorder." In fact, learning problems constitute the major reason for referral of school-aged children for psychological diagnosis and psychotherapeutic treatment (see Kessler, 1966; Clarizio & McCoy, 1970).

Definitions of Mental Retardation

The American Association of Mental Deficiency (AAMD) has published a manual on terminology and classification in which mental retardation is defined as sub-average general intellectual functioning that originates during the developmental period and is associated with impairment in adaptive behavior. In a scholarly and highly regarded book, *The Mentally Retarded Child*, Robinson and Robinson (1965) list five dimensions on which this recent AAMD definition differs from previous, more traditional formulations. First, it is specifically developmental in approach. Whereas older definitions stressed standards appropriate to adult behavior, in this newer definition the retarded child is judged in terms of his success with age-appropriate developmental tasks. Second, this definition focuses on a description of present behavior and disavows the notion of potential intelligence. Thus, it should help to avoid the kinds of past errors that have sometimes been made in predicting adult functioning of persons diagnosed as mentally subnormal in childhood. Third, this AAMD definition places specific reliance on objective measurement of general intelligence using information derived from standardized tests and supplementary evaluations of personality and motivational attributes. A fourth characteristic of the AAMD definition is that it avoids attempting to differentiate between mental retardation and other childhood disorders such as psychosis or organic brain damage. According to this view, a child may legitimately be called mentally subnormal regardless of whether the retardation is primary or secondary to emotional or organic disorders. Finally, the AAMD definition is not limited to the severely retarded but includes a much wider range of subnormality, encompassing those who previously have been considered borderline. According to this definition, all those who on a standard test of intelligence fall more than one standard deviation below the general population mean are regarded as mentally subnormal.

Prevalence of Mental Retardation

With this newer terminology, which includes people who formerly would be regarded as showing borderline intellectual functioning, approximately one-sixth of the United States population, or five out of every 30 pupils in the average classroom, can be considered mentally subnormal. As Robinson and Robinson have pointed out, this change in usage could lead to both positive and negative effects. An advantage of this terminology is that it encourages recognizing even mild retardation, which, in our highly urbanized competitive culture, can be a serious handicap calling for professional help in the form of special education, social agency support, and guidance. A main disadvantage of this new definition is that, traditionally, research on the retarded has dealt only with the markedly handicapped; consequently, this newer view is apt to lead to misinterpretations. After reviewing its pros and cons, Robinson and Robinson adopted this new definition in their book since they felt that it stressed both the uncertainty of current knowledge and the heterogeneity of maladies exhibited by mentally subnormal children.

Robinson and Robinson also discuss the many problems encountered in attempting to determine the actual prevalence of mental retardation. Not only is it extremely difficult to compute exact statistical indices in this country, but in world-wide comparisons, proportions of children regarded as mentally subnormal in different countries vary greatly according to the criteria used. Cultural factors that affect prevalence of perceived mental retardation include attitudes of the community toward the retarded and standards of evaluation related to the individual's age, sex, race, and geographical residence (Robinson & Robinson, 1965). In most large cities in the United States, families of low socioeconomic status are ill-equipped to care for their mentally handicapped children. On the other hand, the Hutterites of the Dakotas, Montana, and Manitoba have a communal form of living that enables them to share in caring for children, widows, and the disabled. Intensive study of a Hutterite community revealed that of the several people who could qualify for admission to an institution for mental defectives, not a single person had ever been institutionalized, even in the case of the most severe mental abnormalities.

Concerning the influence of the child's age, surveys have consistently shown increased diagnosis of retardation during the school years, particularly during early adolescence, and a decrease during late adolescence and adulthood. In considering racial differences, Robinson and Robinson mention that most studies find lower intelligence test scores in black children in comparison with white children. They also refer to the higher incidence of premature births and complications of pregnancy among blacks and state that these factors are found to be associated with relatively high incidence of mental subnormality. Robinson and Robinson favor an environmental interpretation of these findings, citing such factors as depressed living conditions, poor health care, and complex motivational factors in parent-child interactions. They, do, however, conclude with the statement that "Whether or not all such differences can be explained in this way is probably still open to question, although most psychologists in the United States lean toward this view" [1965, p. 47].

Whatever the causes, almost all studies show a much higher incidence of mental deficiency in males than in females. Possible explanations range from hereditary factors involving recessive characteristics carried by the sex chromosomes to social factors that establish stricter standards of economic self–sufficiency for males.

Geographically, there are marked variations in the availability and utilization of institutional facilities for the mentally retarded. Some years ago, census figures revealed 14 retarded individuals institutionalized for every 100,000 persons residing in Arkansas, while the comparable figure was 135 per 100,000 in New York. This is not to suggest that these figures indicate actual differences in rates of retardation in different geographical regions of the country; they merely show the ability and readiness of different locales to provide institutional beds for the handicapped.

Institutional Treatment of Retardates

In their book, *Christmas in Purgatory: A Photographic Essay on Mental Retardation* (1966), Blatt and Kaplan vividly convey the pathos and even horror engendered by a visit to most institutions for the retarded. They report: "we were amazed by the over-crowdedness, by the disrepair of older buildings, by the excessive use of locks and heavy doors, and by the enormity of buildings and numbers of patients assigned to dormitories." Describing these dormitories for severely retarded residents, they state: "The facilities often contribute to the horror. Floors are sometimes wooden and excretions are rubbed into the cracks, leaving permanent stench. Most day rooms have a series of bleacher benches, on which sit unclad residents, jammed together, without purposeful activity, communication, or interaction. In one such dormitory with an overwheming odor, we noticed feces on the wooden ceilings and on the patients as well as the floors." Blatt and Kaplan are convinced that these patients could be taught to wear clothes, to engage in purposeful activities, and to control their bowels if staff members believed that each of these residents is a human being who can learn.

Upsetting as Blatt and Kaplan found the adult facilities, they described the infant dormitories as even more depressing. Among their observations were "Very young children, one or two years of age, lying in cribs, without interaction with any adult, without playthings, without any apparent stimulation ... forty or more unkempt infants crawling around a bare floor in a bare room ... very young children lying, rocking, sleeping, sitting—alone. Each room without toys or adult human contact, although each had desperate-looking adult attendants 'standing by.' " Referring to the "special education" observed in these dormitories for young children, they report, " ... it was certainly not education. But it was special. It was among the most especially frightening and depressing encounters with human beings we have ever experienced."

A more recent report in *Time* magazine (1972), entitled "Human Warehouse," also presented a most depressing picture of the lives of severely retarded individuals residing in a large state-supported institution. Both this report and the one by Blatt and Kaplan are accompanied by photographs that reveal the sickening conditions even more vividly than do the written descriptions. The *Time* report focuses on Willowbrook State School on Staten Island in New York, describing it as " ... a grim repository for those whom society has abandoned." According to this article, what sets Willowbrook apart from similar facilities in other states is the sudden exposure resulting from public attacks against this institution stemming from parents, legislators, and newsmen. They have shown how hopeless and archaic is the custodial approach to treatment of mental retardation. All who have looked into living conditions at Willowbrook reached the conclusion that they were intolerable.

According to *Time*, "For most of Willowbrook's residents, the institution is a warehouse, a place capable of providing only shelter and the barest essentials, for those whose families are either unwilling or unable to care for them. ... Training of any kind is non-existent. ... The room is redolent of sweat, urine, excrement—and despair."

Describing the profoundly retarded children, many of whom have physical handicaps, *Time* reports " ... they sit strapped into special chairs, recline in two-wheeled wagons that look like peddler's pushcarts or lie listlessly on mats on the floor. ... Some of the youngsters weep or grunt unintelligibly; most make no sound at all."

Other wards hold seriously disturbed adults, some of whom are violent, under conditions that "would have made Bedlam look inviting." Greatly understaffed, the attendants caring for large numbers of these agitated patients have all they can do to prevent them from hurting themselves or each other. A rather revolting statistic indicative of the lack of sufficient staff is the fact that of 125 patients who died of various causes in 1970, nine choked on their own vomit before attendants could reach them.

In attempting to account for the tremendous overcrowding in this institution and others like it, *Time* reports that most of the patients are there because there is no place else for them to go. Most experts argue for small centers where patients can receive intensive attention from teachers, therapists, and physicians. Moreover, they recommend that the vast majority of mental retardates be treated in day schools while living at home with their families. In most states, however, such facilities do not exist. This report closes on the futile note that "Willowbrook, despite its well-advertised horrors, has a list of 1,000 awaiting admission."

The Myth of Mental Retardation

In their recent book *Hansels and Gretels: Studies of Children in Institutions for the Mentally Retarded*, Braginsky and Braginsky (1971) describe the ways labels such as "mentally retarded" or "mentally ill" are used to exonerate parents and society for putting these children away in "warehouses for human debris." In their view, most people found in institutions for the mentally retarded are not stupid or inadequate but instead are quite resourceful and competent human beings. Extensive surveys of the backgrounds of institutionalized children revealed that most of them were sent to institutions mainly because of family disintegration and rejection rather than because of their own mental defects. These authors conclude that "the concept of mental retardation must be discarded entirely." According to them, this concept is actually a myth used to camouflage the true picture and to enable society to avoid facing the real problems that must be resolved.

While very critical of present institutional treatment of retardates, Braginsky and Braginsky recognize that many of these unwanted children need some form of living arrangement other than their own homes. They propose the establishment of "cooperative retreats" that would be very different from the impersonal understaffed institutions currently designed to care for masses of unfortunate people in a manner that now ensures perpetuation of the myth of mental deficiency.

The Issues

In the powerful opening paper in this chapter, George W. Albee recommends rehabilitative training, not medical treatment, for the majority of today's retardates. This past president of the American Psychological Association believes that federal funds are misappropriated when spent for bigger, medically oriented facilities for the masses of people who become institutionalized for most of their lives. According to Albee, the lack of emphasis on training retardates to become self-sufficient is largely attributable to the tragic misconception that mental retardation is an inherited or acquired disease.

The paper by Christopher Connolly is concerned with much broader issues than those restricted to problems of mental retardation. It is devoted to children who experience learning difficulties and fail in school for varied reasons. While some of these school failures may be attributable to intellectual deficits, there are also many others who possess adequate intelligence but suffer from other difficulties. A specific issue in this paper pertains to the relationship between learning disabilities and emotional disturbance. Most writers assume that they are positively associated, but Connolly disagrees with this. He points to the difficulties in conducting research on this topic and reports that few studies have attempted to validate the opinions presented in the literature. Connolly also describes inadequacies of the traditional psychiatric model used in studying children with learning problems.

Thus, this paper provides considerable food for thought for those who work with learning-disabled children.

The topic of special education is directly pertinent to the concerns of this chapter; much of the impetus for the development of this specialty stems from the nation's rather belated recognition that education of the retarded had been sorely neglected. In recent years, the federal government and most state governments have passed legislation requiring that educable retardates be taught in public schools, thus requiring the training of teachers who should be specially qualified for working with these and other exceptional children.

In the final paper in this chapter, Lloyd M. Dunn, a past president of The Council for Exceptional Children, presents his view that special education for the educable mentally retarded has been morally and educationally wrong. After devoting more than 20 years to promoting special classes for exceptional children, Dunn reached the conclusion that educators should stop the expansion of special education programs that have proved to be undesirable for many of the children they are dedicated to serve. The issues raised by Dunn are concerned not only with the retarded but with special education of children labeled emotionally disturbed, perceptually impaired, brain injured, and learning disordered.

Additional issues pertaining to treatment of children with learning difficulties and school adjustment problems are included in Chapter Eight, on drug therapy. It is hoped that reading this controversial material will make those who now work in the field or those who are contemplating careers as teachers realize that educators of exceptional children have a long way to go, probably in directions quite different from those followed in the recent past.

References

Blatt, B., & Kaplan, F. *Christmas in purgatory: A photographic essay on mental retardation*. Boston: Allyn & Bacon, 1966.

Braginsky, D. D., & Braginsky, R. M. *Hansels and Gretels: Studies of children in institutions for the mentally retarded*. New York: Holt, Rinehart & Winston, 1971.

Clarizio, H. F., & McCoy, G. F. *Behavior disorders in school-aged children*. Scranton, Penn.: Chandler, 1970.

Human Warehouse. *Time*, 1972, February 14, 67, 69.

Kessler, J. W. *Psychopathology of childhood*. Englewood Cliffs, N. J.: Prentice-Hall, 1966.

Kirk, S. A. Illinois Test of Psycholinguistic Abilities: Its origins and implications. In J. Hellmuth (Ed.), *Learning disorders*. Vol. 3. Seattle, Wash.: Special Child Publications, 1968.

McDonald, C. W. Problems concerning the classification and education of children with learning disabilities. In J. Hellmuth (Ed.), *Learning disorders*. Vol. 3. Seattle, Wash.: Special Child Publications, 1968.

Myklebust, H. R., & Johnson, D. Dyslexia in children. *Exceptional Children*, 1962, **29**, 14–25.

Robinson, H. B., & Robinson, N. M. *The mentally retarded child: A psychological approach*. New York: McGraw-Hill, 1965.

18. A Revolution in Treatment of the Retarded

George W. Albee

Nearly 6,000,000 Americans are mentally handicapped. By 1970, the number will reach almost 6,500,000. A retarded child is born every four minutes; 126,000 will be born this year.

Largely because of the deep personal interest of President Kennedy, in recent years there has been considerable activity to help the retarded. Since 1963, federal funds for research and training have increased at an unprecedented rate. Unfortunately, most of these funds are not being used to help the majority of the retarded—those who are normally slow, not victims of inherited or acquired diseases. Instead, money is being poured into costly biomedical research centers and "treatment" clinics to help a minority—those who are retarded because of organic reasons, like injuries, trauma, infections and biochemical imbalances.

The majority of the retarded need, not medical treatment, but rehabilitative training—so they can use their maximum potential. While every promising research lead should be pursued, and every significant effort in the whole field of retardation should be supported, a truly generous part of the new federal funds ought to be invested in research aimed at helping the retarded lead lives as normal as possible. And more funds should be spent to train people who will, in turn, help train the majority of the retarded.

At the root of this error in priorities is a tragic misconception—namely, that mental retardation is an inherited or acquired disease. Recently, for example, the National Institute of Child Health and Human Development announced that it was allocating new funds for research centers whose purpose will be to 1) discover organic causes of retardation and 2) mount medical efforts to reduce its incidence. The Institute's press release went on: "Inherited diseases are among the leading causes of mental retardation." On May 16, 1967, the U.S. Public Health Service announced a grant for the construction of a $2.2 million center for medical research at a Midwestern university. Its press release stated:

> Several research studies will be aimed at identifying metabolic abnormalities in patients with unknown causes of mental retardation. Through biochemical studies of the urine, blood, and tissues of retarded patients, defects or absences of necessary biologic metabolic enzymes may be uncovered, paving the way for new attacks on mental retardation.

Between the lines of both statements is the promise that the incidence of retardation, because of such medically oriented research, may be significantly reduced. This promise is based on ignorance—or on a distortion of reality.

The truth is that most retardation is *not* an inherited disease. Quite correctly, President Kennedy's Panel on Mental Retardation emphasized the fact that

> ... about 75 percent to 85 percent of those now diagnosed as retarded show no demonstrable gross brain abnormality. They are, by and large, persons with relatively mild degrees of retardation.... Unfavorable environmental and psychological influences are thought to play an important contributory role among this group. Such influences include interference with normal emotional and intellectual stimulation in early infancy, unfavorable psychological or emotional experiences in early childhood, and lack of normal intellectual and cultural experiences during the entire developmental period.

More basically, brightness and dullness are a reflection of inherited capacities—the result of the interaction of a large number of genes operating in a perfectly normal, nonpathological way. While intelligence is thus genetically determined, so is a person's height—and neither stature *nor* mental retardation is an illness.

People are born retarded simply because intelligence is distributed normally throughout the entire population. A certain percentage of all children—slightly more than 2 percent, as it happens—will be born without defect and yet have I.Q.s below 70. Similarly, a certain percentage—also 2 percent—will be born with an I.Q. as high as that of the average graduate student.

Edward Zigler of Yale put it this way:

> We need simply to accept the generally recognized fact that the gene pool of any population is such that there will always be variations in the behavioral... expression of virtually every measurable trait or characteristic of man. From the polygenic model advanced by geneticists, we deduce that the distribution of intelligence is characterized by a bisymmetrical bell-shaped curve....
>
> Once one adopts the position that the familial mental retardate is not defective or pathological but is essentially a normal individual of low intelligence, then the familial retardate no longer represents a mystery but, rather, is viewed as a particular manifestation of the general developmental process.

This point has crucial implications. It illuminates the inappropriateness of our present priorities, whereby 90 to 95 percent of the federal construction funds for retardation centers will be used to house research and training on biomedical approaches. It says the large majority of retarded children and adults are *not* retarded because of an acquired physiological abnormality, or because of a defect in their metabolism, or because of brain injury, or because their mothers had German measles, or because of the effects of any other infectious disease, or because of any other discovered or undiscovered exogenous or biomedical defects.

Rather, the majority of retarded children and adults are produced from the more or less accidental distribution of polygenic factors present in the entire human race. Each parent transmits—often untouched—a large and varied set of genetic potentials from his myriad ancestors to his descendants. Thus each human is potentially the parent or grandparent or great-grandparent of a retarded child. Because of various forms of gene linkage, "familial" retardation is somewhat less common in bright families than in dull families. It occurs most commonly in "average" families—because there are many more of them.

The cold, but realistic, fact must be faced: It is no more likely that medical research findings will raise the intelligence of most retardates than it is that research will raise the intelligence of college students.

Let me make it very clear that I am not opposing medical research, or deprecating the triumphs of biology and medicine in uncovering the causes of several (albeit rare) forms of retardation in the past decade or so. What I am arguing against is the almost exclusive investment of federal monies in medically-oriented research. For the plain truth is that, even after all the post-conception organic causes and all the metabolic and chromosomal defects are discovered and prevented or corrected, at least 2 percent of the general population will *still* be born retarded. And this situation will prevail for the indefinite future.

I believe, therefore, that it is not only unfair but unreasonable that almost every new federally funded, university-affiliated center to train people and to engage in research in this field is in a medically-dominated and biomedically-oriented center. Even in the Mental Retardation Research Centers being funded by the new National Institute of Child Health and Human Development, the major efforts are biomedical. Instead, at least half of these centers should be designed for research in special educational methods and rehabilitation; others should be designed primarily for research in the social and behavioral-science approaches to helping the retarded.

Why is the emphasis, both in research and in treatment, on organic approaches to retardation? One reason: the academic medical institutions' insatiable need for research money. Because of the enormous federal funds recently made available for constructing research and training facilities in the area of retardation, medicine—particularly psychiatry and pediatrics—has discovered and promulgated compelling arguments why these research centers should be placed in medical settings. Almost exclusive emphasis has been on all of the external causes of retardation—the metabolic, the infectious, the undiscovered causes of brain damage. In addition, by controlling the advisory committees that rule on applications for construction funds to build the university-affiliated facilities, the doctors have controlled the character of these centers still further.

Another reason: The powerful citizens' committees in the field of retardation are composed largely of well-informed parents of retarded children. But in these families, normal garden-variety retardation is relatively rare. These parents, from the numerically small but politically advantaged upper-middle classes and upper classes, are more likely to have children who are retarded because of *exogenous* damage than because of normal polygenic inheritance. Their retarded children are more likely to be represented in the below-50 I.Q. group of the seriously-handicapped than among the much more common 50–70 I.Q. group. As a consequence, these citizens' committees militate for biomedical discoveries that will prevent, or cure, exogenous retardation. Their aspirations coincide with the eagerness of academic medicine to have large, expensive research labs. Both groups push legislation—and the rules implementing legislation—in the direction of an overwhelming emphasis on biomedical research.

There are still other reasons to explain the over-emphasis on biological or injury explanations of retardation.

In child-worshipping American society, and particularly in the great sprawling suburban areas, parents are gravely concerned about the academic success of their children. Their children's scores on intelligence tests are therefore exceedingly important to these parents. And when a parent is told that his child tests at the 135-I.Q. level, his response is a feeling of pride, even elation. It means that Johnny can go far, that a society that rewards intellectual success (not necessarily achievement) will eventually be at his feet.

But consider the parent who is told that his child is functioning at a 65-I.Q. level and must be placed in a special class for slow-learners. After his original shock and panic have subsided somewhat, the parent begins to cast about for an explanation. What could have happened? What accident, injury or disease could have caused this terrible thing?

Now, two currently popular diagnoses for mentally deficient children are *minimal brain damage*, or *maturational lag*. The trouble is that the neurological and psychological tests upon which these diagnoses are based leave much to be desired. Nevertheless, one or the other of these diagnoses is made with increasing frequency, perhaps because they are very useful to give to parents who somehow feel personally responsible for a retarded child and seize upon such a diagnosis as an exculpation.

It is difficult for a pediatrician, a psychiatrist or a consulting psychologist to tell parents their child is just slow mentally, and not because of illness, disease or exogenous damage. Similarly, one of the most difficult diagnoses for parents in our society to accept is that their child is normal and has a limited intellectual capacity. No special explanation is required for a child who is bright—he "just comes by that naturally." But when a child is slow intellectually, something must have happened. Thus the diagnosis of minimal brain damage, or maturational lag, has great psychological appeal. Most parents can recall an illness or accident at some point in the child's life, or in the expectant mother's. This is certainly an easier explanation to accept, in an extremely painful situation, than garden-variety, normal retardation. Nor is it hard to understand that such a parent's desire to "do something" leads to still more support of biomedical research.

Whatever the reasons for its origin, the imbalance in the field of mental retardation should be remedied swiftly—if our society truly believes that everyone should have the opportunity to develop his potential to the maximum. We need social and educational research into retardation as much—or more—than we need biological and medical research. What follows is just one example of a recent significant study involving teachers, children and intelligence (Robert Rosenthal and Lenore Jacobsen, 1967).

At the beginning of the school year, intelligence tests were given to children in a city school of 18 classrooms (three at each grade level from first to sixth). By pre-arranged plan, the teachers in the school were told that the tests measured potential for "intellectual blooming." One child in five—chosen at random—in each classroom was said to have scored high on the test. This child, the teacher was told, very probably would show marked intellectual improvement within the next several months.

Eight months later, at the end of the school year, another intelligence test was given. The specially-identified children in the first and second grades had made dramatic improvements. In first grade, the average gain was more than 15 points; in the second grade, more than ten points. In actuality, these children had been randomly chosen for identification. Yet, by some mysterious alchemy, the teachers had behaved in such a way toward these young children, who were designated as special, as to elicit more of their basic potential.

This study illustrates how research can clarify a point that is of crucial importance in planning educational experiences for intellectually handicapped youngsters. The point made in the study is that teachers with the right attitudes and expectations are of critical importance—and can have a significant effect on the development of the child's capacity to its fullest. This is the sort of research we need more of!

Too often we approach the task of teaching retarded children with the expectation that they will not, or cannot, learn. We have not yet begun to tap much of the potential of these children, a potential that might be unlocked not only with new techniques but with new expectations. Such insights and progress, of course, will *not* result from our exclusive reliance on biological research.

But it is not only research efforts that are out of balance. So are efforts at rehabilitation.

For example, the Children's Bureau of the Department of Health, Education and Welfare has struggled painfully—for 11 years—to develop 134 clinics across the nation for the retarded. These clinics ostensibly are operated to demonstrate the value of biomedically-oriented treatment that uses a so-called multi-disciplinary approach. As J. William Oberman (technical adviser on Medical Aspects of Mental Retardation for the Children's Bureau) notes somewhat plaintively, these 134 clinics are able to offer only a very small fraction of the amount of care needed by the retarded and their families. He estimates that each year some 30,000 individuals are served by these clinics and that perhaps "other multidisciplinary clinics under medical direction" provide care for an additional 10,000 retarded children. But this is a trifle compared with the needs of the 6 million retarded children and adults in the United States. Dr. Oberman notes that even 2,500 new clinics (as impossible to staff as 2,500 new major-league baseball teams!) could barely handle the present demand. And the demand keeps increasing. Unmet needs grow. Of what profit is it to demonstrate that an expensive treatment clinic, expertly staffed with high-priced professionals, can see a handful of children a year with modest effectiveness, when it is impossible ever to duplicate such clinics? How long will Congress stand still for this nonsense?

The justification for these clinics having medical direction and treatment (largely unavailable full-time) rests on two highly emotional arguments. One, as we have seen, stresses the pathological or accidental—and theoretically preventable—causes of a high percentage of the severely retarded. The second stresses the concomitant additional physical handicaps, which are alleged to require continuing diagnostic follow-up and medical care.

The truth is that 85 percent of the retarded, after thorough medical evaluation, ordinarily require no more medical care than many other handicapped groups in society. The associated physical complications that are correctable, in a majority of cases, are visual and auditory—outside the competence of the ordinary psychiatrist or pediatrician. A significant number of retardates also have speech problems, and these demand the special skills of a speech therapist rather than a physician.

The kind of professional manpower required for effective and functional care of the retarded is not more physicians, nurses and psychologists with highly specialized training in this field. These people do not spend any significant amount of their professional time working with the retarded anyway. More than anything else, we need teachers and vocational-guidance specialists.

According to the President's Panel, a very large majority of the retarded "can, with special training and assistance, acquire limited job skills and achieve a high measure of independence; they represent 85 percent of the retarded group." Yet many states even now do not provide any classes for the "trainable" retarded, and no state has enough classes for the "educable" retarded. Only one of every five retarded children is now being reached by any kind of special-education program. The President's Panel found 20,000 special-education teachers across the nation, many of them poorly trained, where 55,000 were needed. The panel predicted that by 1970 the need for special teachers will reach 90,000. And state vocational agencies that provide urgently-needed vocational rehabilitation for the mildly retarded are currently reaching only 3 percent of them.

In one investigation in Massachusetts, Simon Olshansky studied over 1,000 children whose families were receiving aid for dependent children. He found that 6.7 percent were retarded. Virtually none were getting any significant help. The mothers were "too immobilized" to recognize the problem, or to seek help. Social agencies, as is frequently the case, had no workers to reach out and seek cases that would add to their excessive caseloads.

To provide adequate help to the 110,000 children born each year with mild but handicapping retardation, and to provide care and rehabilitation for the other 5,500,000 mildly retarded people in our society, we need teachers, teachers and more teachers—and then taxes to support a massive educational effort. Among teachers in this context I include all those specially trained and devoted professional people willing to spend hours and hours in daily and patient interaction with retarded children, unlocking and strengthening whatever skills and abilities are in them. Also included are the vocational-rehabilitation workers and those in occupational therapy, in recreational therapy and in nonprofessional but patient and warm interaction therapies that the retarded yearn for.

Needed desperately, in addition to teachers, are skilled caseworkers, sheltered-workshop personnel, vocational-guidance counselors, speech therapists, and all of the range of other people who have chosen careers that make them their handicapped brother's keeper. Many of these people could be trained in bachelor's or even two-year junior-college programs.

But, first and foremost, it is essential to escape the biomedical orientation that controls our efforts. Fourteen university-affiliated facilities for the retarded, all devoted to research and training, have now been approved for construction with federal funds. The federal government already has allocated the millions of dollars to build these research centers. Every last one of them is in a medical setting where most of the research, the research training, and the education of professionals will be relevant to a small minority of retarded children. What have these huge new research centers to do with training special-education teachers and vocational counselors? The answer: next to nothing.

There *is* a place where medical care is truly needed to prevent retardation, and where it has not been available—in the prenatal and perinatal care of "medically indigent" expectant mothers in our large cities. A significant number of their children are born prematurely, and the prematurity rate is two to three times greater in low-income families where prenatal care is haphazard. Almost 500,000 indigent mothers deliver babies each year in our tax-supported city hospitals. At least 100,000 of these need special medical services for complications in pregnancy and birth. Most of them do not get it.

Here is an area for good medical research and action, because mental retardation that may well have an organic base is associated with prematurity and low birth weight. Among infants who weigh below three pounds at birth, nearly three-quarters subsequently develop physical or mental defects. In an average big-city hospital, the baby girl born to a Negro mother on the "staff service" (free service) weighs nearly a pound less than the baby born to a suburban white mother on the private service of the general hospital. A large percentage of urban indigent Negro mothers are "walk-ins" who receive little or no prenatal care, no special instructions on diet, and no medical guidance until labor pains begin. The retardation rate in infants born to these indigent mothers is ten times the white rate.

If American medicine were to turn its massive resources to the solution of these problems—adequate medical care for the poor—many more cases of retardation could be prevented than will result from the present emphasis on research into esoteric causes. Unfortunately, the growing shortage of physicians, the fee-for-service philosophy of American medicine, and the high prestige of complex research activities in academia all combine to make this significant prevention effort unlikely.

At the root of our double standard of care and intervention with the retarded is the fact that the nice people—the people who do the planning, the governing, the writing, the reading and the decision-making in our society—are members of the economically favored group. Most of them have arranged their lives in such a way as to be sealed off—geographically and socially—from the have-not groups, the disadvantaged and the dispossessed.

But parents of the retarded—parent-citizen groups in particular—are, for the most part, prosperous, and they at least have the advantage of some special insights into some of the darker social forces in our society. Most of them know from personal experience the hardships and heartaches that are the lot of the child or adult in our society who has limited intellectual capacity. Such citizen groups must take the lead in demanding that at least half of the tax dollars be spent for educational and rehabilitative approaches for all our intellectually-handicapped children and adults.

Our efforts are out of balance and out of joint. It is only an informed citizenry that can study the facts and act on them. The retarded cannot speak for themselves.

19. Social and Emotional Factors in Learning Disabilities

Christopher Connolly

Every culture has an unwritten list of valued traits, beliefs and motives that it expects its members to possess (Mussen, Conger, and Kagan, 1969). Among the most highly valued of these traits in contemporary American society are success and achievement. If an individual desires to reap the greatest rewards our culture bestows on its members—recognition, wealth, and power—it usually is necessary for him to achieve high goals and to surpass the expectations that society holds for him.

The goals a person strives for are determined largely by his role, which defines what behaviors are expected of him. For example, the role of father traditionally involves being head of the family and bread-winner. Tasks are structured clearly for him: he is supposed to hold a job, provide sustenance, make major decisions, protect the family, and so forth. The mother's position has evolved in recent years, but in the immediate past she was expected

From H. R. Myklebust (Ed.) *Progress in Learning Disabilities*. Vol. II. Copyright 1971 by Grune & Stratton, Inc. Reproduced by permission.

to be in the home, to raise children, and to provide strength for her husband and nurturance for her children. The child also has a role, which varies according to age; but perhaps his major task, at least between the ages of 5 and 16, is to attend school and to achieve, to succeed and to bring credit on himself and on his family. The child's role demands that he master the basic school subjects and that he learn certain skills as required in American society. The acquiring of these academic skills is thus one of the primary problems facing him.

During the first years of life the family is the main instrument in the child's education and socialization. At age five, though, he leaves his home and enters school; from that time until midadolescence this institution plays an essential role in shaping his total development. Parents retain considerable influence over their children, but now share with the school the responsibility for educating and socializing their offspring to an almost immeasurable degree.

This institution's role has expanded due to the advent of compulsory education laws mandating that all youths must be exposed to formal education for most of their childhood and adolescence. Hence, during the 11-year period covered by most state laws, a child is required to attend school. Because his education involves such an extensive period of time, the school experience becomes a tremendously vital factor in a child's life. How a youngster fares here, both academically and socially, is most influential in determining his later life style. If he fails to master basic subjects we can say with a high degree of probability that he will not hold an esteemed position in our societal structure; he will neither attain high status nor achieve substantial material rewards.

In an achievement-oriented culture, in which successful performance of one's role is paramount, the effects of nonsuccess can be both extensive and intensive. For members of any society, failure can have far-reaching consequences that may become permanent. To illustrate, the child who is chronically defeated in school, who drops out at age 16 after completing only seventh grade, is likely to have an awesome task in reaching high adult goals and in satisfying high adult needs. His academic failure as a child thus limits his future attainments as an adult and, more than likely, predetermines that he will live a life far different from that which he and his family originally had hoped for. In a real sense, then, the child who fails in school is denied an education and all of the economic and cultural benefits that follow. He is deprived of many of the rewards of society because he has been defeated by his school experience.

The child with a learning disability fails in school and, not infrequently, is thoroughly defeated by his academic endeavors. Due to his inability to function satisfactorily in his role as a student, many of his drives are frustrated and many of his needs go unmet. Because this youngster does not conform to societal expectations, he may experience grave difficulties that go far beyond academic learning. The following discussion examines some of the emotional problems and needs that the child with a learning disability encounters.

Difficulties in Researching the Topic

When reviewing the literature concerning the relationship between learning disorders and emotional problems, an interesting phenomenon becomes apparent. Many authors have addressed themselves to this topic, and the consensus is that a positive relationship exists between the two variables. "It has long been recognized that reading disabilities are accompanied by special behavior disorders" (Bender, 1956, p. 134). "Few cases of learning disorders are without emotional difficulties" (Bryant, 1966, p. 271). "The individual who fails constantly . . . is in a chronic state of emotional upset" (Fernald, 1943, p. 7). "Among cases of severe reading disability, about 75% show personality maladjustment" (Gates, 1941, p. 83). "Insofar as children with learning disabilities have poor perceptual or other organic problems, the child by definition has an ego defect" (Giffen, 1968, p. 76). "Among (severe) reading disability cases . . . close to 100% showed maladjustment of some kind" (Harris, 1970, p. 265). "Almost all children with reading disabilities suffer from some kind of personality difficulty" (Natchez, 1968, p. 26). "It is evident that children with marked incompetence in an area so vital (as reading) . . . will suffer inordinately" (Rabinovitch, 1962, p. 78).

However, despite the numerous statements concerning this issue, relatively few writers have attempted to validate their opinions. Furthermore, of those who have sought to provide hard research data to verify their beliefs, many have obtained primarily nonsignificant findings when comparing personality variables of an experimental group of learning-disability subjects with a control group of normals (Connolly, 1969; Myklebust and Boshes, 1969; Goldstein, 1970). Thus, the majority of writers in the field seem to believe that learning disorders and emotional problems are related, yet there is a paucity of research evidence to substantiate these beliefs. Harris (1970, p. 265) summarizes the situation by noting that "While case studies of children often reveal intimate connections between the child's emotional difficulties and his reading difficulties, research studies comparing the personalities of poor readers with good readers have failed to reveal any consistent group differences."

One aspect of the difficulty in researching this topic lies in the semantic confusion. An investigator encounters a dilemma when attempting to employ such classifications as "emotional disturbance" or "psychosocial adjustment." These terms are difficult to define because the conditions designated do not lend themselves to precise quantitative determination. We have no exact means of ascertaining when a child is conflicted or disturbed and when he is not. Emotional malfunctioning is largely an intangible and relative condition based on social norms. The term *emotionally disturbed* actually is derived from a statistical not a psychological concept. In our society normality is distributed along a bell-shaped curve and anything that deviates excessively from the median is considered abnormal. Thus a well-adjusted American youngster of today might be thought disturbed if he were living in a primitive African society, or even in nineteenth-century America. In other words, patterns of behavior and thought cannot be judged as either well adjusted or emotionally disturbed in and of themselves. It is necessary to take a broad view and to consider the youngster and his behavior in the context of his social milieu and culture.

Maladjustment is a subjective phenomenon and as such it connotes different meanings to different people at different times. This lack of agreement may be a major cause of erroneous diagnoses and ineffectual treatment, resulting in minimal therapeutic value. Because of the semantic confusion, or perhaps in addition to it, we often do not have valid criteria for determining emotional difficulties. The problem of obtaining suitable criteria is a formidable one and is shared by many other areas of psychology. Associated with the obstacles of semantics and criteria is the awesome task of assembling a homogeneous sample of learning-disabled subjects. Children with these disorders are, in many ways, an exceedingly heterogeneous group. They do possess some similarities, such as academic deficiencies, but in many instances they are very unlike one another and hence defy neat, accurate classification. Gross errors may occur when children with learning disabilities are all squeezed into a pigeonhole and then studied experimentally. Sample selection is a difficult chore and undoubtedly has contributed to some of the confusion found in the literature.

Another serious obstacle in researching this area is that our instruments for determining adjustment are poorly developed. The best of these measures are subjective and traditionally have received much criticism, frequently violent but unfortunately often justified. This predicament is partially a result of the subject matter we are attempting to examine. Man's emotional condition is largely an amorphous entity, constantly changing, developing, and being altered in an intangible fashion. We must expect our instruments, therefore, to be less than perfect because of the nebulous characteristics of that which we purport to measure. The literature provides little verification for the experimental effectiveness of the Rorschach, Thematic Apperception Test, Human Figure Drawings, and other popular personality tests. It does seem possible that an experienced clinician, working with a single child, can derive useful and valid information from projective methods. However, attempting to utilize these same techniques experimentally, when much of the clinician's experience, subjective judgment, and "feel" for his tests are negated because he is working with experimental groups instead of individuals, has proved to be a largely fruitless effort. At the present time, though, these are the best instruments we have and hence the ones we must employ.

In summary, the general impression received from a review of the literature is that a positive correlation exists between emotional problems and learning disabilities. This position is not held by all authorities, although it appears as the majority view. Because of the obstacles involved in conducting sound research in this area, it is not surprising to find contradictory opinions and studies whose results are inconclusive or unclear. Few definitive statements can be made because the percentage of emotional problems and maladjustment reported by a particular investigator varies with the standards he uses, as well as with the type of population studied. In considering the literature, perhaps Orton (1937, p. 132) summarized it best more than

30 years ago when he said, "No generalization is possible concerning the appearance of emotional disturbance."

Inadequacy of the Traditional Psychiatric Model

Children have been failing in school for as long as these institutions have existed. Children also have been experiencing learning disabilities for as long as they have been failing, although it is not until recent years that we have begun to apply this diagnostic term. To paraphrase Ebbinghaus's famous statement concerning psychology, "Learning Disabilities has a long past but only a short history." Although an infant in terms of scientific specialties, this discipline has made important contributions to the general area of child study and has provided a vital new framework from which to view children.

In the past a youngster of average intelligence who failed in school usually was thought to have an emotional problem. Even today the majority of cases who come to child guidance clinics are referred because of a school problem (Rabinovitch, 1959; Hatton, 1966). Hence, for years, in practice, even if not in theory, there has been a tacit assumption that learning disorders and emotional problems are related. Clements and Peters (1962, p. 185) report:

> For many years it has been the custom among child guidance workers to attribute the behavioral and learning deviations seen in children almost exclusively to the rearing patterns and interpersonal relations experienced by such youngsters. In many clinics it has become habitual to assume psychogenicity when no easily recognizable organic deviation can be found.

Today, however, more children who previously were thought to be emotional problems or slow learners are being considered differently. Behavioral scientists have broadened their scope and understanding and have come to realize that these youngsters are neither disturbed nor retarded but rather are handicapped as a result of a learning disability associated with minimal brain dysfunction. The cerebral dysfunction frequently is of a relatively minor nature neurologically, so it does not draw attention to itself. Though the child with this deficit appears normal in most respects, he is unable to learn as well or as rapidly as his parents and teachers believe he should. In the past he might have been diagnosed as a behavior problem or as a youngster who could not achieve because of some psychological factor that interfered with the learning process. It might have been said that the child was rebelling against his parents by refusing to read, or showing his insecurity in peer relationships by failing to master arithmetic. Alternative explanations might have emphasized inadequate instructional methods, inferior teaching, or mental subnormality.

It is assumed and verified, both clinically and experimentally, that learning problems can arise from all these causes. However, during recent years evidence has been accumulating that illustrates the gross inadequacy of conceptualizing learning disorders as simply a manifestation of an underlying emotional disturbance. Instead of sending a youngster off to a child guidance clinic as the first referral for school failure, there is now a distinct trend to consider organic factors, in addition to psychological ones. Hatton (1966) feels that a sizable proportion of children who are referred to a typical guidance facility for emotional problems show evidence of minimal brain dysfunction. Boder (1966) states that more children are being referred to pediatric neurologists today rather than being sent directly to psychiatrists. Natchez (1968) adds that whereas psychodynamic etiology was prevalent in the recent past, neurological explanations have increased in popularity of late.

In light of recent discoveries in the field, the inaccuracies and limitations of the traditional psychiatric framework have become apparent. An example of the explanations put forth to explain reading difficulties in psychodynamic terms is found in Sylvester and Kunst (1943). These authors feel that if parents thwart an infant's early curiosity and exploratory behavior he may learn to perceive these activities as threatening to his acceptance and love. Therefore, in order to maintain his parental relationship he shuts off these drives. Consequently, in the future any exploration of new situations may become mixed with danger and anxiety. When he enters school, then, the new experience of reading can become associated with similar anxiety, and thus the child feels safer in avoiding the unknown (that is, reading) rather than in dealing with it. These authors feel that the youngster's fear of losing his parents' affection causes his fear of learning to read. They go on to explain hesitations in reading as being caused by the desire of the child to cling to his present position (the last word he read) and his fear of moving on to the next unknown position (the following word). Similarly, reading that is too rapid is seen as an attempt to take the "dangerous position" by storm and with a shout.

A traditional psychoanalytic viewpoint of learning problems interprets them as resulting from the child's failure to identify with his parents, peers, or teachers (Pearson, 1954). Under this framework the youngster may hate or fear someone in his environment so much that he cannot learn. In other cases, a child may feel too inadequate to risk competition, he may secretly wish to retaliate against those who exploit him, or he may manifest a need not to know.

It is granted that some children who exhibit learning deficiencies are conflicted and do possess the neurotic fears and traits described in the psychodynamically oriented literature. However, to assume that all, or even most, of the children with learning disabilities fit into this conceptual framework is inaccurate at best, and grossly dangerous and unjust at worst. An example of the hazards involved in this type of thinking is found in Daniels (1964). This psychoanalyst writes of a child with a learning disability: "Usually, too, he shows himself quite capable of learning outside the classroom; only *he chooses* the time, the place, and the subject matter. . . . Whatever his outward behavior, *he tenaciously refuses* to avail himself of the opportunities afforded by formal education" (italics added).

Here lies the danger of the psychoanalytic model. The child is seen as refusing to achieve and as choosing when and what he will learn. Daniels's description of the situation implies that the youngster has a choice between achieving and failing; he infers that the child's attainment is under his own control. What must be the consequences of viewing a true learning disability from this framework? How do parents react when presented with this explanation of their child's problems? The indiscriminate application of this psychoanalytic model must evitably lead to frustration, anxiety, guilt, and hostility. It is little wonder that the cure rate for psychotherapy is so unconvincing and unimpressive (Eysenck, 1961).

A second drawback to this model is that learning problems due to psychological factors may clear up as soon as the emotional difficulty is cured, but disabilities arising from minimal brain dysfunction do not go away so quickly. Because of this important difference, people who send a child with a learning problem to a child guidance clinic, with the hope that the emotional block to learning will be removed, often are disappointed when the youngster does not show rapid academic gains. Rabinovitch (1962, p. 73) feels the unrealistic expectancy that the emotional block will be eradicated has "been fostered in part by the attitude of some of our colleagues in child psychiatry and related fields who have been prone to overgeneralize dynamic formulations."

Another psychiatrist has some relevant comments based on his own personal experiences while consulting in a psychiatric setting (Stein, 1969, pp. 458–461):

> Here I met adolescents who could not be considered mentally retarded or schizophrenic, but who had gross deficits in language, number concepts, and marked difficulties in perceptual-motor functions. Here were phenomena that I could not readily consider under the more familiar rubric of intrapsychic or interpersonal dynamics. These problems were so far removed from what I felt to be the psychodynamic sphere that I could not even label them as broadly as I have done here, let alone define or conceptualize them. . . .

> I felt quite inadequate to the task of understanding these phenomena which had such obvious relevance to emotional maturity and well-being. There was no provision for this situation in my psychiatric training. The analytic framework . . . seemed too general and not readily applicable to the specific phenomena I was witnessing. . . .

> I wondered how many learning problems I had missed, or what, to the children, were the emotional consequences of those problems which I had squeezed to fit the dynamic model of intrafamilial relationships, and which I had treated accordingly, achieving in many instances only questionable results.

The purpose here is not to discredit the work of Freud and others in the field. Freud's emphasis on the importance of childhood experiences in influencing later adult personality, his work with the defense mechanisms, and his unsurpassed contributions to personality theory and psychopathology need not be belabored here. Nonetheless, the grave dangers of trying to fit all children with learning disabilities into a strict psychodynamic mold must be pointed out. Child psychiatry since Freud has developed a traditional and very strongly psychoanalytic bias (Kurlander and Colodny, 1969). Thus, it is neither unreasonable nor unexpected that professionals trained in psychodynamics will tend to find dynamically oriented problems in their patients. This points to the real need to educate professionals and parents to recognize the signs of a learning disability. Hatton (1966) stresses that teachers, for example, are inclined to categorize all disorders as emotional though experimental evidence for the organic basis of many of these disorders continues to accumulate from all directions. Likewise, parents at the earliest sign of serious trouble think first of the psychiatrist and only much later consider alternatives such as learning disabilities or speech and hearing problems as the source of their child's condition. There is a need for professionals and parents to realize that many childhood anomalies have organic, not simply psychological, elements.

In summary, the traditional psychiatric framework is believed to be inadequate for learning disabilities; furthermore, this model can produce harmful effects in some cases. The phenomenon of self-fulfilling prophecies and the results of therapy in which there is little relationship between disorder and treatment method are well known. This is not to say that psychiatry has no role in the field of learning disabilities. Some of these youngsters do require psychiatric intervention, just as do some members of any population, whether it be comprised of deaf, retarded, culturally deprived, or "normal" individuals. The majority of disabled children could profit from exposure to certain select psychotherapeutic methods, as will be described later, but relatively few require the traditional psychiatric effort....

Responses to Several Critical Problems

Need for Understanding: Family

It would seem that one of the greatest unmet needs of the child with a learning disability is the need to be understood. Many people in his environment, himself included, are not aware of the source of his disorder and mistakenly believe him to be a behavior problem, or of limited intelligence, or simply lazy and unmotivated. Because of the total lack of understanding that frequently surrounds the learning problem, many unfortunate consequences may arise that affect the child's social and emotional functioning. Parents become angry with the youngster and develop guilt feelings, school personnel give up on him and place him in the slowest track, the child himself develops a poor self-image and becomes frustrated and anxious.

This pervasive lack of understanding is a serious problem and one that inevitably leads to less than optimal treatment. In clinical work it is typical to find families who have been making the rounds of local clinics, agencies, and assorted private "experts" for years in their search for answers and guidance. The parents often are bewildered, and it is not unusual to discover a great amount of confusion and helplessness. They have been living with a serious problem for many years and usually have been unable to find competent help or, as in many cases, even to determine what the primary problem is. To exist year after year in a state of confusion and uncertainty is an exceedingly anxiety-provoking condition. This manner of existence burdens a family with chronic pressure and not infrequently, contributes to an unhappy and tense home environment.

Although the field of learning disabilities is young, although much is not known concerning these disorders, and although remedial facilities often are not available even if the problem is diagnosed correctly, there still remains a great need to know and to understand on the part of all concerned. Kurlander and Colodny (1969) write that even a disability that our present knowledge cannot correct, or one that may be found too late for optimal remediation, does far less psychological harm if it can be defined and understood than if it remains a nameless, pervasive anxiety. If the child and his family are not even aware of the nature of his handicap, the conditions are set for the development of gross misunderstanding and all its harmful emotional concomitants.

The unsatisfied need for understanding points to the importance of a thorough diagnostic evaluation. To diagnose the learning disability and to interpret the problem to the parents is the first and perhaps most essential aspect of treatment (Hatton, 1966). The family often is relieved simply to learn that the child's disorder has a name and that it perhaps might be alleviated with remediation.

Most of the energy expended in discussing and diagnosing learning problems is focused on the child who sustains these handicaps. However, this is only one aspect of the total situation, albeit probably the most important. In our achievement-oriented society, a youngster failing in school frequently reflects badly on his parents. Thus, his deficiencies have a direct effect on them. If they identify closely with him, his academic failure may cause them to feel that they are failures, also. This is especially true if the child is firstborn. The parents question their child-rearing methods and search for the causes of their offspring's problems. Guilt feelings are a typical reaction; it is not difficult for them to find instances in which they have been less than perfect and in which they have erred in some way. Adding to these guilt feelings are the numerous magazine articles that describe various ways in which parents can help their children become an intellectual giant, learn to read at age three, and so forth—or conversely, how they can stunt their child's development and retard his progress by committing any of a multitude of errors.

After a while many parents become angry—angry at their child for failing and letting them down, angry at themselves for their real or imaginary contributions to the problem, and angry at the school for its inability to solve their youngster's difficulties. They feel helpless because they do not have the training necessary to understand a learning disability or to do anything about it. Furthermore, too often they receive little or no help from the school and outside professionals. They are told their child has a visual-perceptual problem, a neurological anomaly, or an inability to decode visual symbols, but they do not understand these terms nor can they translate this jargon into language that would provide comprehension of the disorder and suggestions for home management. Thus the parents develop feelings of frustration, helplessness, and anger, although these reactions often are hidden from the clinician or misinterpreted by him. Their child's learning disability has an emotional effect on them, too. They could profit from some clear explanations and guidance on the part of school officials and other professionals.

The concern of the parents is great, and they sometimes require as much help as the disabled child himself. This suggests the value of parental counseling and group meetings. Counseling is advisable because it helps parents to understand their child's disorder and their own emotional involvement in the situation. Because learning disabilities tend to run in families, counseling also is useful and efficient; when parents are helped to understand one of their children they automatically are helped to become aware of their other offspring who may experience this same disorder. Group meetings are productive in that they lessen parental feelings of helplessness and inadequacy and enable parents to share information and home management techniques. Furthermore, these meetings show parents they are not unique or alone and frequently lead to the development of effective pressure groups that act to make better educational facilities in the schools available.

Need for Understanding: School

Along with the need for learning-disabled youngsters and their parents to understand the problem, there is also a crucial and largely unmet need for teachers and other school officials to have some awareness of this disorder. It is estimated that at least 5 percent of all children sustain learning disabilities (Myklebust, 1964), yet many educators know nothing about this handicap. The estimated incidence of this disorder indicates the magnitude of the problem and the extent of its occurrence. At a very minimum, it should be required that teachers, counselors, and school psychologists at least be aware of the nature of learning problems and the symptoms that point to this disorder. This requirement is not unrealistic. Enrolling for a single university course, even attending a single good workshop or reading one authoritative text, would help to make more school authorities cognizant of this problem.

It should be mandatory that teacher-training programs in universities require all students to be exposed to course work in learning disabilities, exceptional children, and abnormal psychology. It is unthinkable for a university that alleges to prepare elementary schoolteachers not to expose them to the factors that precipitate school failure. Most children will progress through their education with little difficulty and probably will achieve well, despite mediocre teaching. However, those youngsters who do experience trouble, such as the learning-disabled group, desperately need first-rate teaching and adequate educational facilities. For them the difference between overcoming their disability and leading a productive life, as opposed to becoming ensnared in the failure-behavior problem pattern, may simply be the opportunity for exposure to high quality, well-trained teachers. The plight of the learning-disabled child, and the emotional difficulties and obstacles he encounters, would be far less formidable if he were better understood by those responsible for his education.

As mentioned previously, children with learning disorders are not necessarily disturbed. Yet it is apparent that they face difficulties with which they could benefit from guidance, and they frequently have certain basic needs that remain unfilled. In an ideal setting these children would obtain remediation from an educator and counseling from a psychologist, while at the same time parents would receive help from a social worker. In an ideal world the child's emotional needs would receive more attention; we would have the time and manpower available to deal with social and emotional issues that arise. No one denies the importance of the child's personality development and adjustment, but too often no one really does anything about it. Schools do not have the facilities and funds to work with these problems.

This produces a dilemma. We cannot simply ignore the problem and look only at academic skills while stating that emotional issues are not our concern. Emotional attitudes and feelings are too interrelated with academic endeavors to separate them completely. The only feasible solution seems to be that school personnel and parents must take on part of the role of a counselor or psychotherapist. This idea may sound unrealistic at first encounter, but let us evaluate it more closely. What is psychotherapy? It is the developing of a relationship in which the client can feel free to grow and to change; the establishing of an arrangement in which the client is accepted by the therapist, the atmosphere is warm and friendly, and the client does not have to be afraid of making mistakes and showing his weaknesses. Psychotherapy is basically a helping relationship. It is sometimes defined as a learning process in which the therapist serves as a guide, tutor, model and primary source of reward. What is a teacher or parent if not a guide, tutor, model, and rewarder?

A teacher usually does not think of herself as a psychotherapist, but if she likes a child and this feeling is reciprocated, if she respects him and he trusts her, in short, if she treats him as a human being, she has developed a therapeutic relationship with this youngster. She may not conceptualize the situation in these terms. She may feel more comfortable saying, "I have good rapport with this child" or "We get along well and he seems to enjoy working with me." If the teacher or remedial specialist can make statements such as this, she has formed a therapeutic relationship. The school personnel must become counselors or therapists if the child's needs are to be met; no one else is going to fill this role. They must take up the slack and involve themselves with the emotional and social aspects of the child's functioning.

Clements (1966, p. 7) writes that "in order to provide the proper educational environment, the teacher must be able to function as a therapist. Her attitude toward children in general, and 'the difficult' child in particular, is the most important single factor in working with handicapped youngsters." Abrams (1969, p. 575) adds that, "perhaps the most important factor in teaching is the quality of the interpersonal relationship established between teacher and child." Harris (1970, p. 294) notes that, "Good remedial teaching has some of the characteristics of good psychotherapy. It is based on the development of a friendly, warm, comfortable relationship between teacher and pupil. It strengthens the child's self-respect and builds his confidence."

> Alan is a sixth-grader who was reading at a first-grade level. In the course of following up the diagnosis, his reading tutor was describing his skills and their remedial activities. When asked how the boy was getting along in class and whether he seemed happy or not, she replied that this was none of her business, and she had no idea what was going on in class or if he was happy. How could she work three times a week with this boy and not get some idea of his feelings? She appeared to have no awareness that Alan's academic difficulties were related to his emotional status. She did not have to be a trained psychotherapist to ask the boy how he was getting along, or to notice he never made eye contact, that his shoulders were always stooped and his gait slow, that he slumped in his chair and his speech was very hesitant and soft.

It happens that at this time Alan was becoming a serious behavior problem. He was disruptive in class, fought continually on the playground, and was disliked universally by teachers and peers. After eight months of working with Alan, in which he progressed very little, the reading tutor resigned to accept another position. Alan's new tutor took a more active interest in his feelings and attitudes. She developed a warm, personal relationship with the boy and showed him her interest and affection. After two months his behavior had changed markedly. He was more cooperative in class, related better with his peers, and generally reflected a more stable and mature adjustment. After 18 months of remediation, this severely dyslexic child still had a gross reading problem, but his skills were beginning to improve more rapidly and, significantly, he now evidenced no behavior problems. The pattern followed by Alan is found fairly frequently among the most severely disabled youngsters: An improvement in behavior precedes an improvement in academic skills. Orton (1937, p. 135) notes that "the greatest profit from such a program (remediation) comes not so much in the reading advance, which at best must be slow, as in the effect which this improvement brings about in the child's personality." Thus, behavioral change can sometimes be effected more quickly than significant improvement in school skills. Furthermore, with some children their behavior and attitudes must be altered before any noticeable growth in learning will occur.

What can a teacher or, more specifically, a reading specialist, do to make use of the therapeutic relationship she has developed? (1) She can spend a few minutes each session and simply talk with the child. She can ask him about his classes, what he thinks about his reading problem, how his parents feel about the situation. In short, she might encourage the child to talk about his feelings and attitudes associated with learning. (2) She should try to be understanding and let him know she is making this attempt. She might use expressions of empathy and support, such as "You must feel terrible if your friends laugh when you read," or "It must be frustrating to try so hard and still not be able to read very well." She can try to reflect the child's feelings and let him know he is not all alone. If he says, "I hate reading!" the teacher might respond, "I would hate it, too, if it caused me so much trouble." (3) She might talk about his specific problem with him. She could explain as clearly as possible why he is having trouble: "You are a pretty bright guy but you seem to have difficulty remembering what sounds go with what letters. We are going to work on that and see if you can begin to sound out words a little better." The youngster may feel better if he knows he is not unique; the experienced teacher can tell him that she has worked with many children who are smart but who cannot seem to get the knack of reading. (4) The educator should spend some time with the child's other teachers and his parents. She should inform them if the youngster is improving and, if so, encourage them to reinforce his progress by stating, for instance, "Your reading seems to be a little better; six months ago I don't think you could have read that sentence."

It is felt that the emotional problems confronting the learning-disabled child could be coped with more successfully if adults in his environment were more willing to act as psychotherapists or counselors. The frustration, anxiety, and lowered self-image discussed previously would not be such formidable threats to a youngster's psychosocial adjustment if those responsible for his education and welfare would more actively use their relationship with him to effect positive change and to minimize the possibility of emotional disturbances arising. To illustrate, when a teacher or parent makes the effort to tell a child that they understand his problem, that they accept him and value him despite his disorder, the child's positive self-image stands a better chance of surviving. His frustration from goal-blockage and his anxiety from failure will not disappear completely, but they may be alleviated enough to enable the child to function more normally and to avoid developing secondary emotional problems.

Special Needs of the Inner-City Child

The final problem area to be discussed concerns learning disabilities as they relate to socioeconomic level and juvenile delinquency. The relationship between emotional disorders and such forms of maladaptive behavior as delinquency is unclear, but vitally important to both the individual child and to society as a whole. This issue is contained within a broader sociological problem, one aspect of which concerns the necessity for society to respond more adequately to the needs of its school population, especially those of the inner city.

It is a recurrent theme that there are insufficient facilities for educating children with learning handicaps. Most school systems do not have enough staff or space to accommodate this population; many systems do not contain a single learning-disability classroom or employ even one teacher trained for work with this group. It is apparent that our educational institutions are not meeting the needs, both academic and emotional, of this population. This unfilled need is most evident in the ghetto areas where special education classes are sparce and professional staff and materials invariably insufficient. Learning disabilities often seem to be considered primarily a middle and upper class phenomenon. However, there is a distinct possibility that the incidence of this disorder is greatest in lower socioeconomic areas (Eisenberg, 1966). Furthermore, it is possible that the high incidence of disabilities in these areas may be contributing factors to social and emotional problems such as high unemployment, delinquency, and criminality.

Learning disabilities are associated with minimal brain dysfunction, and this impairment may be expected more frequently in a group in which precipitating factors such as inadequate prenatal and postnatal medical care are common. It is estimated that one-fifth of the indigent mothers who deliver babies in tax-supported hospitals have complications during pregnancy and birth that require special medical services, and that these services are seldom received (Tarnapol, 1969). The frequency of these complications in the pre- and postnatal periods of development strongly suggests the possibility that the highest rate of minimal brain dysfunction is to be found in the lowest income group. This population incurs a larger proportion of infant mortality and premature and complicated births than any other socioeconomic group. For instance, in 1964 statistics from the U.S. Census Bureau (1967) revealed that the rate of infant mortality for white children was 21.5 per 1,000 while for nonwhites it was 40.3.

Thus, medical and statistical evidence that suggests that children living in deprived socioeconomic conditions have a higher probability of sustaining neurological dysfunctions than any other group of youngsters is accumulating. Furthermore, it is verified that children in inner-city schools often achieve more poorly than those in other areas (New York State Department of Education, 1968; Vellutino and Connolly, 1971). It seems not unreasonable to conclude that a number of these children, perhaps a substantial minority, are experiencing learning disabilities.

Although the relationship between juvenile delinquency and learning disorders remains unclear, there is the feeling that a correlation exists between the two. Poremba (1967, p. 145) reports, "I have had occasion to spend some ten years as chief psychologist of the Denver Juvenile Court. In my experiences there I have come to feel very strongly that as many as fifty percent of the children we were seeing were exhibiting specific learning disabilities." Among those tested by the psychiatric unit of the Children's Court in New York City in 1955, 75 percent were found to be two or more years retarded in reading, while more than half of these were at least five years below grade level (Margolin, 1955). Critchley (1964) adds that the same percentage has been found in France, where in a group of young offenders the proportion of nonreaders was at least 75 percent. These figures indicate that there appears to be a connection between such forms of maladaptive behavior as juvenile delinquency and the presence of learning problems. However, to say that there exists a correlation between the two variables is not to claim a cause-and-effect relationship. Despite the fact that the connection is indefinite at this time, it is probable that there are a number of delinquents who sustain learning disorders.

The evidence that links disabilities, low socioeconomic level, and emotional and social inadequacies points to the great need to provide more and better services to the inner-city population. If we are to eliminate the cycle involving learning disorders—academic failure, school dropout, juvenile delinquency—we must provide improved educational facilities and medical care for the population that perhaps sustains the highest incidence of disorders. The learning-disabled youngster with the greatest unmet needs undoubtedly is the child who lives in the inner city. Along with encountering the same obstacles faced by his suburban counterpart, this child's situation is intensified severely by the addition of a deprived environment.

Conclusion

A youngster with a learning disability is first, and most important, a child; only secondarily should he be viewed as an individual with a handicap. In many ways he is very similar to other children. He lives in the same society, shares the same needs, and progresses through the same stages of development as his peers. Owing to his disorder, however, he is confronted with certain obstacles and pressures that other children do not face. These sometimes impair his adjustment and contribute to psychological problems of varying degree.

The viewpoint advocated in this chapter has not presented the learning-disabled group as being emotionally disturbed. The personality types and behavioral patterns found in this population are diverse, just as they are with any other large group of human beings.

References

Abrams, J. An interdisciplinary approach to learning disabilities. *Journal of Learning Disabilities,* 1969, 2:575–578.

Bender, L. *Psychopathology of Children with Organic Brain Disorders.* Springfield: Charles C. Thomas, 1956.

Boder, E. A neuropediatric approach to the diagnosis and management of school behavior and learning disorders. In *Learning Disorders*, vol. 2. Seattle: Special Child Publications, 1966. pp. 15–44.

Bryant, N. Clinic inadequacies with learning disorders: the missing clinical educator. *In* J. Hellmuth, ed., *Learning Disorders,* vol. 2. Seattle: Special Child Publications, 1966. pp. 265–279.

Clements, S. *Some Aspects of the Characteristics, Management and Education of the Child with Learning Disabilities.* Arkansas: Arkansas Association for Children with Learning Disabilities, 1966.

Clements, S., and Peters, J. Minimal brain dysfunctions in the school-age child. *Archives of General Psychiatry,* 1962, 6:185–197.

Connolly, C. The psychosocial adjustment of children with dyslexia. *Exceptional Children,* 1969, 36:126–127.

Critchley, M. *Developmental Dyslexia.* Springfield: Charles C. Thomas, 1964.

Daniels, M. The dynamics of morbid envy in the etiology and treatment of chronic learning disability. *Psychoanalytic Review,* 1964, 51:45–56.

Eisenberg, L. The epidemiology of reading retardation and a program for preventive intervention. *In* J. Money, ed., *The Disabled Reader.* Baltimore: Johns Hopkins Press, 1966. pp. 3–19.

Eysenck, H. *Handbook of Abnormal Psychology.* New York: Basic Books, 1961.

Fernald, G. *Remedial Techniques in Basic School Subjects.* New York: McGraw-Hill Co., 1943.

Gates, A. The role of personality maladjustment in reading disability. *Journal of Genetic Psychology,* 1941, 59:77–83.

Giffen, M. The role of child psychiatry in learning disabilities. *In* H. Myklebust, ed., *Progress in Learning Disabilities,* vol. 1. New York: Grune & Stratton, 1968. pp. 75-97.

Goldstein, S. A study of the self-concepts of selected boys with learning disabilities. Unpublished master's thesis, University of Kansas, 1970.

Harris, A. *How to Increase Reading Ability: A Guide to Developmental and Remedial Methods* 5th ed. New York: McKay, 1970.

Hatton, D. The child with minimal cerebral dysfunction. *Developmental Medicine and Child Neurology,* 1966, 8:71–78.

Kurlander, L., and Colodny, D. Psychiatric disability and learning problems. *In* L. Tarnapol, ed., *Learning Disabilities: Introduction to Educational and Medical Management.* Springfield: Charles C. Thomas, 1969, pp. 131–153.

Margolin, J. Roman, M., and Harris, C. Reading disability in the delinquent child: a microcosm of psychosocial pathology. *American Journal of Orthopsychiatry,* 1955, 25: 25–35.

Mussen, P. Conger, J., and Kagan, J. *Child Development and Personality,* 3d ed. New York: Harper & Row, 1969.

Myklebust, H. Learning disorders: psychoneurological disturbances in childhood. *Rehabilitation Literature,* 1964, 25:35–360.

Myklebust, H., and Boshes, B. *Minimal Brain Damage in Children.* Washington, D.C.: U.S. Department of Health, Education and Welfare, 1969.

Natchez, G. ed. *Children with Reading Problems.* New York: Basic Books, 1968.

New York State Department of Education.*Educational Disadvantage in New York State.* Albany: New York State Department of Education, 1968.

Orton, S. *Reading, Writing and Speech Problems in Children.* New York: Norton, 1937.

Pearson, G. *Psychoanalysis and the Education of the Child.* New York: Norton, 1954.

Poremba, C. The adolescent and young adult with learning disabilities: what are his needs: what are the needs of those who deal with him? *In* J. Arena. ed., *Selected Papers on Learning Disabilities,* Third Annual International Conference of ACLD. California: Academic Therapy Publications, 1967, pp. 142–148.

Rabinovitch, R. Reading and learning disabilities. *In* S. Arieti, ed., *American Handbook of Psychiatry,* vol. 1. New York: Basic Books, 1959. pp. 857–869.

Rabinovitch, R. Dyslexia: psychiatric considerations. *In* J. Money, ed., *Reading Disability: Progress and Research Needs in Dyslexia.* Baltimore: Johns Hopkins Press, 1962. pp. 73–79.

Stein, S. The child psychiatry resident: innovations in training and treatment of learning disabilities. In J. Arena, ed., *Selected Papers on Learning Disabilities,* Fifth Annual International Conference of ACLD, California: Academic Therapy Publications, 1969. pp. 458–462.

Sylvester, E., and Kunst, M. Psychodynamic aspects of the reading problem. *American Journal of Orthopsychiatry,* 1943, 13:69–76.

Tarnapol, L. Delinquency and learning disabilities. *In* L. Tarnapol, ed., *Learning Disabilities: Introduction to Education and Medical Management.* Springfield: Charles C. Thomas, 1969. pp. 305–330.

U.S. Census Bureau. *Statistical Abstracts of the United States.* Washington, D.C.: U.S. Government Printing Office, 1967.

Vellutino, F., and Connolly, C. The training of paraprofessionals as remedial reading assistants in an inner-city school. *The Reading Teacher,* 1971, 24:506–512.

20. Special Education for the Mildly Retarded—Is Much of It Justifiable?

Lloyd M. Dunn

A better education than special class placement is needed for socioculturally deprived children with mild learning problems who have been labeled educable mentally retarded. Over the years, the status of these pupils who come from poverty, broken and inadequate homes, and low status ethnic groups has been a checkered one. In the early days, these children were simply excluded from school. Then, as Hollingworth (1923) pointed out, with the advent of compulsory attendance laws, the schools and these children "were forced into a reluctant mutual recognition of each other." This resulted in the establishment of self contained special schools and classes as a method of transferring these "misfits" out of the regular grades. This practice continues to this day and, unless counterforces are set in motion now, it will probably become even more prevalent in the immediate future due in large measure to increased racial integration and militant teacher organizations. For example, a local affiliate of the National Education Association demanded of a local school board recently that more special classes be provided for disruptive and slow learning children (Nashville *Tennessean,* December 18, 1967).

The number of special day classes for the retarded has been increasing by leaps and bounds. The most recent 1967–1968 statistics compiled by the US Office of Education now indicate that there are approximately 32,000 teachers of the retarded employed by local school systems—over one-third of all special educators in the nation. In my best judgment, about 60 to 80 percent of the pupils taught by these teachers are children from low status backgrounds—including Afro-Americans, American Indians, Mexicans, and Puerto Rican Americans; those from nonstandard English speaking, broken, disorganized, and inadequate homes; and children from other nonmiddle class environments. This expensive proliferation of self contained special schools and classes raises serious educational and civil rights issues which must be squarely faced. It is my thesis that we must stop labeling these deprived children as mentally retarded. Furthermore we must stop segregating them by placing them into our allegedly special programs.

The purpose of this article is twofold: first, to provide reasons for taking the position that a large proportion of this so called special education in its present form is obsolete and unjustifiable from the point of view of the pupils so placed; and second, to outline a blueprint for changing this major

From *Exceptional Children,* 1968, **35,** 5–22. Reprinted with permission of The Council for Exceptional Children.

segment of education for exceptional children to make it more acceptable. We are not arguing that we do away with our special education programs for the moderately and severely retarded, for other types of more handicapped children, or for the multiply handicapped. The emphasis is on doing something better for slow learning children who live in slum conditions, although much of what is said should also have relevance for those children we are labeling emotionally disturbed, perceptually impaired, brain injured, and learning disordered. Furthermore, the emphasis of the article is on children, in that no attempt is made to suggest an adequate high school environment for adolescents still functioning as slow learners.

Reasons for Change

Regular teachers and administrators have sincerely felt they were doing these pupils a favor by removing them from the pressures of an unrealistic and inappropriate program of studies. Special educators have also fully believed that the children involved would make greater progress in special schools and classes. However, the overwhelming evidence is that our present and past practices have their major justification in removing pressures on regular teachers and pupils, at the expense of the socioculturally deprived slow learning pupils themselves. Some major arguments for this position are outlined below.

Homogeneous Grouping

Homogeneous groupings tend to work to the disadvantage of the slow-learners and underprivileged. Apparently such pupils learn much from being in the same class with children from white middle class homes. Also, teachers seem to concentrate on the slower children to bring them up to standard. This principle was dramatically applied in the Judge J. Skelly Wright decision in the District of Columbia concerning the track system. Judge Wright ordered that tracks be abolished, contending they discriminated against the racially and/or economically disadvantaged and therefore were in violation of the Fifth Amendment of the Constitution of the United States. One may object to the Judge's making educational decisions based on legal considerations. However, Passow (1967), upon the completion of a study of the same school system, reached the same conclusion concerning tracking. The recent national study by Coleman et al. (1966) provides supporting evidence in finding that academically disadvantaged Negro children in racially segregated schools made less progress than those of comparable ability in integrated schools. Furthermore, racial integration appeared to deter school progress very little for Caucasian and more academically able students.

What are the implications of Judge Wright's rulings for special education? Clearly special schools and classes are a form of homogeneous grouping and tracking. This fact was demonstrated in September, 1967, when the District of Columbia (as a result of the Wright decision) abolished Track 5, into which had been routed the slowest learning pupils in the District of Columbia schools. These pupils and their teachers were returned to the regular classrooms. Complaints followed from the regular teachers that these children were taking an inordinate amount of their time. A few parents observed that their slow learning children were frustrated by the more academic program and were rejected by the other students. Thus, there are efforts afoot to develop a special education program in D.C. which cannot be labeled a track. Self contained special classes will probably not be tolerated under the present court ruling but perhaps itinerant and resource room programs would be. What if the Supreme Court ruled against tracks, and all self contained special classes across the nation which serve primarily ethnically and/or economically disadvantaged children were forced to close down? Make no mistake—this could happen! If I were a Negro from the slums or a disadvantaged parent who had heard of the Judge Wright decision and knew what I know now about special classes for the educable mentally retarded, other things being equal, I would then go to court before allowing the schools to label my child as "mentally retarded" and place him in a "self contained special school or class." Thus there is the real possibility that additional court actions will be forthcoming.[1]

Efficacy Studies

The findings of studies on the efficacy of special classes for the educable mentally retarded constitute another argument for change. These results are well known (Kirk, 1964) and suggest consistently that retarded pupils make as much or more progress in the regular grades as they do in special education. Recent studies such as those by Hoelke (1966) and Smith and Kennedy (1967) continue to provide similar evidence. Johnson (1962) has summarized the situation well:

> It is indeed paradoxical that mentally handicapped children having teachers especially trained, having more money (per capita) spent on their education, and being designed to provide for their unique needs, should be accomplishing the objectives of their education at the same or at a lower level than similar mentally handicapped children who have not had these advantages and have been forced to remain in the regular grades [p. 66].

Efficacy studies on special day classes for other mildly handicapped children, including the emotionally handicapped, reveal the same results. For

---

[1]Litigation has now occurred. According to an item in a June 8, 1968, issue of the *Los Angeles Times* received after this article was sent to the printer, the attorneys in the national office for the rights of the indigent filed a suit in behalf of the Mexican-American parents of the Santa Ana Unified School District asking for an injunction against the District's classes for the educable mentally retarded because the psychological examinations required prior to placement are unconstitutional since they have failed to use adequate evaluation techniques for children from different language and cultural backgrounds, and because parents have been denied the right of hearing to refute evidence for placement. Furthermore, the suit seeks to force the district to grant hearings on all children currently in such special classes to allow for the chance to remove the stigma of the label "mentally retarded" from school records of such pupils.

example, Rubin, Senison, and Betwee (1966) found that disturbed children did as well in the regular grades as in special classes, concluding that there is little or no evidence that special class programing is generally beneficial to emotionally disturbed children as a specific method of intervention and correction. Evidence such as this is another reason to find better ways of serving children with mild learning disorders than placing them in self contained special schools and classes.

Labeling Processes

Our past and present diagnostic procedures comprise another reason for change. These procedures have probably been doing more harm than good in that they have resulted in disability labels and in that they have grouped children homogeneously in school on the basis of these labels. Generally, these diagnostic practices have been conducted by one of two procedures. In rare cases, the workup has been provided by a multidiscipli-nary team, usually consisting of physicians, social workers, psychologists, speech and hearing specialists, and occasionally educators. The avowed goal of this approach has been to look at the complete child, but the outcome has been merely to label him mentally retarded, perceptually impaired, emo-tionally disturbed, minimally brain injured, or some other such term depend-ing on the predispositions, idiosyncracies, and backgrounds of the team members. Too, the team usually has looked for causation, and diagnosis tends to stop when something has been found wrong with the child, when the why has either been found or conjectured, and when some justification has been found for recommending placement in a special education class.

In the second and more common case, the assessment of educational potential has been left to the school psychologist who generally administers —in an hour or so—a psychometric battery, at best consisting of individual tests of intelligence, achievement, and social and personal adjustment. Again the purpose has been to find out what is wrong with the child in order to label him and thus make him eligible for special education services. In large measure this has resulted in digging the educational graves of many racially and/or economically disadvantaged children by using a WISC or Binet IQ score to justify the label "mentally retarded." This term then becomes a destructive, self fulfilling prophecy.

What is the evidence against the continued use of these diagnostic prac-tices and disability labels?

First, we must examine the effects of these disability labels on the attitudes and expectancies of teachers. Here we can extrapolate from studies by Rosenthal and Jacobson (1966), who set out to determine whether or not the expectancies of teachers influenced pupil progress. Working with elementary school teachers across the first six grades, they obtained pretest measures on pupils by using intelligence and achievement tests. A sample of pupils was randomly drawn and labeled "rapid learners" with hidden potential. Teachers were told that these children would show unusual intel-lectual gains and school progress during the year. All pupils were retested late in the school year. Not all differences were statistically significant, but the gains of the children who had been arbitrarily labeled rapid learners were generally significantly greater than those of the other pupils, with especially dramatic changes in the first and second grades. To extrapolate from this study, we must expect that labeling a child "handicapped" reduces the teacher's expectancy for him to succeed.

Second, we must examine the effects of these disability labels on the pupils themselves. Certainly none of these labels are badges of distinction. Separating a child from other children in his neighborhood—or removing him from the regular classroom for therapy or special class placement— probably has a serious debilitating effect upon his self image. Here again our research is limited but supportive of this contention. Goffman (1961) has described the stripping and mortification process that takes place when an individual is placed in a residential facility. Meyerowitz (1965) demonstrated that a group of educable mentally retarded pupils increased in feelings of self-derogation after one year in special classes. More recent results indicate that special class placement, instead of helping such a pupil adjust to his neighborhood peers, actually hinders him (Meyerowitz, 1967). While much more research is needed, we cannot ignore the evidence that removing a handicapped child from the regular grades for special education probably contributes significantly to his feelings of inferiority and problems of acceptance.

Improvements in General Education

Another reason self contained special classes are less justifiable today than in the past is that regular school programs are now better able to deal with individual differences in pupils. No longer is the choice just between a self contained special class and a self contained regular elementary classroom. Although the impact of the American Revolution in Education is just beginning to be felt and is still more an ideal than a reality, special education should begin moving now to fit into a changing general education program and to assist in achieving the program's goals. Because of increased support at the local, state, and federal levels, four powerful forces are at work:

Changes in school organization. In place of self contained regular classrooms, there is increasingly more team teaching, ungraded primary departments, and flexible groupings. Radical departures in school organization are projected—educational parks in place of neighborhood schools, metropolitan school districts cutting across our inner cities and wealthy suburbs, and, perhaps most revolutionary of all, competing public school systems. Furthermore, and of great significance to those of us who have focused our careers on slow learning children, public kindergartens and nurseries are becoming more available for children of the poor.

Curricular changes. Instead of the standard diet of Look and Say readers, many new and exciting options for teaching reading are evolving. Contemporary mathematics programs teach in the primary grades concepts formerly reserved for high school. More programed textbooks and other materials are finding their way into the classroom. Ingenious procedures, such as those by Bereiter and Engelmann (1966), are being developed to teach oral language and reasoning to pre-school disadvantaged children.

Changes in professional public school personnel. More ancillary personnel are now employed by the schools—i.e., psychologists, guidance workers, physical educators, remedial educators, teacher aides, and technicians. Furthermore, some teachers are functioning in different ways, serving as teacher coordinators, or cluster teachers who provide released time for other teachers to prepare lessons, etc. Too, regular classroom teachers are increasingly better trained to deal with individual differences—although much still remains to be done.

Hardware changes. Computerized teaching, teaching machines, feedback typewriters, ETV, videotapes, and other materials are making autoinstruction possible, as never before.

We must ask what the implications of this American Revolution in Education are for special educators. Mackie (1967), formerly of the US Office of Education, addressed herself to the question: "Is the modern school changing sufficiently to provide [adequate services in general education] for large numbers of pupils who have functional mental retardation due to environmental factors [p. 5]?" In her view, hundreds—perhaps even thousands—of so called retarded pupils may make satisfactory progress in schools with diversified programs of instruction and thus will never need placement in self contained special classes. With earlier, better, and more flexible regular school programs many of the children should not need to be relegated to the type of special education we have so often provided.

In my view, the above four reasons for change are cogent ones. Much of special education for the mildly retarded is becoming obsolete. Never in our history has there been a greater urgency to take stock and to search out new roles for a large number of today's special educators.

A Blueprint for Change

Two major suggestions which constitute my attempt at a blueprint for change are developed below. First, a fairly radical departure from conventional methods will be proposed in procedures for diagnosing, placing, and teaching children with mild learning difficulties. Second, a proposal for curriculum revision will be sketched out. These are intended as proposals which should be examined, studied, and tested. What is needed are programs based on scientific evidence of worth and not more of those founded on philosophy, tradition, and expediency.

A Thought

There is an important difference between regular educators talking us into trying to remediate or live with the learning difficulties of pupils with which they haven't been able to deal; versus striving to evolve a special education program that is either developmental in nature, wherein we assume responsibility for the total education of more severely handicapped children from an early age, or is supportive in nature, wherein general education would continue to have central responsibility for the vast majority of the children with mild learning disabilities—with us serving as resource teachers in devising effective prescriptions and in tutoring such pupils.

A Clinical Approach

Existing diagnostic procedures should be replaced by expecting special educators, in large measure, to be responsible for their own diagnostic teaching and their clinical teaching. In this regard, it is suggested that we do away with many existing disability labels and the present practice of grouping children homogeneously by these labels into special classes. Instead, we should try keeping slow learning children more in the mainstream of education, with special educators serving as diagnostic, clinical, remedial, resource room, itinerant and/or team teachers, consultants, and developers of instructional materials and prescriptions for effective teaching.

The accomplishment of the above *modus operandi* will require a revolution in much of special education. A moratorium needs to be placed on the proliferation (if not continuance) of self contained special classes which enroll primarily the ethnically and/or economically disadvantaged children we have been labeling educable mentally retarded. Such pupils should be left in (or returned to) the regular elementary grades until we are "tooled up" to do something better for them.

References

Bereiter, C., & Engelmann, S. *Teaching disadvantaged children in the preschool.* Englewood Cliffs, N.J.: Prentice-Hall, 1966.

Coleman, J. S., et al. *Equality of educational opportunity.* Washington, D.C.: USGPO, 1966.

Goffman, E. *Asylums: Essays on the social situation of mental patients and other inmates.* Garden City, N.Y.: Anchor, 1961.

Hoelke, G. M. *Effectiveness of special class placement for educable mentally retarded children.* Lincoln, Neb.: University of Nebraska, 1966.

Hollingworth, L. S. *The psychology of subnormal children.* New York: Macmillan, 1923.

Johnson, G. O. Special education for mentally handicapped—a paradox. *Exceptional Children,* 1962, **19,** 62–69.

Kirk, S. A. Research in education. In H. A. Stevens & R. Heber (Eds.), *Mental retardation.* Chicago, Ill.: University of Chicago Press, 1964.

Mackie, R. P. *Functional handicaps among school children due to cultural or economic deprivation.* Paper presented at the First Congress of the International Association for the Scientific Study of Mental Deficiency, Montpellier, France, September, 1967.

Meyerowitz, J. H. Family background of educable mentally retarded children. In H. Goldstein, J. W. Moss & L. J. Jordan. *The efficacy of special education training on the development of mentally retarded children.* Urbana, Ill.: University of Illinois Institute for Research on Exceptional Children, 1965. Pp. 152–182.

Meyerowitz, J. H. Peer groups and special classes. *Mental Retardation,* 1967, **5,** 23–26.

Passow, A. H. *A summary of findings and recommendations of a study of the Washington, D.C. schools.* New York: Teachers College, Columbia University, 1967.

Rosenthal, R., & Jacobson, L. Teachers' expectancies: Determinants of pupils' IQ gains. *Psychological Reports,* 1966, **19,** 115–118.

Rubin, E. Z., Senison, C. B., & Betwee, M. C. *Emotionally handicapped children in the elementary school.* Detroit: Wayne State University Press, 1966.

Smith H. W., & Kennedy, W. A. Effects of three educational programs on mentally retarded children. *Perceptual and Motor Skills,* 1967, **24,** 174.

Part III

Therapeutic Approaches

Chapter Eight

Drug Therapy

A news report appearing in the *Washington Post* in the summer of 1970 provoked a storm of controversy throughout the nation. According to this account, between 5 and 10 percent of the school children in Omaha, Nebraska, were being administered drugs to modify their classroom behavior and increase their potential for learning in public schools. It seems that the story originated from a protest lodged by a concerned parent at a meeting of the local school board. School officials in Omaha denied many aspects of the accusations, but public concern was actively aroused by this news, which soon appeared in newspapers and on radio and television newscasts across the country. This publicity, however, only brought to a head a troublesome problem that had been festering for quite some time.

Many pediatricians and child psychiatrists have prescribed drugs for hyperactive children and others with learning disabilities. Recently, this use of medication has increased. Consequently, parents and educators have become much more aware that medications can be, and often are, used for purposes of controlling impulsive behavior and enhancing scholastic performance.

Bradley's Pioneering Studies

In 1937, Charles Bradley, who was then the Medical Director of the Bradley Home in Rhode Island, first published "The Behavior of Children Receiving Benzedrine." This was followed by "School Performance of Children Receiving Amphetamine (Benzedrine) Sulfate," written in collaboration with a registered nurse (Bradley & Bowen, 1940). These early workers had discovered quite by accident that amphetamines which serve as stimulants to "normal" people somehow have a reverse reaction when given to hyperkinetic children. This pioneering research with child psychiatric patients in the mid-1930s revealed that overactive youngsters who received this form of medication became better able to concentrate and cope with the demands encountered in the classroom. In fact, staff members who worked with Bradley in the early days recall that he referred to this medication as "arithmetic pills."

Hyperkinetic Disorder

The term hyperkinesis refers to children who show the following characteristics: hyperactivity, short attention span and poor powers of concentration, variability, impulsiveness and inability to delay gratification, irritability, and explosiveness. This cluster of traits has been referred to as forming the "hyperkinetic impulse disorder" in children's behavior problems (Laufer, Denhoff, & Solomons, 1957). Children who display these behavioral characteristics are usually unable to perform up to expectations in the ordinary school setting and consequently often show various forms of learning disabilities. Rating scales for assessing characteristics of the hyperkinetic disorder have recently been developed by Davids (1971) and can be used by teachers and investigators who are engaged in practical work or research with hyperkinetic children.

Increasing Usage and Growing Concern

In the 1950s, educators became increasingly aware of the uses of psychopharmacological agents in the modification of children's problem behaviors, and they more often encouraged parents to seek the help of the child's physician in treating learning disabilities and other difficulties in school adjustment. It became evident that drugs were being over-used and were sometimes prescribed merely because a parent or teacher described a child's behavior at home or in school as troublesome. Recently, many parents, educators, and physicians have administered this form of medication without sufficient awareness of the necessary safeguards or critical problems of differential diagnosis. That is, they did not concern themselves with the very important differences that exist and must be recognized between the hyperkinetic impulse disorder and other types of problem behavior in which overactivity is also a predominant feature.

Recent Attempts at Clarification

The controversy pertaining to hyperactive behavior led the National Institute of Health to organize a panel to explore the issues. This resulted in subsequent description of children with "minimal brain dysfunction," and publication of a comprehensive list of guidelines to be followed in diagnosis and treatment of such children. In January 1971, the Office of Child Development and Department of Health, Education, and Welfare sponsored a conference on the use of stimulant drugs in treatment of behaviorally disturbed school children. While the report of the experts who served on this panel does help to highlight the problems involved, it also reveals the many areas of ignorance that await research attention.

As a further step toward increased understanding, the *Journal of Learning*

Disabilities devoted its November 1971 issue to the role of medication in treatment of learning disabilities and related disorders. This special issue, produced under the guest editorship of Eric Denhoff, was composed of several independent papers focusing on various aspects of problems encountered in diagnosis, treatment, and research on hyperkinesis and psychomedications. In his editorial, "To medicate—to debate—or to validate?," Denhoff (1971), a leading pediatric neurologist, stated:

> When does an accepted medical treatment become a controversial problem and a subject for national debate? When parents become sophisticated and concerned enough to start asking searching questions demanding clear, explicit answers, and professionals respond only with vague, sometimes arbitrary statements, satisfying no one [p. 467] . . . . We hope the symposium can motivate the scientific minds in this country to devote energy to working on a critical problem in child development—hyperactivity and short attention span. There is an urgent need to clarify the issues of cause, mechanisms, and relationships of medication usage to immediate and long-term outcome. If other ways could be developed to help such a child adjust to home and school, then medication could possibly be eliminated. In sum, the material in this issue of the *Journal of Learning Disabilities* attempts to provide in an unemotional, logical manner the facts demanded by the Omaha parent and his supporters. We hope that the "consumer" continues to demand clear answers and that the professionals are permitted to publish their replies, so that there will be no end to the continuing search for a better way for the "at-risk" children of America to live as acceptable and valued members of their society [p. 469].

The Issues

In general, reports emanating from the government-sponsored conferences and papers published in the Denhoff-edited volume were favorable in their view of uses and effects of medications in treating hyperkinetic children. However, there are still many critics. Two of the more eloquent critics are John Holt and Edward T. Ladd, who have written the first two articles in this chapter. Holt is also the author of *How Children Fail* (1964), *The Underachieving School* (1969), and other widely read books that are critical of how children are treated in most present-day schools. Ladd is a professor of education who has also written extensively on the subject of public school discipline and students' rights. To present a somewhat more balanced view of this controversial situation, we have included a thoughtful statement by Leon Eisenberg, who speaks from years of clinical practice and research conducted in medical settings at Johns Hopkins and Harvard. Thus, papers reprinted in this chapter should convey both sides of the argument.

The controversy is still far from resolved. On two occasions in February 1972, the *Providence* (Rhode Island) *Sunday Journal* published front-page stories concerning these issues, one of them entitled "A Crutch for the Teacher? Many Pupils Given Unneeded Drugs." On another occasion, the feature article was entitled "Drugs for Children—Miracle or Nightmare? Behavior Control Attempt Stirs Rhode Island Debate." These are merely examples of the kinds of stories that are continuing to appear in national magazines and newspapers.

This problem situation is obviously complex, and there is no easy solution in sight. While psychostimulant drugs produce gratifying beneficial effects in many cases, not all hyperactive children respond favorably to this form of medication. Along with medical concerns about negative side-effects, there are important ethical issues pertaining to the rights of children to be free. Some feel that adults do not have the right to restrict the behavior of children by administering medication over which the child himself has no control. On the other hand, others feel that to deprive children of the opportunity of functioning better in school and learning to full capacity during this formative stage is also very wrong; that is, if medication enables a child to be less restless and impulsive, making it possible to concentrate and perform more effectively in school, then it would seem improper to withhold drug therapy.

One fundamental research concern is to discover exactly what biochemical mechanisms are involved in the functioning of these drugs with hyperkinetic children. There is considerable theorizing and speculation about the mechanisms involved but, at this date, there are no satisfactory explanations of why and how these medications achieve what sometimes seem to be almost magical effects with many children. For additional information on this subject, see Paul Wender's (1971) recent book, *Minimal Brain Dysfunction in Children.*

In the closing paper in this chapter, Maurice W. Laufer, a recognized authority in child psychiatry, reports findings from an exploratory attempt to discover long-range outcomes of this kind of drug therapy administered in early childhood. Surprisingly, in spite of the widespread prescription of these drugs by physicians, there are practically no published reports of studies assessing the adult status of individuals who were subjected to these medical manipulations during their developmental years. There is obviously great need for investigation of this multi-faceted problem, with increasing attention devoted to follow-up studies.

References

Bradley, C. The behavior of children receiving benzedrine. *American Journal of Psychiatry,* 1937, **94,** 577–585.

Bradley, C., & Bowen, M. School performance of children receiving amphetamine (benzedrine) sulfate. *American Journal of Orthopsychiatry,* 1940, **10,** 782–788.

Davids, A. An objective instrument for assessing hyperkinesis in children. *Journal of Learning Disabilities,* 1971, **4,** 499–501.

Denhoff, E. To medicate—to debate—or to validate? *Journal of Learning Disabilities,* 1971, **4,** 467–469.

Holt, J. *How children fail.* New York: Pitman, 1964.

Holt, J. *The underachieving school.* New York: Pitman, 1969.

Laufer, M. W., Denhoff, E., & Solomons, G. Hyperkinetic impulse disorder in children's behavior problems. *Psychosomatic Medicine,* 1957, **19,** 38–49.

Wender, P. H. *Minimal brain dysfunction in children.* New York: Wiley-Interscience, 1971.

21. Quackery

John Holt

In a story in the July 3 *New York Times* I read, "According to the best estimates, from 5 to 20 percent of American children suffer from ... a complex and little-understood learning and behavior disorder sometimes called 'minimal brain dysfunction' ... such children, usually boys, are all too evident in almost every classroom. They jump up and down, throw paper airplanes at the teacher, fight and shove on the lunch line, can concentrate for only a short time, frustrate easily, etc. etc." I then read that many doctors are treating this so-called disorder by dosing the children with amphetamines.

It is most unfortunate that the *Times* should have given this much support to this currently fashionable quackery, which blames on the nervous systems of children the stupidities and inhumanities of our schools, recently described by Charles Silberman in detail in an all too aptly titled article, "Murder in the Schoolroom."

We take lively, curious, energetic children, eager to make contact with the world and to learn about it, stick them in barren classrooms with teachers who on the whole neither like nor respect nor understand nor trust them, restrict their freedom of speech and movement to a degree that would be judged excessive and inhuman even in a maximum security prison, and that their teachers themselves could not and would not tolerate. Then, when the children resist this brutalizing and stupefying treatment and retreat from it in anger, bewilderment, and terror, we say that they are sick with "complex and little-understood" disorders, and proceed to dose them with powerful drugs that are indeed complex and of whose long-run effects we know little or nothing, so that they may be more ready to do the asinine things the schools ask them to do.

It would seem reasonable and prudent, to say nothing of scientific, to ask ourselves a few questions about this "complex and little-understood disorder" that supposedly afflicts as many as 20 percent of our children. If indeed it has something to do with injuries incurred during or soon after birth, how is it possible that it affects mostly boys? Is it not a hundred times more likely that boys have a harder time in school because their women teachers do not like and cannot deal with the kind of behavior that boys have grown up to think of as being appropriately boyish? Might it not be wise to see whether there is as great an incidence of this "disorder" in classes that are taught by men, or in schools where the children are *not* forbidden to move or talk? Might it not also be wise to see whether there is some correlation between the incidence of this disorder and the age of the teacher, or the rigidity of the classroom? If this is indeed a defect induced at birth, births being about the same everywhere, might it not be wise to inquire whether other countries have also noticed this strange "disorder"? Given the fact that some children are more energetic and active than others, might it not be easier, more healthy, and more humane to deal with this fact by giving them more time and scope to make use of and work off their energy?

It is not surprising that the schools in many places should have given their support to this practice of doping children to make them quiet and docile in school, but that so many doctors and psychiatrists have joined them in doing so seems to me shocking and disgusting beyond words. And finally we must ask ourselves what can be the effect on a child of being told that he is so incurably bad that only a powerful pill can make him good?

Someone may suggest soon that the easiest and surest way to solve the problems of our schools may be to give all children a pre-frontal lobotomy at birth, or plant some behavior-controlling electrodes in their heads. We seem to me to be dangerously close to such horrors.

22. Pills for Classroom Peace?

Edward T. Ladd

Last Fourth of July, after a day of celebrating their inalienable rights to liberty and the pursuit of happiness, Americans were jolted to learn from the Huntley-Brinkley program that doctors in Omaha, Nebraska, are giving hundreds of school children so-called behavior modification drugs, to "make them behave better in school." This report drew the nation's attention to a practice first reported in a Washington *Post* scoop five days before. Already a violent controversy was under way. Does giving hyperactive children drugs to improve their classroom behavior free them for the better pursuit of happiness? Or does it infringe on their liberty?

The Omaha story brought to the public's attention that for well over a decade physicians increasingly have been using drugs to treat children for certain difficulties they have in school. Why and how the practice started helps to explain the issues in the controversy over it.

Originally, psychiatrists and psychologists had become interested in the

From *Saturday Review,* November 21, 1970. Copyright 1970 Saturday Review, Inc. Reproduced by permission.

study of learning difficulties through their work with children who were institutionalized or were visiting clinics because of emotional disturbance or delinquency, most of whom have trouble with learning of one kind or another. Later they broadened out to work with learning difficulties as such. They established that many learning disabilities—which may involve from 5 percent to 20 percent of our children—can't be attributed to low intelligence, emotional disturbance, or overt physical handicaps, but seem to reflect something abnormal about the workings of the children's central nervous systems (CNS), the parts of their brains where, so to speak, messages come in and get sorted out. The intensive work of first-rate investigators in several academic disciplines has still failed to reveal just what is wrong with these children's CNS, whether its cause is genetic, a result of injury, or both, and what is best to do about it. If the new terms—specific learning disability, dyslexia, cerebral dysfunction, minimum brain damage, neurological handicaps, and perceptual handicaps—have confused laymen who follow educational developments, the confusion reflects in part this continuing lack of agreement among the experts themselves.

Soon, concern with learning troubles came to be intertwined with concern with "behavior disorders"—a term that is unhappily ambiguous. The intertwining was natural, since learning and behavior themselves are closely related, not only in the obvious ways, but through their common source in the CNS. The way a child's CNS works, it was concluded, can interfere with both his learning and the conduct of the class he is in, by making him compulsively responsive to stimuli from within or without, and hence compulsively hyperactive. Apparently, what happens in such a case is that the instructions the child sends his CNS more or less deliberately are superseded or swamped by other messages coming in from elsewhere in his brain, his body, or his environment, and, as a Canadian researcher has put it, "the child tries to react to everything at once." Fidgety Phil cannot sit still, however much he may want to. This phenomenon has the medical name hyperkinesia, but is often simply called hyperactivity, the latter being another ambiguous term, the use of which has helped to confuse the issue.

As physicians have known for years, hyperkinesia can be controlled by amphetamine and amphetamine-like drugs. These drugs are not tranquilizers; in fact, for a person whose CNS functions normally, they are the opposite: By blocking out messages about fatigue, discomfort, or hunger that would normally interfere with his concentrating on an activity, they pep him up. In the case of the medically hyperactive child, it seems, the blocking-out of messages that make him fidgety enables him to be quieter and to do better work. Incidentally, the effect they have of speeding up some persons and quieting down others, often called paradoxical, provides a pretty good guarantee that they will make children more subdued only if the hyperactivity is involuntary. Such hyperactivity has been helpfully treated with a number of drugs in this category, including three reported as being used in Omaha: dextroamphetamine, Ritalin, and Deaner.

A more familiar group of drugs that also control hyperactivity and "behavior disorders" but are given less frequently is the tranquilizers. One of these, Raudixin, a strong drug derived from the *Rauwolfia serpentina* root, was mentioned in one Omaha report. Tranquilizers, as is commonly known, can dilute the strength of a child's emotions, and they can thus combat temper tantrums, destructiveness, and boisterousness.

Tofranil and Aventyl, the other two drugs mentioned as being given in Omaha, are mood-changing drugs of a third kind: anti-depressants. Their main use is for treating neurotic depression, which may make children irritable and restless.

It is drugs of these different kinds that in laymen's language are called behavior modification drugs. Both the American Medical Association's Council on Drugs and a panel of the National Academy of Science have evaluated them, and, while caution is still recommended, the medical support for their use is impressive.

The use of drugs to improve school performance by controlling hyperactivity and disabling emotions is now so well established it is not surprising that, even in the face of violent criticism, Omaha physicians and school officials stood their ground. The pediatrician in the middle of the controversy said he felt like a Ping-Pong ball, but insisted that he and other physicians were circumspect about what they were doing and were following good medical practice. Apparently, most parents of children being treated were behind it. An article on the science page of *The New York Times* entitled "Drugs That Help Control the Unruly Child" cited distinguished support, as did a major story on the Omaha affair in the AMA's *American Medical News.* The latter journal, interviewing pediatricians and child psychiatrists across the nation, summed up their attitude as being "What's all the fuss about?"

School officials appeared equally unperturbed. To them, it seems, the use of drugs for modifying behavior was strictly a medical matter. Quite apart from the fact that for teachers to administer drugs to children would have been illegal, by Board of Education policy, educators were not to be involved in behavior control through medication "in any manner whatsoever." Officials apparently saw no reason for concern about the school system's efforts to build communication between parents and physicians, the presence of school personnel at meetings addressed by representatives of drug companies, the reported practice of having teachers identify children they think can benefit from drugs, the screening of children for referral to private physicians by the school system's health and psychological services, teachers' holding drugs in safe-keeping for children and on occasion probably reminding children to take them, or the convincing evidence that some teachers have approached parents about getting their children put on drugs in a way that made the parents feel they were being badgered.

These practices are not unique to Omaha but are common throughout the United States and, indeed, abroad. Most educators believe that such practices give no grounds for concern. They seem pleased, in fact, to be working alongside physicians as fellow professionals. They share with physicians a devotion to helping children and know they are in a particularly good position to spot those who have special medical needs, refer them for help, and then observe them intensively. What *is* all the fuss about?

The real fuss is about the fact that using drugs to influence classroom behavior entails at least five serious risks, four of which the professionals take far too lightly, even though parents and politicians, in their intuitive and sometimes inarticulate way, have recognized them with some dismay.

Two of the five risks are medical, the most dramatic being that of producing undesirable physiological side effects, known or as yet unknown, possibly including addiction—in the physiological sense. Although some of the drugs mentioned can have bad side effects, the danger of such effects is one the physicians in question are well aware of, have studied, and keep very much in mind. The drugs being used are prescription drugs, they are not physiologically addictive for children, and the pediatricians who prescribe them no doubt feel that if they give them to children only with the informed consent of their parents, and then with care, the safeguards are adequate. Since pediatricians are conscientious, dedicated people, and there is fairly good reason to accept their assurances on this score, and since, anyway, the Food and Drug Administration polices their behavior, this risk need not concern us further.

The other medical risk to be considered is that of faulty diagnoses. While physicians seem to feel that they have avoided this risk, too, it is probable that they have not. When the drug is Ritalin or another of the amphetamine types, as it most often is, an error may correct itself: If the child isn't suffering from clinical hyperactivity, his pills will probably make him livelier. This is not true, however, for the tranquilizers.

The real reason why physicians are confident of their diagnoses seems to lie in the cooperation they have from school people who observe their patients' behavior day in, day out. The physicians working in this area lean on teachers very heavily, frequently giving as a reason for doing so their belief that teachers' judgments about children are objective.

In their great desire to help, however, physicians are inclined to trust teachers' judgments too much. One distinguished physician who has done a great deal of research in this area has used a check list for identifying children with an "emotional disturbance," which defines "deviancy" as doing anything disapproved by the teacher; it lists as abnormal behavior a child's dismantling his ballpoint pen, propping up his desk with his pencil, or stopping on the way back from the pencil sharpener to talk with someone or to look at things on the teacher's desk. When teachers' evaluations of children's behavior are that questionable (the reasons for this will be explained below), diagnoses based on their reports are questionable, too.

The three non-medical risks, though less tangible, are at least as serious. The first of these is the risk of contributing to the drug culture. As one Omaha parent remarked, "I don't want my child to grow up believing that as soon as things aren't right, they can take a pill to make it better." The risk of disposing children psychologically toward drugs in general is in a sense an educational one. Since no one yet knows how to deal with it, and since at the same time medical people might be a bit overinclined to resort to medication, it would make sense for physicians themselves, parents, and school people who might influence a decision to put an overactive child on drugs, to keep this risk very much in mind.

The other two risks arise when the purpose of the drug is specifically the modifying of classroom behavior. The first has directly to do with education, one aim of which is to help children learn to regulate their behavior for themselves. For them to do this requires that they come to grips with their natural dispositions and learn to use in a certain way what Philip Jackson at the University of Chicago has nicely called their own "executive powers." Any form of intervention that relieves a restless or unruly child of the need, or deprives him of the opportunity, to use his executive powers deprives him to that extent of the chance to develop insight and skill in self-control. True, this is a price we constantly pay and have to pay so that school and life can go on. Still, for each child these opportunities are finite, and beyond a certain point interfering with his governing his own behavior jeopardizes his growth in independence.

The fifth risk is that of infringing on children's legal rights or their civil liberties. Recent court cases have brought to light a number of things school children do that teachers and principals think disruptive, but that the children are legally entitled to do, such as refusing to pledge allegiance to the flag, distributing political pamphlets, and, in many cases, wearing long hair and saying nasty things in school newspapers. There ai e no doubt other kinds of behavior that children have a right to engage in, and that are just as repugnant to teachers and principals, but on which the courts haven't yet ruled. Actually, according to legal theory, the only objectionable behavior the school has a right to control is that which it *must* control in order to accomplish its job and protect persons and the institution. Going still further, civil libertarians and some educators hold that over and above behavior protected by law, there are many other things a child should be free to do, however objectionable they may be. For legal reasons, then, and perhaps educational and moral ones, too, the kinds of behavior the school tries to bring under control should be limited. Whether the school's effort along this line is aimed directly at the student or channeled through his parent or doctor, there is always the risk of its pushing beyond that limit.

Neither school people nor physicians concerned with "children with special problems" show much concern about any of these non-medical risks. Why? Since they have to do with learning and the conduct of schools, it seems fair to attribute the physicians' obliviousness of them to the educators' not having pointed them out. Who could be expected to know as much as educators do about ways of helping children develop mental health, about the classroom conditions under which children can best learn self-control, and about the proper extent of their rights and liberties? Who should be more able to gauge the extent to which a child's behavior in school is productive, legitimate, disruptive, or dangerous?

Unfortunately, while educators are aware of the issues in a general way, most are themselves as oblivious of the practical risks as physicians. This is why they are satisfied that control of classroom hyperactivity through drugs is strictly a medical matter. The root of the trouble is that they have no rationally thought-out criteria for disciplinary practice in general, so that their decisions about it can only be intuitive and subjective. Thus, behavior that some teachers regard as healthy, constructive, and within children's rights causes others great concern.

As long as this remains so, physicians, parents, and teachers themselves should not look upon teachers' negative assessments of children's behavior as informed professional judgments but take them with a grain of salt. Several grains, indeed, because of a number of factors tending to distort those assessments in the direction of repressiveness. These factors have been studied so little that most people are hardly aware of them. Four are particularly important to understand.

First, a special ideology about discipline holds sway in most American schools. One aspect of it is the idea that children will not only behave best but learn best how to regulate their behavior later on if they are kept under tight control; control produces self-control. This is a view inherited from Puritan days, cultivated by school boards, and enshrined for decades in American school law, a view that contrary findings of psychology have weakened only in part. Another aspect, paradoxically, is a very optimistic idea derived indirectly from Rousseau, Dewey, and the mental hygienists, and promoted by schools of education: Children's behavior is naturally good, a good teacher shouldn't have to be concerned with regulating it, and any behavior the teacher finds objectionable is an abnormal phenomenon, a "discipline problem," a form of pathology having some specific cause. Hence the belief—the third aspect of the ideology—that any misbehavior can be stopped if one can just pinpoint its cause and find the right cure. Taken together, these notions lead teachers and principals to believe that objectionable behavior must never be countenanced, and that if it occurs something is seriously wrong; so, since it always does occur, "classroom control" may come to be an obsession. (European educators are often surprised to find American school children very orderly, yet American teachers greatly concerned nonetheless about disorder.) More often than not, obviously, a teacher looks for the presumed cause of a conflict between the child and the school, not in a disturbing school setting or an inappropriate demand made on the child, but inside the child himself.

Second, public school systems in America are monopolistic, classical, government bureaucracies, in which the students, for most purposes, compose the bottom echelon. Although some children are glad to attend school, and it wouldn't be right to call their membership in this bureaucracy unwilling, they can hardly ever forget that it is compulsory. When it comes to children's behavior, these facts are important in two ways. For one thing, the form of organization cannot but greatly restrict children's freedom: The superintendent is responsible for *everything* that goes on in the school, and the teacher for *everything* that goes on in his classroom, and responsibility must, of course, be accompanied by control. Then, too, when teachers or other professional school personnel are caught in conflicts between their professional standards and the preferences of their administrators, they tend to follow the latter. So, because principals, for several reasons, usually insist on a high degree of order, teachers are forced to do the same. Administrators' pressure on teachers to sit on children is described by a team of Yale psychologists as "most intolerant."

Ironically, however, our public schools provide teachers quite inadequate means for performing the task. Organizations characteristically regulate behavior through rewards and punishments, and most provide supervisors with persuasive repertoires of both. The one great power the school gives the teacher, his say over children's academic futures, is too remote to have much effect on most children's behavior. Otherwise the typical school affords the teacher practically no rewards to dispense and arms him with at most five kinds of punishment—extra work, physical hitting and beating, detention, referral to the principal or the parent, and barring from extracurricular activities—each of which may be so disadvantageous to the teacher or the child that its usefulness is limited. The contrast is stark between the disciplinary situations in ordinary public schools and in schools where researchers or private entrepreneurs are allowed to reward children with money, trading stamps, transistor radios, field trips, or free time.

Lacking resources supplied by the school, teachers are forced to try to regulate children's behavior almost exclusively with more personal ones, their skill in manipulating, their smiles and frowns, encouragement and praise, expressions of disapproval, reproaches, humiliation, and the like. Up to a point, a personal approach to children is normal and proper. But when it is almost the only one a teacher can use, and the pressure to keep the class under tight control is great, any obstreperous child is likely to become a personal threat. In this situation the idea that there is something wrong with the child that someone might fix up by doctoring his internal mechanisms, whether through psychotherapy or chemotherapy, may become irresistible. And, because misbehavior is defined as abnormal anyway, changing the child so that he will behave is easily justified as being in the child's own interest.

Fourth, teachers have unrecognized power over parents, stemming from the strong position they are in to favor or harass children day by day, as well as to influence their futures. This power teachers themselves overlook, probably because the parents who catch their special attention are those who are intransigent. Parents who are uneducated or poor or lack political clout are particularly vulnerable to pressure. So when teachers make suggestions, many parents take them as recommendations, while recommendations, in turn, are often taken as witting or unwitting threats.

It is because these aspects of the typical public school teacher's ideology and role are likely to color his judgment that his judgment is no adequate protection against the risks. At least until teachers' situations and their thinking change, then, other protections must be established. If the dedicated Omaha people who were battered by controversy last summer have been the vehicles for educating us on this score, they have served us well.

What might be realistic safeguards? Following are a few suggestions:

—It would be useful for school officials, pediatricians, and parents of children with behavior difficulties to explore *all* the risks in behavior modification through drugs openly, thoroughly, and continuously.

—School systems would do well to draw up policies to guide teachers' and administrators' activities in educational associations that concern themselves with influencing classroom behavior and that include parents and physicians. These policies should take account of the conflict of interest that may arise between a teacher's personal desire to help an individual child and his obligation as a functionary of the state's school system to enforce that system's policies.

—When a teacher or someone else in a school system finds a child's behavior intolerable and suspects a medical cause, the school system might well follow a different procedure from that for ordinary medical cases and allow only school personnel whose relationship with the child is a strictly professional, confidential one, and who are not in a position to reward or penalize him directly or indirectly, to approach a parent about possible medical treatment. (This sort of safeguard might well apply to psychotherapeutic treatment, too.)

—It would be a good policy to allow school personnel to do nothing in regard to the referring of a child with behavior problems to a physician or clinic or the treating of such a child, except as requested in writing by the parent.

—When physicians receive reports that children behave badly in school, they should remain skeptical until they have obtained independent evidence.

—It is important that each state make its proper contribution to the health and education of the young. Drugs have a part to play in both. But it is important, too, that the state be restrained in the limits it sets on deviancy. Drugs, perhaps more than any other instrument for controlling children's behavior, may endanger both of these ideals. Eternal vigilance has no substitute.

23. Principles of Drug Therapy in Child Psychiatry with Special Reference to Stimulant Drugs

Leon Eisenberg

Let me state at the outset what pride of authorship constrains me to call Eisenberg's First Law of Psychopharmacology: the less the evidence on which an opinion is based, the firmer the conviction with which it will be maintained. Once this fundamental concept has been mastered, one will be better prepared for the polemics, the obfuscations, and the personal vendettas that beset the field. But I would prefer to emphasize issues rather than persons. It seems to me appropriate to begin by considering four dilemmas: the therapeutic "orphaning" of children; the problem of long-term effects; the issue of who is being treated; and the problem of social cost. Let us consider them seriatim, before turning to an outline of principles of treatment.

I. Therapeutic Orphans

The Canadian pediatrician, Harry Shirkey,[22] coined the term "therapeutic orphans" to refer to the anomalous situation in which the reluctance to test drugs in children results in insufficient data on efficacy and safety so that the drugs are labelled in a fashion that precludes their use in many children who might be expected to benefit from them; hence, children become the orphans of pharmacology. Since about 1962, the drug package insert approved by the Food and Drug Administration has contained the clause "not to be used in children, since clinical studies have been insufficient to establish recommendations for its use." This statement, it should be noted, is to be distinguished sharply from labelling that contains the phrase: "contraindicated in infants or children on the basis of studies showing it to be unsafe or ineffective." The latter is based upon data that make prescription unwise; the former reflects *lack* of data as of the time the package insert was prepared. Most pediatricians would agree with the position of Modell[17] that the insert is a useful guide, but nothing more; its recommendations should be evaluated together with other information available to the physician. What remains unclear, however, is the legal status of prescribing a drug not yet approved for use with children. While official "approval"

From *American Journal of Orthopsychiatry*, 1971, **41**, 371–379. Copyright © 1971, the American Orthopsychiatric Association, Inc. Reproduced by permission.

of a drug does not protect the physician from liability for consequences subsequent to its use, there is considerable uncertainty, in the absence of recorded test cases, as to whether a physician who prescribed a drug in good faith (based upon available clinical evidence) might be placed in jeopardy, should an undesired effect occur, precisely because of the influence of the language of the package insert on judge and jury. It is likely that many physicians, as well as clinical investigators, are reluctant to innovate with drugs in children because of the putative danger arising from this warning. Such physician behavior can only result in denying useful medications to children.

At the heart of the problem lies the dubious ethic of experimenting with drugs in normal children. Whereas it would appear legitimate to secure adult volunteers who are willing to undergo a potential hazard after being informed of the risk because of their conviction that they are contributing to medical knowledge, few of us are convinced that parents should be asked to "volunteer" their children under similar circumstances. My department, for one, has never seen its way clear to such an undertaking despite our very great interest in the information that might be so obtained. The fact that stimulant drugs reliably produce enhanced attention and diminished purposeless motor activity in hyperkinetic children permits no informed conclusion as to what such drugs would do in normal children. Such knowledge would give us a better basis for interpreting the findings in the disturbed child. Nonetheless, we have not undertaken such studies; nor has anyone else, to our knowledge. Investigation has been limited to to the use of a drug in children with a behavior disorder thought to be responsive to its administration.

Thus, the usual sequence has been thorough testing in a variety of animal species followed by investigative use in the sick child. That situation has as its corollary the necessity to gather as much information as possible in studies with pediatric patients. The problems of inter-specific comparison and the remarkably different effects related to developmental age point to the necessity for far more extensive programs in pediatric clinical pharmacology than are now in existence. The child, it should not need pointing out here, is not a miniature adult. Differences, both quantitative and qualitative, in drug response distinguish the developing organism from the adult; these differences are greatest in the youngest epochs—fetal, premature, neonate (first month) and infant (up to two years) but also characterize children and adolescents.

The relevant variables are multiple and complex. *Rate of absorption* is influenced by the efficiency of transport across the intestinal villi, the time of transit as affected by the length of the GI tract, the recumbent posture and differences in diet and GI contents. *Body distribution* is influenced by differences in the percentage of lean body mass as opposed to fat and water, by the relatively greater body surface area in the infant, by the immaturity of the blood-brain barrier and by kinetics of protein binding. As one example of the latter, the injudicious use of sulfonamides displaces bilirubin from protein thus rendering it far more toxic at the same total blood level.[18] Further, *detoxification mechanisms*, in particular conjugation with glucuronic acid, are far less effective in the newborn, thus altering the effective half-life of ingested drugs. *Excretion* of drugs is affected by the fact that the immature kidney is relatively low in glomerular filtration rate and tubular clearance so that a substance such as penicillin G persists in the circulation for a period considerably longer than in the adult.[2] Finally, one anticipates differences in *end-organ responsiveness.* These topics have been reviewed in detail elsewhere;[4] it will suffice to call them to attention as a backdrop for further deliberations.

II. Long-Term Effects

The immediate problem for the toxicologist in both adult and in child therapeutics is the here and now toxicity of a new drug; that is, what are its immediate consequences for morbidity and mortality? In the adult, if the period of administration is brief, there is usually little reason for concern about subsequent effects. However, in the child, what is given even briefly at a particular developmental period may have unforeseen long-term consequences. As one example, consider the effect of tetracycline on children even to the age of eight in producing dental staining in deciduous and permanent teeth. The chronic use of drugs raises many problems in adults as well, but in children we have particular concern with drug effects on growth and development, as evidenced by the growth retardation produced by the long-term use of steroids.

What we do not know, but all of us fear, is the possibility of behavioral long-term consequences. Animal data suggest that the administration of sedatives to pregnant animals or to the newborns themselves alter the behavior of the offspring when they are mature at a time when the drug is no longer detectable.[13] We are all aware of the potent effects of miniscule doses of sex hormones given at birth on the sexual behavior of the mature animal.[16] It is not likely that human development is so readily influenceable, given the much longer periods available for learning and the lack of phenomena strictly comparable to "imprinting."[8] Nonetheless, we are becoming ever more aware of how widespread are drug actions on the biology of the organism at points far removed from the target of their administration. The effect of phenobarbital on liver enzyme systems or of many drugs on the adenyl cyclase system (the so-called second messenger) are cases in point. For most of the issues with which this paper is concerned, few relevant data are available on long-term effects, but by analogy to what is known, the available data urge caution upon us.

III. Who is Being Treated?

The third of our dilemmas refers to the issue of patienthood. The adult generally volunteers himself as the psychiatric patient. He may at times be an unwilling "volunteer" coerced by family, community or court but most often it is he who suffers the discomfort that leads him to consult the physician. Although exceptions do exist, the child rarely volunteers; ordinarily, he is brought by his parents, sometimes at the behest of his teacher or the courts. Is the child designated as "patient" because his mother is anxious about behavior that on a normative scale would be considered average? Is he brought for treatment because his teacher is angered by normally assertive behavior that threatens her authority? Does the court designate his problem "psychiatric" simply because alternative ways of dealing with it are unavailable even though the pathology is social (as is all too often the case in children found to be neglected or delinquent)?

While mothers may be unduly anxious, teachers insecure and courts at a loss, there is evidence that children designated as patients are indeed deviant. Shula Wolff[23] has shown this in a comparison of patients with the general child population. Lee Robins's[19] followup of child guidance cases into adulthood indicates clearly that former patients are at significant risk for adult psychopathology when compared with classroom controls. Rutter[21] and his co-workers have carried out an epidemiologic study on the Isle of Wight that indicates that clinicians can reliably identify children in need of help.

This is not to deny the possibility of abuse. It does serve to emphasize the importance of a careful clinical evaluation before starting *any* treatment program. Psychiatrists should not allow themselves to become the agents of disturbed mothers, inadequate teachers or uninformed judges. If they adhere to the basic tenets of their professional training, they will not be. The risks of abuse can be contained only if drug administration is recognized to be a medical responsibility and if the physicians empowered to use drugs are appropriately trained and ethically responsible.

IV. Social Cost

Pharmacology is accustomed to weighing risk against benefit. Benefit is assessed in terms of the condition being treated, the outcome in the absence of treatment and the differences produced by the treatment. Risk is measured in terms of morbidity and mortality from drug action. In the case of children, one has to consider both the risk and the benefit in terms of long-term consequences as well as immediate ones. The behavior disorder may appear to be time-limited (as in the overactivity of the hyperkinetic child) but the risk of other and more serious subsequent disturbance has also to be weighed. If the apparent overactivity and distractibility do fade with time (even in the absence of treatment), must we not also take into account the cost to the child of not having learned during that time span because of the interference with learning produced by the symptoms? And what of the secondary consequences, both of being labelled as "bad" and of being blamed for failing to learn: the poor self-concept and the antisocial behavior that may well result?

A hidden component of cost is the problem presented by any effective treatment; namely, the possibility that its very success will diminish the social zeal for prevention. For example, the availability of methods for treating lead poisoning *may* have been a factor in the failure of the medical profession to take the leadership it should have exerted in public campaigns to remove lead-containing interior paints. It is not so much that physicians would not wish to see this hazard removed as that they have not been as aggressive in social action as they might have been. I am not arguing that any are completely satisfied with available treatments (which fall far short of reversing the patient's illness) but rather that preoccupation with treatment and its refinement has absorbed energy that might more effectively be aimed at removing causes. There are major research problems still to be solved in treating lead poisoning but there is no lack of data about the source of that poisoning; yet physicians put more energy into the refinement of treatment than into preventing the disorder by condemning slum housing.[1]

In like fashion, it is at least arguable that the relative ease with which symptoms of overactive and impulsive behavior can be treated with stimulant drugs might lead to a diminution of efforts to prevent those conditions which, in part, bring it about: complications of pregnancy and parturition; post-natal infection, malnutrition and trauma; crowded homes and crowded schools; poorly trained and poorly motivated teachers; in addition to the unknown factors that require to be searched out.

It has been suggested[15] that ours is a drug oriented society that relies on substance use to alter the sensorium in place of attempts to make life more rewarding for those troubled by it. Whether or not this indictment is correct in all respects, any reader of medical journals can point to pharmaceutical advertisements that imply that unhappy housewives or harassed executives should receive this or that tranquilizer—without even so much as a suggestion that the fundamental problem is the life style that produced the unhappiness or the harassment. To the extent that physicians subscribe uncritically to this philosophy, then, indeed, the cost in toxicity from tranquilizing drugs is likely to be far greater than can be measured by counting what are customarily listed as side effects. The most costly (and uncounted) "side effect" will have been the diversion of effort from a direct attack on the sources of the symptoms, much as the prescription of aspirin for a headache caused by a meningioma allows the tumor to grow unchecked by diminishing the signal warning of its presence. More specific to our topic, restlessness in an inner city classroom can be diminished by feeding the children, since many come to school without breakfast and exhibit restlessness resulting from hypoglycemia. Let there be no misunderstanding of my view: it would be a criminal abdication of medical responsibility to treat such children with stimulant drugs. If drugs are used indiscriminately in response to symptoms rather than to the underlying medical disorder, just such abuses will occur. Moreover, every clinician (and every school teacher, for that matter) knows that behavior in the classroom is a function of the teacher's effectiveness, which, though not the *only* relevant variable, is an important determinant of children's behavior. Were a child to be referred for impulsive and distractable behavior from a class led by an incompetent teacher, drug administration would be counter-productive as contrasted with steps to retrain or replace the teacher. The fact that abuse *can* occur accents medical responsibility for diagnosis; it is a poor argument for abandoning drug use, thus denying treatment to those who might profit from it in order to spare those whom drugs might injure.

The basic clinical problem stems from the fact that behavior symptoms are a final common pathway for the expression of multiple causes. A tremor may result from simple anxiety, from hyperthyroidism or from disorders of the basal ganglia. The appropriate treatment of the same manifest behavior is different in each case. With such symptoms as overactivity and distractibility, diagnostic differentiation is more difficult since we lack pathognomonic signs and symptoms. We can, however, rule out identifiable causes and reserve symptomatic medication for the cases for which no alternative remedy is available.

But what of the accusation that the hyperkinetic syndrome is nothing more than "the normal exuberance of childhood"? This statement was attributed to a distinguished physician in a newspaper account of Senate hearings.[12] Are drugs, as alleged by Congressman Gallagher,[11] "being employed to induce conformity, rather than creativity, in the classroom?" Or, in the words of the Brown-Pembroke SDS,[3] are they used for "stifling rebelliousness and maintaining the status quo" in classrooms for black children?

As I have been at pain to point out, the possibility of abuse does exist. Teachers all too often do prefer conformity; physicians at times do abandon their responsibility for diagnosis and prescribe in response to parental pressure; black children *are* victimized by American society. But none of these admissions constitutes evidence for a nationwide conspiracy to drug children into insensibility nor contravenes the reality of a behavioral syndrome for which proper medication can produce dramatic benefit.

In 1967, the World Health Organization assembled psychiatrists and epidemiologists from France, Japan, Norway, Peru, the United Kingdom, the U.S.S.R., Austria, Italy, Belgium, Switzerland, the Netherlands, Portugal, Spain, Formosa, Australia and the United States to discuss the diagnosis and classification of psychiatric disorders in children. That expert group agreed unanimously on the need for a category termed "hyperkinetic syndrome" whose chief characteristics were described as "extreme overactivity which was poorly organized and poorly regulated by the usual social controls, distractability, short attention span, impulsiveness, and often also, marked mood fluctuations and aggression. Such disorders were much commoner in boys than in girls; there was often a characteristic response to drugs such as amphetamine, and frequently, too, there were associated perceptual difficulties and problems at school. While these conditions were sometimes associated with organic brain pathology, it was generally agreed that this was often not the case and that certainly this could not constitute any part of the diagnostic criteria."[20]

Agreed, the reality of a clinical disorder is not established by vote; it *does* seem noteworthy that a world panel of psychiatrists, trained in different schools of thought, functioning in different cultures, and speaking different languages, all agreed on the existence in their home countries of children who exhibit the hyperkinetic syndrome and who benefit from stimulant drugs. Surely, this is a far cry from the contention that we are dealing with "the normal exuberance of childhood" or that we are employing drugs "to induce conformity" or "to stifle rebelliousness."

This is not the place to review in extenso the reports from our own laboratory on the repeated demonstration of beneficial effects from stimulant drugs in the treatment of children with hyperkinetic behavior and school learning problems.[5] [6] [7] [9] [10] Suffice it to say that these agents have the unique property of diminishing purposeless motor activity and of enhancing attention span with the result of improving learning, all of this at the price of relatively minor side effects. It has been argued recently that, despite these encouraging findings, we may be introducing youngsters to the use of drugs and thus inadvertently making them more vulnerable to drug abuse in adolescence. An unpublished followup of cases treated by Laufer,[14] youngsters put on medication in childhood but surveyed in late adolescence or early adulthood, revealed no known drug abusers. These findings are not surprising. I am aware of no evidence that epileptics who, of necessity, are long-term drug users are thereby at risk for drug abuse with other substances. No such evidence exists for diabetics, for individuals with hypothyroidism, or any of the myriad chronic conditions that require prolonged drug use. What accounts for this phenomenon, I suggest, is that none of these drugs produces a euphoric affect in the pre-adolescent child and thus there is no subjective experience that leads the patient to seek the drug deliberately. Those alarmed by the abuse potential of amphetamines in adolescence, a real and frightening phenomenon, assume that the subjective effect in the child taking amphetamines resembles that in the older user. But the clinical facts are otherwise. Most often, if the child comments at all about subjective effects, it is to complain of dysphoria or sleepiness; some even are subject to unprovoked episodes of crying. The child may feel positive about the social consequences of the effect of the drug on his own behavior; that is, he may feel better *about* himself because his teacher compliments him for learning or his mother no longer complains about his misbehaving, but he obtains no direct "high" from the drug itself.

Any potent drug may be abused—and that includes stimulants. But should we deny diabetics insulin because insulin can be (and has been) used to commit suicide? Should we deny schizophrenics phenothiazines because overworked housewives can be drugged into insensibility instead of being helped to find a more meaningful life role? Should we deny distractible children stimulants that can enhance their ability to succeed at learning because incompetent or even malicious teachers, doctors or parents may mistreat nonconforming or underfed children? The possibility of abuse is an argument for better medical practice, not a return to astrology. Perhaps the greatest source of confusion with stimulant drugs is the use of the descriptive adjective "stimulant" which, while it may accurately reflect drug action in the adolescent or adult, hardly categorizes its effect in children. If we believe words have power, perhaps we should return to the use of the term sympathomimetic. Would that our social problems could be solved so easily!

Principles of Drug Treatment

No drug should be employed without firm indication for its use, without careful supervision of the patient to be treated, and without due precautions for the recognition and control of toxicity. If a drug is to be used, the severity of the presenting condition and the likelihood of benefit must outweigh the risk of toxicity. If the patients to be treated are children, clinical decisions must be based upon data from pediatric studies; we cannot safely extrapolate from adults to children. Surveillance for toxicity must consider long-term as well as immediate consequences.

The second principle might be labelled pharmacologic conservatism: an old and familiar drug is to be preferred to a new drug unless there is preponderant evidence for superiority of the latter. Unexpected toxicity from a new agent may become apparent only after prolonged experience with its use; we should therefore be cautious in using a new agent except when its benefit is so superior as to warrant the putative risk.

Drugs can be useful agents in the management of pediatric psychiatric disorders when chosen appropriately and applied with discrimination. They can control symptoms not readily managed by other means and can facilitate other methods of psychiatric treatment by allaying symptoms that disrupt learning.

Every study reveals the potency of placebo effects; that is, benefits occurring from expectation in physician and patient. These expectations can be used to potentiate drug effects by recognizing that the prescription of medicine is an important communication both to the child and to his family. Drugs can have negative effects if the physician regards them solely as weapons to impose control or as measures of desperation. The meaning of the transaction is determined by the attitudes of all participants: the patient, his family and his physician. Skill in the use of drugs requires, in addition to detailed knowledge of their pharmacologic properties, sensitivity to their psychologic implications.

Drugs should be used no longer than necessary. Dosage should be reduced periodically with the goal of ceasing treatment if symptoms do not return on a lower dosage or after the drug has been discontinued. This applies with particular force to drugs used over long periods in treating chronic conditions. In the case of stimulant drug treatment of hyperkinesis, it has been our practice to discontinue medication at the end of the school term and to allow a child a trial return to school without medication, the drug to be resumed only if it proves to be necessary. Dosage must be individualized. Each patient is metabolically unique. Under-treatment, as well as over-treatment, can result from rigid use of medication without appropriate sensitivity to manipulation of dosage.

Medication should not be used to relieve the physician of the responsibility for seeking to identify and eliminate factors causing or aggravating the underlying disorder. Stimulant drugs treat symptoms, not diseases. Symptomatic relief is not to be disparaged; often, it is the most the physician can offer. However, since symptom suppression can delay appropriate intervention, treatment should follow, not precede, thorough diagnostic evaluation.

With no intent to minimize the importance of alertness to drug toxicity, it is necessary to balance this risk against the cost of doing nothing as well as the cost of alternative treatments. We, then, must ask: what is the natural history of the disorder in the absence of treatment? The greater the immediate and the long-term morbidity, the readier the justification for heroic interventions. We must ask, also: what is the "toxicity" of alternative non-drug treatments? Psychotherapy is not necessarily benign; it can foster dependency, increase self-preoccupation, and produce feelings of futility and hopelessness when used to "treat" a condition for which it is inappropriate.

Our goal is the healthy development of children. Stimulant drugs may be helpful in suppressing symptoms that interfere with learning. But these agents do no more than make it *possible* for the child to learn; in themselves, they teach him nothing. To the extent that he has failed to learn or has developed faulty learning habits, he will require remedial educational measures. Thus, the administration of drugs, an important part of the therapeutic plan when they are given appropriately, constitutes only *one* part of the total treatment program. They must be accompanied by appropriate school plans, parent counselling, recreational programs and other growth-promoting activities that encourage personal development. Pharmacologic methods provide neither the passport to a brave new world nor the gateway to the inferno. With thoughtful selection, careful regulation of dosage and close scrutiny for toxicity, they can add a significant component to total patient care. For all of this, the physician bears a major responsibility as the patient's advocate. To be successful, he will need to enlist the cooperation of teachers, psychologists, parents, and the community as a political body, if he is to create a climate within which each child can attain his human potential.

References

1. Anderson, D. 1971. Public institutions: their war against black youth. Amer. J. Orthopsychiat. 41:65.
2. Barnett, H. et al. 1949. Renal clearances of sodium penicillin G, procaine penicillin G and insulin in infants and children. Pediatrics 3:418.
3. Brown-Pembroke Students for a Democratic Society. 1970. Mimeographed handout.
4. Conference on Pediatric Pharmacology. 1967 (Feb. 19–21). Supt. of Documents, U.S. Government Printing Office, Washington.
5. Conners, C. et al. 1967. Effect of dextroamphetamine on children. Arch. Gen. Psychiat. 17:478.
6. Conners, C. et al. 1969. Dextroamphetamine sulfate in children with learning disorders. Arch. Gen. Psychiat. 21:182.
7. Eisenberg, L. 1966. The management of the hyperkinetic child. Developm. Med. Child Neurol. 8:593.
8. Eisenberg, L. 1969. Persistent problems in the biopsychology of development. Presented at American Museum of Natural History, New York.

9. Eisenberg, L. et al. 1963. A psychopharmacologic study in a training school for delinquents. Amer. J. Orthopsychiat. 33:431.
10. Eisenberg, L. and Conners, C. 1963. The effect of a stimulant drug on impulsivity and learning in disturbed children. Amer. J. Psychiat. 120:458.
11. Gallagher, C. 1970 (Sept. 21). News release. House Office Building, Washington.
12. Hollister, L. 1970 (Nov. 26). Quoted in Associated Press dispatch, Providence Evening Bulletin, Providence, R.I.
13. Kornetsky, C. 1970. Psychoactive drugs in the immature organism. Psychopharmacologia 17:105.
14. Laufer, M., Conners, C. and McCarthy, P. 1970. Unpublished manuscript.
15. Lennard, H. et al. 1970. Hazards implicit in prescribing psychoactive drugs. Science 169:438.
16. Levine, S. and Mullins, R. 1966. Hormonal influences on brain organization in infant rats. Science 152:1585.
17. Modell, W. 1967. FDA Censorship. Clin. Pharmacol. Ther. 8:359.
18. Odell, G. 1959. The dissociation of bilirubin from albumin and its clinical implications. J. Pediat. 55:268.
19. Robins, L. 1966. Deviant Children Grown Up. Williams & Wilkins, Baltimore.
20. Rutter, M. et al. 1969. A tri-axial classification of mental disorders in childhood. J. Child. Psychol. Psychiat. 10:41.
21. Rutter, M., Tizard, J. and Whitmore, K. 1970. Education, Health and Behaviour. Longman, London.
22. Shirkey, H. 1968. Therapeutic Orphans. J. Pediat. 72:119.
23. Wolff, S. 1967. Behavioral characteristics of primary school children referred to a psychiatric department. Brit. J. Psychiat. 113:885.

24. Long-Term Management and Some Follow-Up Findings on the Use of Drugs with Minimal Cerebral Syndromes

Maurice W. Laufer

This report is based upon the concept that there is a major role for medications in controlling the symptomatic manifestations of the behavioral picture known as "hyperkinetic impulse disorder," and that such control is the basic reason for the generally noted improvement in school work. Those medications displaying a favorable effect cause an increase in available norepinephrine at cell surfaces in the central nervous system. The reverse is also true.

Generally the efficacy of the medications is monitored by their effects on overactivity and distractibility, over a period of years, rather than months.

From *Journal of Learning Disabilities*, 1971, **4**, 518–522. Copyright 1971 by The Professional Press, Inc. Reproduced by permission.

Desired Level. The goal is to have activity and attention under the control of the individual, so that he may be active and attentive when and where he desires, neither incapable of such control, nor having excessive control forced upon him.

Excessive Dosage. This may be indicated by over-control (too quiet, too still, fixated upon what he is doing, even put to sleep), or by the appearance of stimulation (overactivity, irritability, tension, tearfulness). These findings require lessening of the dosage.

Side Effects. With the most commonly used medications (amphetamines and methylphenidate), they are fundamentally similar. Though none necessarily occur, the most common are:

1. *Amphetamine look.* A pale, pinched, serious facial expression, with dark hollows under the eyes. This does not represent any serious difficulty and there is no way to alter it.

2. *Anorexia.* This may pass in time, fade with a different medication, be controlled by the use of Periactin before meals, or circumvented by a pre-bedtime snack and giving medication *after* breakfast.

3. *Insomnia.* Actually, there are a number of possible causes for this. One is the persistence of the hyperkinetic picture at night, so that a bedtime dose of medication is required. Another is a rebound effect after the daytime medication has worn off. This may respond to Benadryl before bed. Last, it could be a drug-specific effect, so that switching to another medication may terminate the insomnia.

4. *Headache and abdominal pain.* Observation and impression, rather than scientific study, suggest that these tend to occur together at about noon and are often relieved or prevented by ingestion of a glucose-containing solid or liquid.

Dosage Frequency and Duration. Ideally, the desired effects should last long enough to cover homework-time, without displaying a prebedtime-rebound. With the amphetamines available in both tablet and long-acting form, it is most often possible to achieve this with a single morning dose, though some will require a 3-4 p.m. dose, also. This avoids the handicaps and hazards of administering medication during the school day. Unfortunately, methylphenidate more often displays a shorter span of action, so that frequent administration may be required. With imipramine, it has been reported that a day's dosage may be given the night before.

Specificity. There is often an unpredictable specificity of response, one child doing well with one, several, or all of the medications in current use (amphetamines, methylphenidate, psychic energizers, thioridazine or mesoridazine).

Short-Term Alterations in Response. Though uncommon, it sometimes happens that a previously efficacious medication no longer seems so, but response is renewed when a different medication is used. And there are a few children who characteristically show a good effect for a few weeks and then cease to respond, and they display this pattern with *each* new medication tried.

Long-term Alterations in Response. Over long periods of time (prior to the eventual outgrowing of the condition), previously correct dosages may turn out to be too much or too little. Review every six months has seemed to work well.

Interruption of Medication. As the medications control but do not cure and work only for the day in which given, it is perfectly possible and often desirable to interrupt the medication in a number of ways, for instance, omitting on weekends and school vacations. For those individuals who are disruptive at home, in the neighborhood, and at camp, this would not apply.

Recognition that Condition is Outgrown. There are two possible guidelines for this: The first is to stop the medication and see if the underlying condition is still present. Usually this will immediately become apparent. However, there are some children in whom the medication effect lasts longer than usual, so it may take a week to be sure of this point. Another indicator is that when the condition is outgrown, the child then displays the normal response to stimulants. In other words, a medication which previously has controlled, slowed, and quieted will suddenly begin to stimulate. This is definitely the time to stop.

Concurrent Work with Family. At the outset the family must be enlisted in monitoring the results of medication. They must be helped to recognize that not all the child's problems are necessarily due to hyperkinetic components. The physician must be on the alert for evidence of significant, continuing family dysfunction which may require concurrent family therapy, casework, and other attention.

Concurrent Work with Child. The child often needs psychotherapy for distorted feelings secondary to the problems created for him through his difficulty; or for other problems, to which the presence of hyperkinetic impulse disorder certainly does not make him immune. Experience indicates that the use of medication does not impede psychotherapy. It is imperative to work with the child to ensure his understanding of what we conceive his problem to be and the role of medication in its remediation.

Concurrent Work with School. Of major importance is to clarify for the school exactly what can be attributed to the hyperkinetic condition so that those at the school will understand what this condition has been responsible for and not attribute every kind of difficulty or problem to it. They must, for instance, be helped to see where different teaching methods are indicated. The school also can be very helpful in monitoring the effects of the medication.

Summation. The long-term use of these medications requires constant vigilance, monitoring of effects and adjustment of dosage, as well as recognition where indicated of need for psychotherapy for the child and work with the family, plus alertness to possible need for alteration of educational management.

Follow-Up. The follow-up on the use of drugs with cerebral minimal syndromes, which is reported on here was done by Dr. Paul McCarthy. Preliminary scoring and tabulation was done by Dr. Keith Conners. Further statistical work is necessary before the results are presented in formal, final form. What is presented here is based purely upon inspection of the findings, without attempts at this time to assess statistical significance.

Follow-up was attempted on 100 former hyperkinetic private patients treated with amphetamines or methylphenidate. Responses to a questionnaire were received from 66, but not all questions were answered. The population ranged from age 3 to 13 at onset of medication (mean age 8.00), and at the time of the questionnaire ranged from 15 to 26 (mean age 19.8). As for intelligence (Binet or Wechsler), distribution was very similar to that within the normal population. As for duration of treatment, replies were received from 24 who had taken medication for less than six months and 31 from six months to five years. By the time of follow-up, eight had married and they had six children. Some form of special schooling had been required for 50. Only six had not gone any higher than the eighth grade and 14 reporting had completed high school. At the time of reporting, 13 were in college and one was in graduate school. (This is 14 out of 37 who were 19 yrs. or older = 37%.) Of the ten who reported having military service, only one had a bad conduct record. Of the 56 who reported on subsequent non-psychiatric hospitalizations, 33 had none, but only one more than once. By the time of reporting disappearance of hyperactivity had been noted in 27 and in most (61%) it had disappeared from the 12th to 16th year.

The following figures related to personality and drug status assume particular significance:

Overdose. Out of 57 reporting two had taken an overdose of medication of any kind and 55 (96.5%) had not.

Suicide. Of 50 reporting on this question, there were no suicide attempts.

Continuing Medication. Of 57 reporting, 10 were presently taking any kind of prescribed medication and 47 (82%) were not. Of the 10 taking medication, four were anticonvulsants, two were minor tranquilizers and one a major tranquilizer. *None* was taking cerebral stimulants or antidepressants. Altogether, out of 56 reporting, ten had taken prescribed medication continuously prior to the time of the questionnaire, but subsequent to that time prescribed amphetamines ceased and 46 (80%) had not taken any. Of the 10 who had, two were getting anticonvulsants, one a cerebral stimulant, two were on minor tranquilizers, and none received anti-depressants or major tranquilizers.

Most were described as having good friends, good appearance, pleasant manner and meticulous, while a minority were described as moody, loners, having violent outbursts and subject to feelings of persecution.

Out of 37 who were 19 years or older, 18 were employed, and 14 were in college or graduate school.

Respondents were specifically questioned as to whether there had been any subsequent experimentation with drugs such as "pot" and LSD. Of the 57 respondents, five had and 52 (91.2%) had not. No one reported being "hooked."

Further, respondents were specifically questioned about experimentation with Dexedrine, Benzedrine, "speed," etc. Of 56 respondents, three had and 53 (94.6%) had not. No one reported habitual use of such agents.

As for excessive drinking, out of 50, four were so described and 46 (92%) were not.

As for reckless driving, 17 percent were so classified and 82 percent were not.

Out of 55, there were 16 (30%) listed as having been in some kind of trouble with police, but none were in jail.

As for subsequent psychiatric treatment, of 56 respondents, 20 (35%) reported subsequent help as being needed, most in early adolescence. However, only five (9%) were receiving such treatment at time of reporting. Overall, only three (5%) of the 54 reporting had required psychiatric hospitalization; 51 (95%) had not.

Out of 56 reporting, only one (1.8%) ever reported hallucinations, only three (5%) had seizures after age eight.

Only three of 54 respondents reported similar difficulties in siblings.

Over-view. Within the limitations previously mentioned, this study does not support dire predictions as to the outcome of long-term use of medications for hyperkinetic children.

Chapter Nine

Psychotherapy

Some years ago at a conference concerned with the training of clinical psychologists, psychotherapy was defined as "an unidentified technique applied to unspecific problems with unpredictable outcomes [Raimy, 1950]." This somewhat facetious definition was prompted by the recommendation that in spite of the confusion and disagreement regarding the nature of psychotherapy, in order to practice this little understood treatment, one must undergo rigorous training.

Definitions of Psychotherapy

In a comprehensive critical review of the effects of psychotherapy, Eysenck (1961) includes several serious definitions of psychotherapy, including "treating mental and emotional disorders and diseases through changing ideas and emotions to bring about a more favorable psychic equilibrium"; "almost any method used to alleviate or remove the results of emotional conflict and improve psychic adjustment"; and "relieving symptoms of psychic origin by adjusting attitudes that have led to their development." According to Shoeben (1953), psychotherapy is a certain kind of social relationship between two persons who hold periodic conversations in pursuit of the goal of alleviating symptoms and increasing the patient's effective comfort and social utility. In considering various definitions of psychotherapy found in the literature, one should realize that they are largely determined by the particular personality theory and therapeutic technique adopted by the therapist.

Freud's Psychoanalytic Therapy

Probably the most influential force behind most psychotherapy practiced in this country is the clinical work and theorizing carried out by Sigmund Freud in Vienna more than 50 years ago. There he developed both the psychoanalytic theory of psychosexual development and the therapeutic procedure known as psychoanalysis (Freud, 1943). Briefly, the procedure consisted of a neurotic patient lying on a couch and "free-associating" with the analyst, who would sit quietly in the background, intruding as little as possible into the situation and offering only an occasional "interpretation." More specifically, the troubled patient came to Freud's office five times each week and spent one hour lying on the couch verbalizing whatever thoughts and fantasies came to mind regardless of how bizarre or unsocialized these associations might be. The analyst tried to play the role of a "blank screen" against which the patient could reflect his innermost fantasies, dreams, and uncensored thoughts.

The aim of this procedure was for the patient to express emotional content that had been repressed as a result of traumatic experiences in childhood. Usually this repressed material had an underlying sexual or aggressive connotation, and the conflict involved parent and child. As a result of the anxiety engendered by this conflict, the patient was believed to develop defense mechanisms enabling him to avoid facing the unpleasantness. Thus the unresolved conflict remained repressed in the unconscious. However, it requires psychic energy to keep these conflicts from appearing in consciousness, and the neurotic must devote so much energy to coping with his unresolved conflicts, that he becomes unable to cope adequately with other problems encountered in everyday life. Psychoanalysis is supposed to lead to the "release of the repressed," and through the analyst's interpretations of the meanings underlying the patient's associations, he is supposed to gain insight into his dilemma and thereby overcome the neurosis.

Deviants from Orthodox Psychoanalysis

In the beginning Freud had many devoted followers, but some of them did not agree with certain aspects of his theory or his therapeutic procedure; they developed theories and techniques of their own (see Hall & Lindzey, 1970). Of these, Jung and Adler were the most famous early deviants from orthodox psychoanalysis. More recently, people like Sullivan, Horney, and Fromm developed their own schools devoted to somewhat different forms of psychoanalysis and psychotherapy. Today, orthodox psychoanalysis is practiced much less frequently than it was in the past, mainly because of the time and expense it involves. Patients must be seen several times each week, often for a number of years, paying the analyst $40 to $50 per each 50-minute session. Obviously, only a minute proportion of the population can afford such luxurious treatment.

Psychoanalytically Oriented Psychotherapy

Rather than this orthodox form of psychoanalysis, many of today's therapists practice what is known as "psychoanalytically oriented psychotherapy." With this modified procedure, the therapist adheres to most tenets of psychoanalytic theory and uses certain features of analytic procedure in working with patients. Some important changes from orthodox procedure are that the patient is seen much less frequently, sits in a chair rather than lying on a couch, engages in much more direct verbal interaction with the therapist, and may be seen for only a few weeks or months. Thus, this procedure is briefer, less expensive, and more oriented to reality problems and everyday life situations than to unconscious fantasies.

Rogers' Non-Directive Therapy

Another widely practiced form of psychotherapy is Rogers' (1951) non-directive therapy. With this approach, the patient (referred to as the "client") is free to talk about whatever he wishes in a face-to-face interview with the therapist (sometimes called the "counselor"). The therapist strives to influence the content and process of therapy as little as possible in keeping with Rogers' teaching that it must be "client-centered." The therapist's main function is to provide a non-threatening interpersonal setting in which the client can talk freely about whatever he chooses. Another important therapeutic function is to reflect the feeling behind the client's statements. That is, in response to the client's factual statements the therapist reflects the emotional component that constitutes the essence of what is being expressed.

Bergin's Conclusions Regarding Therapeutic Practice

After surveying the psychotherapy research literature, Bergin (1966) digested the findings into six broad conclusions and implications for psychotherapeutic practice and research. The first of these is that psychotherapy may cause people to become better or worse adjusted than comparable people who do not receive such treatment. The implication here is that those engaged in this field should find out whom they are making worse or better, and how, with all due speed. The second conclusion is that control subjects who do not receive psychotherapy tend to improve with time as a result of informal therapeutic encounters. This is the so-called spontaneous remission effect, and it should be given much more research attention than it has received to date. Third, therapeutic progress varies as a function of therapist characteristics such as warmth, empathy, adequacy of adjustment, and experience. The implication of these particular findings is that therapists should be selected for these qualities and not solely on the basis of academic qualifications and intellectual abilities.

The fourth conclusion is that the only school of interview-oriented psychotherapy that has consistently yielded positive outcomes in research studies is client-centered therapy. Interestingly, the poorest results were obtained from classical, long-term psychoanalysis, with analytically oriented eclectic therapy appearing somewhat more successful. The fifth general conclusion is that traditional therapies are seriously limited in effectiveness and are relevant for only a small minority of the large number of people with emotional disturbances. The implication of these results is that new or modified techniques must be developed for dealing with a vast population whose problems are not amenable to standard psychotherapeutic methods. The final conclusion derived from Bergin's survey is that behavior therapies hold considerable promise for enhancing therapeutic effectiveness and should be used and experimented with more widely.

Play Therapy with Children

Most of what we have considered so far pertains mainly to psychotherapy with adults. In this regard, it is noteworthy that the adult patient usually brings himself to the therapist because he is anxious, unhappy, and disturbed by his mental condition and/or his social behavior. That is, he seeks professional help, and the therapist attempts to provide it through a process of verbalizations in a therapeutic relationship.

With children, several modifications in therapeutic practices are necessary (Haworth, 1964). A fundamental difference is that most young children are unable or unwilling to verbalize about the things that trouble them. Thus the technique of play therapy has been developed to allow child patients to express their needs, desires, fears, and view of their life situation through the medium of play. Rather than sitting in the therapist's office and engaging in 50 minutes of verbal interaction, the child patient and therapist go to a play-therapy room that is usually equipped with paints, clay, water, dolls, puppets, and a variety of other toys, including some of an aggressive nature, such as guns and soldiers. The child and therapist sometimes play a game of checkers or cards or the therapist observes while the child engages himself with whatever toys and play activities he chooses.

The aims of this procedure, when conducted with a psychoanalytic orientation, are the release of unconscious repressed material and, through the therapist's interpretations, the gaining of insight by the child patient. That is, as a result of his expressive play and through his relationship with the non-threatening therapist, the child is supposed to understand better the unresolved conflicts that have led to his emotional disturbance; consequently, the child should progress toward a better state of mental health. Note that children rarely, if ever, bring themselves into a therapeutic relationship. Almost always, they are sent to a therapist by their parents, the school system, or legal authorities. This is a very important difference between psychotherapy with adults and with children.

Psychotherapy with Adolescents

Psychotherapy with adolescents poses some unique problems. These patients are no longer children and therefore are not amenable to treatment via playing with toys, nor are they sufficiently adult, in most cases, to realize they have problems that might be helped through talking with a professional therapist. Adolescents, therefore, are often the most difficult cases to work with since they are (a) likely to have been referred for therapy by some adult authority figure (such as a parent or school official), (b) too mature to play with toys, and (c) unwilling to verbalize freely about their problems with a psychotherapist.

Most forms of psychotherapy recognize that the relationship between patient and therapist is an essential ingredient determining the success of the process. In work with adolescents, establishing rapport is probably even more important than in therapy conducted with young children or with adults. Very often the adolescent does not feel the need for help or the desire to change his personality or behavior. Moreover, he has little desire to confide in some adult stranger who seems to expect him to talk openly about his personal secrets, feelings, and activities. If the therapist is first able to establish some feeling of positive regard between them and conveys the impression of genuineness, warmth, and empathy (Truax, 1963), then they can often proceed to talk about things that may be seriously troubling the adolescent patient.

Group Therapy and Family Therapy

Other forms of therapy currently used with children and adolescents are group therapy and family therapy. In group therapy, several youngsters—usually of similar age and with similar problems—meet in a small group and engage in verbal interaction under the guidance of a professional therapist. In family therapy, the child patient, both parents, and often his siblings meet as a group with a therapist. In this therapeutic setting, all family members can hear each other's verbalizations as well as the therapist's interpretations and recommendations.

The Issues

Studies of the effectiveness of psychotherapy have not indicated great success. Citing numerous studies showing no beneficial effects, Eysenck (1961) stated, "... it seems that psychologists and psychiatrists will have to acknowledge the fact that current psychotherapeutic procedures have not lived up to the hopes which greeted their emergence 50 years ago."

In his book on minimal brain dysfunction in children, Wender (1971) states that despite the absence of supporting data and the presence of data denying the usefulness of psychotherapy, many psychiatrists consistently recommend it for children. In making this point, Wender quotes another physician, Werry (1968), who observed that "child psychiatrists prescribe individual psychotherapy in the same indiscriminate way that surgeons once removed tonsils, teeth, and colons as a cure for all ills and with about as much evidence of efficacy."

While Wender is concerned mainly with treatment of hyperkinetic children similar to those discussed in Chapter Eight, he admits that for treatment of psychological difficulties in the interpersonal sphere, psychotherapy has proved useful with some children. He recommends that such psychotherapy be conducted with limited goals in mind, including such things as helping the child to attain a valid picture of his world, improving his self-concept and attitudes towards significant persons in his life, clarifying inaccurate perceptions and notions formed on the basis of previous experience, and making him better able to understand the dynamics of social interactions.

After indicating the potential good that might accrue from some forms of psychotherapy with some kinds of children, Wender mentions possible "psychonoxious effects." He states that those who practice psychotherapy tend to believe almost universally that psychotherapy has the power to produce only good, when in fact it should be recognized that for many children psychotherapy leads to exacerbation (worsening) of their problems. For example, "release therapy," in which the child is encouraged to express openly and act out his aggressive and other socially unacceptable impulses, sometimes is observed to weaken the child's already inadequate ego controls and to aggravate further his interpersonal problems.

Another often ignored reason for questioning the desirability of traditional psychotherapy, according to Wender, is the possibility that identifying the child as a therapy patient may be demeaning for him and serve to diminish his self-esteem. That is, in his own eyes and among others in his cultural surroundings, the fact of going to a psychiatrist or psychologist for therapeutic treatment may not be viewed as a form of self-actualization but as a sign that one is crazy. Thus, to assume that only good can come from the professional recommendation that a child receive psychotherapy is to ignore the meaning of the situation from the child's viewpoint as well as the lack of evidence that the outcome justifies the investment.

Although we are presenting here the opinions of several clinicians and investigators who take a rather dim view of psychotherapy, both with children and adults, countless other members of the "helping professions" believe very strongly in the value of psychotherapeutic treatment. In practically every child treatment facility in this country there are sincere, dedicated professionals conducting varied forms of psychotherapy with disturbed children and their families. While the published findings do not provide much support for the validity and utility of psychotherapeutic practices, case studies presented at staff conferences in most child guidance clinics and residential treatment centers seem to reveal noteworthy benefits from psychotherapy.

Speaking against the critics of psychotherapy, Kubie has said "We will soon be ashamed of the extent to which we may have been turned against the term by the recent flood of ignorant, naive, and biased attacks on psychotherapy as a field. While pretending to be scientific, these studies have violated important principles of research design. Certainly a precise investigation of the psychotherapeutic process . . . is urgently needed. But we do not yet have reliable techniques by which to make meaningful evaluations of results. Anyone who pretends today that he is making accurate evaluations or comparisons is merely exhibiting naiveté, bias, and ignorance [1971, p. 23]." The author of these comments is an internationally famous psychiatrist, psychoanalyst, and former professor at Yale University who has made significant contributions to many aspects of the field of psychiatry. These opinions were voiced by Kubie in the course of stressing the need for a new profession and calling for establishment of innovative academic programs awarding a doctorate in psychotherapy.

In a related publication, Littner and Schour (1971), a psychiatrist and a social worker, discuss special problems in training psychotherapists to work with children. According to these authors, well over one million children in the United States need psychiatric care, and only about one-third receive it. In Chicago alone, more than 100,000 children of school age are sufficiently disturbed to warrant direct treatment for their emotional problems, but relatively few receive therapeutic help. These authors make the interesting observation that very few disturbed children in this country are actually treated by child psychiatrists, while the vast majority receive their therapeutic treatment from non-medical personnel, especially social workers.

Reviewing the facts and figures, these authors conclude: "It is virtually certain that in the foreseeable future enough child psychiatrists to meet the need cannot and will not be trained." In view of this, they advocate a new profession known as "child psychotherapy," which would be taught to college graduates in a four-year, full-time program in a graduate school of psychotherapy as part of a university. They describe the curriculum, which would be psychoanalytic in orientation, and discuss the pros and cons of training young people who would enter this program directly from their undergraduate education and would not obtain prior professional degrees as is currently required.

The specific details of this proposed program are not our main concern here, but we should realize that the status of child psychotherapy is very unsettled; some prominent researchers are attempting to show that traditional psychotherapy is usually ineffective and sometimes even harmful, and other clinicians and educators are expounding the great value of psychotherapy and emphasizing the need for many additional young people to become specialists in psychotherapy.

At this point, let us turn to the article by Eugene E. Levitt and then read the thoughtful discussion of therapy presented by James O. Palmer. After reading these papers and those on behavior therapy in the next chapter, your overall view of this controversial situation should become somewhat more clarified. However, this material is not designed to provide final answers to these perplexing questions.

References

Bergin, E. E. Some implications of psychotherapy research for therapeutic practice. *Journal of Abnormal Psychology.* 1966, **71,** 235–246.

Eysenck, H. J. The effects of psychotherapy. In H. J. Eysenck (Ed.), *Handbook of abnormal psychology.* New York: Basic Books, 1961.

Freud, S. *A general introduction to psychoanalysis.* New York: Garden City Publishing, 1943.

Hall, C. S., & Lindzey, G. *Theories of personality.* New York: Wiley, 1970.

Haworth, M. R. (Ed.) *Child psychotherapy.* New York: Basic Books, 1964.

Kubie, L. S. A doctorate in psychotherapy: The reasons for a new profession. In R. R. Holt (Ed.), *New horizons for psychotherapy.* New York: International Universities Press, 1971.

Littner, N., & Schour, E. Special problems of training psychotherapists to work with children. In R. R. Holt (Ed.), *New Horizons in psychotherapy.* New York: International Universities Press, 1971.

Raimy, V. (Ed.) *Training in clinic..l psychology.* New York: Prentice-Hall, 1950.

Rogers, C. R. *Client-centered therapy: Its current practice, implications, and theory.* Boston: Houghton, 1951.

Shoeben, E. J. Some observations on psychotherapy and the learning process. In O. H. Mowrer (Ed.) *Psychotherapy: Theory and research.* New York: Ronald Press, 1953.

Truax, C. B. Effective ingredients in psychotherapy. *Journal of Counseling Psychology,* 1963, **10,** 256–263.

Wender, P. H. *Minimal brain dysfunction in children.* New York: Wiley, 1971.

Werry, J. S. Developmental hyperactivity. *Pediatric Clinics of North America.* 1968, **15,** 581–598.

25. Research on Psychotherapy with Children

Eugene E. Levitt

The entire child guidance movement in this country in 1909 comprised one psychiatrist, one psychologist, a secretary, and three small rooms on the ground floor of the juvenile detention home in Chicago. From this tiny inception, The Idea, as Healy (1948) once called it, was to grow in three score years to an established community force, operating with a corps of twelve hundred clinics, replete with "training centers and professorships in leading universities, specialized periodicals, national and international societies and conventions... and intensive research activities" (Kanner, 1967).

This spectacular burgeoning reflected a reasonable hope that dealing with the young was the ultimate solution to all of the nation's mental health problems. The rationale was invitingly simple and seemed unchallengeable.

The untreated, emotionally disturbed child is expected to become, eventually, an emotionally disturbed adult, an axis that Lewis (1965) has called "the continuity hypothesis." Effective intervention at the child level should not only improve the child's immediately subsequent adjustment, but ought also to effect a noticeable reduction in the future incidence of adult disorders. Lewis (1965) refers to this prediction as the "intervention hypothesis."

The value of child guidance, or more fashionably, child psychotherapy, is now being seriously questioned from within the movement for the first time (for example, Simmons, 1963; Hersch, 1968; Sonis, 1968) on the grounds that after 60 years, the intervention hypothesis is not yet conclusively demonstrated. Evaluation research fails to show unequivocally that child psychotherapy is effective. Six decades of child guidance do not seem to have reduced either the demand for mental health services to children, or the incidence of emotional illness among adults. As Hunt (1958) remarked sadly, "Our hopes of preventing mental illness by mental health education and child guidance clinics have been disappointed, and there is no convincing evidence that anyone has ever been kept out of the state hospital by such measures."

The failure to demonstrate the effectiveness of child psychotherapy is reflected in the data of Table 1. These have been aggregated from two reviews (Levitt, 1957a, 1963), and represent 47 reports of the outcome of child psychotherapy spanning a 35-year period up to around 1960. Nine-thousand, three-hundred and fifty-nine cases are involved, including 5,140

TABLE 1. SUMMARY OF REPORTS OF OUTCOME OF PSYCHOTHERAPY WITH CHILDREN*

Diagnostic Group	N	Per cent Improved
Neurotic at close	4539	67.4
Psychotic at close	252	65.1
Acting-out at close	349	55.0
Total at close	5140	66.4
Neurotic at follow-up†	4219	78.2

*Data from Levitt (1957a, 1963).
†Estimated median interval of 4.8 years after close.

cases evaluated at the close of treatment and 4,219 evaluated at follow-up. The findings may be summarized as follows:

1. About two-thirds of all cases are seen as improved to a noticeable extent at close of treatment.

2. This figure holds, approximately, for children classified as psychotic as well as those who are seen as having "neurotic" disorders.[1]

3. Children with acting-out symptoms have an improvement rate of only 55 percent.

4. At follow-up, nearly 80 percent of all cases are regarded as improved.

The improvement rate reported in Table 1 is approximately the same as that found in groups of treatment "defectors" or "terminators," that is, emotionally disturbed children who were offered formal clinic treatment but failed to take advantage of the opportunity (Levitt, 1957a; Levitt, et al., 1959). Defectors appear to be the most appropriate medium for estimating the so-called spontaneous remission rate, provided that the group is properly selected. It should consist of cases which (a) have been subjected to the same diagnostic procedures as the treated cases; (b) have been accepted for treatment, and; (c) have never had any formal therapy sessions.

The use of defectors as a base line control is the salient hypostasis of the case for the unproven efficacy of child psychotherapy. The defector control has been sharply criticized, primarily on the grounds that defectors and treated cases are originally dissimilar on certain dimensions, such as intensity of disturbance, which render the defectors a biased control group (Hood-Williams, 1960; Heinicke and Goldman, 1960; Eisenberg and Gruenberg, 1961). However, when the defector sample conforms to the description in the previous paragraph, objective comparisons reveal no meaningful differences between treated and defector children (Levitt, 1957c, 1958; Williams and Pollack, 1964).

Requirements of methodology demand that a treated group and its control group should be selected from the same population. With few exceptions, outcome studies are carried out by the staff of an agency or institution, which ordinarily has access only to those persons who have voluntarily sought services at that agency or institution. The investigators are thus

[1]Diagnostic categories based on adult patients do not hold clearly for children and adolescents. For purposes of rough communication, "neurotic" refers to a child who has not been diagnosed as psychotic, or as having a primary behavior disorder or a special symptom.

restricted to a particular population, within which the defector control group appears to be the most reasonable method of estimating spontaneous remission rate.

One of the rare outcome studies that employed a different sampling method was done as part of the Buckinghamshire Child Survey in England between 1961 and 1964 (Shepherd et al., 1966). The treated sample consisted of 50 randomly chosen "neurotic" children between the ages of 5 and 15, seen at child guidance clinics in the county for the first time in 1962 (27 percent of the total clinic population at that time). A control sample matched for age, sex, and symptoms was selected from a random sample of more than 6,000 children who had never obtained or sought psychiatric assistance.

Outcome ratings were made by clinicians based on interviews with parents in 1962 and again in 1964. Sixty-five percent of the treated sample was rated as improved, compared to 61 percent of the controls. Sixteen percent of the treated children and 9 percent of the controls was rated as worse, and the rest of both groups was rated as unchanged. The percentages of improvement, which do not differ significantly, are strikingly similar to those in Table 1.

The Buckinghamshire investigation is impressive, despite the relatively small samples, as a rare instance of true random sampling. Its results suggest strongly that the so-called spontaneous recovery rate lies somewhere between 60 and 70 percent, no matter how it is estimated.

A comparison of improvement rate with treatment against spontaneous remission rate assumes a condition suitable for a one-tailed test. It is presumed in physical medicine that, though a treatment may not result in symptomatic improvement, it will certainly not harm the patient. *Primum non nocere;* chemical therapies undergo exhaustive experimentation with infrahuman mammals to insure that there are no noxious side effects before administration to humans.

The assumption of no harm was also made for many years by psychotherapists and psychotherapy researchers, despite the absence of an animal research analog. Until very recently, rating scales used to evaluate treatment outcome did not include a category labelled Worse. A therapist, no matter how bumbling or webfooted he might be, could not possibly be inferior to no therapist at all. Currently, however, the concept of the "psychonoxious" therapist (Truax, 1963) or what Bergin (1967) calls "the deterioration effect," is now readily accepted by most psychotherapy researchers as the most probable explanation for the apparent failure of psychotherapy.[2]

Truax and Wargo (1966) suggest that there are individual differences in therapy effectiveness among clinics and treatment institutions as well as among therapists. Apparent support for this position is reflected in 18 reports of outcome of psychotherapy with children from various treatment sources (Levitt, 1957a). Improvement rates at close showed a statistically significant variation from 43 percent to 86 percent. The standard deviation of the dis-

---

[2]"In fact, four children viewed their psychotherapeutic experiences negatively, voiced some dislike of their therapist (3 of the 4 had the same therapist)" (Weiss and Burke, 1967).

tribution is 11.4, and the range is 1.6 standard deviation units above and 2.2 standard deviation units below the mean. These characteristics strikingly resemble those of a distribution of scores from any small sample drawn from a normal population. This is exactly what would be expected according to the hypothesis of effective-ineffective treatment agencies.

A survey of play-therapy practices (Ginott and Lebo, 1961, 1963) suggests that there is considerable variation in the specific behaviors of child therapists in the therapy situation, and that these differences may be unrelated to theoretical orientation. This type of finding has been reported in a number of studies of adult patients. It underscores the possibility that there is a broad variation in effectiveness among therapists.

The concepts of the psychonoxious therapist and the deterioration effect have turned the attention of psychotherapy researchers from unadorned outcome studies to investigations that seek to discover "what specific therapeutic interventions produce specific changes in specific patients under specific conditions" (Strupp and Bergin, 1969), that is, the conditions under which the intervention hypothesis may be valid or invalid. This quest has instigated much therapist-patient-process research in the adult psychotherapy field in recent years. Unfortunately, it has stimulated little additional research in child psychotherapy, where the volume of objective investigations has always been much smaller than in the adult field. Only six of the reviewers of psychotherapy research in the *Annual Review of Psychology,* since its inception in 1950, found it necessary to employ a subheading for research with child patients. These six groupings encompassed only 2.2 percent of the pages in the 19 chapters. One explanation of this neglect is the extra methodological difficulties involved in child psychotherapy research (see below). Another is the general reluctance of administrators, parents, and other concerned adults to sanction experimentation with disturbed children. The prepotent reason, however, is that child guidance is perennially dominated by two notoriously anti-research forces: psychoanalysis and social work. Their exclusive emphasis on service and training has effectively kept research out of the country's child guidance clinics.

Hopefully, the reader, now forewarned, will not be disappointed by the sparseness of references in this chapter and by its repeated substantive gaps.

Special Problems of Psychotherapy Research with Children

The multitude of slippery methodological problems that plague the psychotherapy researcher have been detailed in a number of thoughtful articles during the past 15 years. Child therapy research faces several unique problems, though they may have analogs in the adult field. These problems and their implications for findings are often entirely ignored by investigators. They are presented here briefly for identification only; no solutions are proposed.

1. Because the child is a developing organism:

(a) *The many symptomatic manifestations in children who are basically normal tend to disappear in time as a function of development,* that is, are subject to so-called spontaneous remission. There is a substantial incidence among normal children of behaviors usually considered to be symptoms of emotional disturbance—temper tantrums, sleep disturbances, enuresis, hyperactivity, specific fears, and the like (Macfarlane, et al., 1954; Lapouse and Monk, 1959). Apparently, there is some reality in the common-sense notion that children "grow out" of symptomatic behavior, that is, learn to cope with the stresses that cause them as their capacities to adjust improve with maturation. But an alarmed mother may bring a symptomatic child to the guidance clinic, where developmental remission may be recorded as therapeutic success.[3] Identical remission is likely to occur in the comparable child who remained untreated, which will then suggest that treatment was not effective. A more significant inference would be that *treatment may have been unnecessary*, a conclusion advanced by Shepherd and his associates (1966). They found that

> ... referral to a child-guidance clinic is related chiefly to parental reactions. The mothers of clinic-children were more apt to be anxious, depressed and easily upset by stress; they were less able to cope with their children, more apt to discuss their problems and to seek advice.

The clinic children themselves were not more disturbed than non-referred children.

(b) *Symptoms that are pathognomic of an underlying emotional illness may also disappear as a function of development, but will then be replaced by other symptoms.* This *developmental symptom substitution* is not really a spontaneous remission. It simply reflects the finding that certain symptoms are more likely to occur at particular ages. School phobia is most common in the elementary school years, while the behaviors usually categorized as delinquent occur most frequently in adolescence. An emotionally disturbed child may "grow out" of one symptom and grow into another. Developmental symptom substitution seems to be fairly common. A follow-up of treated children (Levitt, 1957b) disclosed that 22 percent had developed new symptoms since the close of treatment. The phenomenon is suggested by Gardner's (1967) investigation of child guidance patients who were later hospitalized with a diagnosis of schizophrenia.

Consider the methodological problem. An eight-year old child is treated for enuresis and nightmares with subsequent remission of these symptoms. Therapy, evaluated at close, evidently has been effective. Later on, the child is found to be manifesting severe obsessive-compulsive behavior, or aggressive acting-out. Can the researcher still be confident that treatment was effective, that the disappearance of the original symptoms was due to intervention and not to developmental factors?

2. *Persons other than the child patient may be a direct focus of treatment.* In most child clinics, an effort is made to involve at least the mother in treatment. Some clinics give priority to cases in which both mother and

---

[3]The improvement rate with treatment for various compartmentalized symptoms is reported as higher than for diffuse psychopathologies (Levitt, 1963).

father are willing to be seen in treatment. Treatment focus is thus a variable, one not found in adult therapy. The research problem is to separate effects. For example, a successful treatment effort involves mother and child with separate therapists. Is success due to the child's therapist, the mother's therapist, to both therapists, equally or in what proportions, or is it possible to separate effects or to determine relative weights?

A Variety of Therapeutic Approaches

Inpatient Milieu

Segregated inpatient services for younger age groups are still comparatively rare, and inpatients under the age of 18—mostly adolescents—are commonly hospitalized on adult wards. The adolescent on the adult ward ordinarily has access to appropriate educational and recreational stimulation, so that the only important difference from the segregated ward is segregation itself.

Clinicians disagree about which milieu is more therapeutically effective. Beskind (1962), in a review of the earlier literature, refers to some of the advantages and disadvantages of each environment. On adult wards, adolescents are faced by poor adult models, lack proper social relationships, and may be poorly tolerated by patients and staff.[4] On the other hand, severely disturbed adolescents, especially those manifesting aggressive and destructive behavior, tend to disrupt segregated wards, are more easily managed on adult wards, and may receive more attention from doctors and from adult patients. Adolescents normally live surrounded by adults; this situation is desirably approximated by the adult-adolescent ward.

Two recent investigations (Hartmann et al., 1968; Warren, 1965a, 1965b) furnish a somewhat labored comparison of outcome as a function of milieu. The studies are fairly comparable in terms of samples (institutionalized adolescents averaging about 15 years of age) and method of evaluating outcome (ratings based on interviews by psychiatrist and social workers). The data, in percentage of patients improved compared with status at admission, are summarized in Table 2. The Hartmann sample of adolescents treated on adult wards was evaluated at close, a half to one year later, and again one to two years later. The Warren sample, which was treated on a special ward for adolescents, was evaluated six years after discharge.

The Hartmann sample does well at the time of discharge; three out of four were rated as improved. Backsliding must begin almost immediately. Within a year after discharge, more than 15 percent of those rated as improved at close are now no better off or worse than they were on admission. At the end of the second year, more than 10 percent more have regres-

---

[4]In a follow-up of a small group of institutionalized children (Weiss and Burke, 1967), half the expatients stated that the "most help in the hospital" had been provided by "living with other children."

TABLE 2. PERCENTAGE OF IMPROVED CASES AMONG ADOLESCENTS TREATED ON ADULT AND SEPARATE WARDS

	Treated on Adult Wards*		Treated on a Separate Ward†	
	At close	½–1 year later	1–2 years later	6 years later
Improved	75	59	48	54‡
No change	25	20	42	18
Worse	—	22	10	28

*Data from Hartmann et al. (1968).
†Data from Warren (1965b).
‡Percent improved at close was at least 65.

sed, a total loss of 27 percent in the improvement rate in a relatively short time after discharge.

In contrast, the Warren sample reports an improvement rate of 54 percent after six years. This, too, represents a regression, since at least 65 percent of the cases were reported improved at close. (Unfortunately, the data are not presented in a form that permits a precise statement of outcome at close.)

Both samples were worse at follow-up than at close, but more of the patients treated on a separate ward maintained improvement for a longer period of time. At the same time, however, there were more cases who were worse at the longer follow-up of the separate ward group.

Peculiarly, in both studies, status at discharge did not predict status at follow-up. This absence of correlation may be the result of a subgroup of patients who improve symptomatically upon institutionalization but regress upon discharge, and another subgroup that does not manifest favorable effects of treatment until some time after discharge. Or it may merely reflect the accidental circumstance that most of the evaluations at close were performed by psychiatry residents, and most of the follow-up evaluations were done by social workers.

Beckett et al. (1968) contrast the effects of a conventional inpatient adolescent service with a permissive milieu in which patient behavior was partly controlled by self-government. A one-year follow-up showed no differences between the effects of the two milieus on six of seven variables, including rehospitalization, contact with an outpatient facility, and overall adjustment rating. The patients who had been subjected to the more permissive milieu did, however, manifest considerably fewer aggressive and antisocial behaviors. The authors suggest that this may be due to the fact that the permissive milieu tended to be selectively more effective with patients whose antisocial symptoms had a neurotic rather than a sociopathic basis.

The Day Treatment Center

The day treatment center is a relatively new conception in the structure of psychological care. Temporally, it stands midway between the residential treatment center where the child patient spends the 24-hour day, and the conventional child guidance clinic with its weekly one-hour visit. The patient of the day treatment center is considered to be living at home. He is brought to the center in the morning by his parents and returns home each evening.

The day treatment center lies between the clinic and residential center on a structural dimension, but may not differ from the residential center along other dimensions. For example, there does not appear to be a high correlation between structure and degree of disturbance of the children admitted to the three types of treatment units. The children treated at the Children's Day Treatment Center and School in New York City (La Vietes, et al., 1960) seem no less disturbed, either in degree or intensity, than Project Re-ED children (Hobbs, 1966) or those of any other residential treatment center. In effect, the day treatment center is probably a less expensive substitute for the scarce residential treatment center.

The day treatment center therapy program of the La Vietes group includes a required treatment of both parents for a minimum of one session per week, group counseling of all mothers, and therapy sessions with the individual child from one to three times weekly. This "comprehensive family treatment program" has "a dynamic psychoanalytic orientation," and is considered essential because the child is still regarded as living at home.

The La Vietes group attempted an evaluation of 38 children treated during the first seven years of the existence of the Children's Day Treatment Center and School (La Vietes et al., 1965). The evaluation is incompletely reported. It indicates that about three-quarters of the treated children were considered at least moderately improved, whether the criterion is ability to function outside of center, clinical impression, or psychological tests. Interestingly enough, intellectual measures did not reveal statistically significant improvement (Reens, 1965). The finding is strikingly similar to that reported by Project Re-ED (Weinstein, 1969). Despite the marked attention paid to formal education by the treatment agency, improvement occurs along behavior-emotional dimensions, but not in the academic sphere. Is this paradoxical outcome a function of program emphasis, or a reflection of an unequitable investment or preparation of teachers, or selection of patients, or is there some other explanation? Again, the objective research, because of its paucity, raises more questions than it answers.

The Special Class

The school room, where a child spends about as much time during the week as he does in his own home, is a stressful environment for many emotionally disturbed children. Psychopathological manifestations seem more prone to erupt in the school than in the home. Acting-out behaviors such as destructiveness, assaultiveness, and hyperactivity disrupt the class, interfere with teaching, and threaten the teacher's control. The child whose pathology is expressed through such symptoms is seldom tolerated in the classroom for very long. His withdrawal is likely to be enforced by school authorities, a certain indication to parents that special measures must be taken in order to continue the child's education. Institutionalization is, of course, one possibility. Another is the special class for emotionally disturbed children, a service provided by some school systems.

There must be a sizeable number of such special classes around the country, but a study by Haring and Phillips (1962) is a rare instance of an attempt to objectively evaluate the effect of this type of facility. They set up three groups of elementary school children rated as emotionally disturbed, with specific symptoms of the type that usually necessitates removal of the child from a regular class. Group I had a highly structured atmosphere characterized by rigid limits on behavior and by isolation as a disciplinary technique. Group II children were simply left in their regular classrooms with regular teachers receiving extensive professional consultation about the disturbed children. Group II may be regarded essentially as a control. Group III was relatively permissive, especially compared to Group I, with the intent of encouraging freedom to express feelings.

Evaluation at the end of a school year was based on before-and-after scores on The California Achievement Test and the Behavior Rating Scale, an ad hoc instrument developed by the authors, which uses the class teachers as raters. On the CAT, Group I showed a mean gain of 1.97, compared to 1.02 for Group II and 0.70 for Group III. Unfortunately, these difference scores are perfectly negatively correlated with the pretreatment scores, apparently due to nonrandom assignment of subjects to groups. It is plausible that the Law of Initial Values prevented Group III (pretreatment mean 5.36) from advancing as far in the school year as Group I (pretreatment mean 2.19). The only safe conclusion is that Group I caught up with Group II by the end of the year, but both were still functioning at an academic level considerably below that of Group III.

The BRS data shows an identical situation with respect to pre-treatment scores. The difference scores, however, are not perfectly correlated. Group I again achieved the largest gain, but Group II made almost no improvement, while Group III progressed moderately.

If we overlook the highly questionable use of class teachers as raters and the absence of any independent ratings on the BRS, the findings of the Haring-Phillips study suggest that any type of segregated class with a specially trained teacher is likely to be more therapeutic than the regular class. A highly structured environment in which aberrant behavior is systematically negatively reinforced appears to be more therapeutic than a permissive milieu that emphasizes expression of affect. The latter comparison should delight the behavior therapists and dismay the traditionalists.

Foster Home Care

The vast majority of children who do not live with their natural parents are the victims of illegitimacy, broken homes, and absent parents. They are drawn largely from among the underprivileged, are below average in intelligence, and will probably have had more than one foster home placement before reaching adulthood (for example, Eisenberg, et al., 1958; Maas and Engler, 1959). They are, in Eisenberg's (1962) bitterly concise words, "children of the lower depths, children mistreated before they came into care and treated not too well afterward."

In many cases, there is an implicit assumption that placement has psychological implications, either therapeutic or preventive. In an unknown, but probably quite small, number of cases, the child is placed in a foster home for explicit psychotherapeutic reasons. It has been clinically determined by a public agency that the home atmosphere is so malignantly psychopathogenic that the prognosis for the child is zero unless he is transferred to a healthier environment. This judgment is made with extreme reluctance; placement is usually viewed by the agency as a desperate measure. It seems to follow that placed children will be severely emotionally disturbed, and that there will be a minimum of concern with the psychotherapeutic effectiveness of the foster home, such as led to the project reported by DeFries et al. (1964, 1965).

Fifty-two emotionally disturbed children in foster home placements were evaluated over a three-year period by means of psychiatric interviews. Half of the children had been subjected to concurrent, intensive, weekly psychotherapy. At the end of the treatment phase, 40 percent of the placed children were labeled as improved, 33 percent as worse, and the remainder as unchanged. Outcome was not materially affected by psychotherapy. Evidently, the effectiveness of foster home care in conventional terms is less than that of other forms of treatment. Its average effectiveness is practically nil. DeFries et al. (1965) conclude:

> The foster family care concept carries with it the sentimental view that there is the need to simulate family life for the dislocated, neglected, and abused child. This view had been propounded partly in order to counteract the widely proclaimed ill effects of institutionalization on children, often discussed in the psychoanalytic literature. That it is possible to simulate a family for the disturbed foster child is an unrealistic and outdated concept, however, that must be critically examined before further progress can be made.

Foster home care appears most clearly to be a psychotherapeutic failure, on the average. The data also clearly suggest that there are psychotherapeutic foster homes and psychonoxious ones. Some of the potentially relevant "therapist" variables are indicated by DeFries et al. (1965). A majority of their foster parents were middle-aged, below average in intelligence and educational level, from lower income brackets, and had an average of three other children in the home. It would be prudent to investigate the "therapist" factor before concluding finally that foster home care is unrealistic and outdated.

Mother as the Therapist

There are divergent ideas as to how to come to grips with the national shortage of therapists, such as the training of nonprofessional therapists (Rioch et al., 1965; Truax, 1968) and Schofield's (1964) conception of the friend as a therapist. In the child area, recent attention has been paid to the possibility of the mother—a logical candidate—as a therapist. Thinking comes from two disparate sources: the behavior therapists, and the Rogerians, represented by the pioneer work of Guerney (1964).

The theoretical considerations underlying these two approaches appear, at first glance, to be entirely different. Guerney's technique consists primarily of training the mother to develop an empathic relationship with the child. The behavior therapy method places emphasis on determining the factors of parent behavior that maintain deviant child behavior. There is some overlap, however, in that Guerney allows that the behavior to be modified was *"learned* in the presence of, or by the influence of, parental attitude," and can therefore be "more effectively *unlearned,* or *extinguished* [my italics], under similar conditions . . . (Stover and Guerney, 1967). Perhaps, as Truax (1966) suggested, client-centered therapy and behavior modification do have common elements.

Stover and Guerney (1967) present some evidence that suggests effectiveness of the latter's technique. Among the behavior therapists, Wahler et al. (1965) were apparently successful in altering deviant behavior in two of three children using the mother as a behavior therapist, and single-case successes are reported by Zeilberger et al. (1968) and Hawkins et al. (1966).

There is, perhaps, a question of how training a mother-therapist differs from parent counseling in the conventional child guidance or family service setting. Both share a common basic ingredient: a professional person evaluates the home situation and instructs the mother how to behave toward her child. The professional does not have direct contact with the child. The important difference is a diagnostic rather than a therapeutic one. The mother-therapist trainers observe the home situation *directly* and make an effort to record *systematically* the interaction of child and parent behaviors. The prescriptions that change the mother from erring parent to behavior therapist are thus based on much sounder evidence than is customarily available in the conventional clinic.

Child development theory indicates that the mother-therapist will be maximally effective with the preschool child. The handful of reports cited here suggest that the psychologists involved in training mother-therapists agree.

Presumably, a mother becomes a therapist for her own child only, whether the technique is Rogerian or learning-theory oriented. Unlike other approaches to training nonprofessional therapists, "filial" therapy does not seem to save much time for the professionals involved, and may, in fact, be more time-consuming than traditional techniques. Its practicality in a world of professional scarcity, as well as its efficacy, remain to be demonstrated.

Newer Therapeutic Techniques

Outcome studies like those in Table 1 have been repeatedly criticized on methodological grounds. Defector or other kinds of untreated control groups are actually individuals undergoing minimal treatment or are otherwise inappropriate; measuring instruments are insufficiently sensitive to detect changes in treated cases; percentage of cases improved is a misleading index because it can conceal more rapid improvement by treated cases; etc. These criticisms, like the concepts of the psychonoxious therapist and the deterioration effect, are essentially alternative hypotheses that seek to explain why the aggregated outcome reports fail to demonstrate that psychotherapy is effective. The primary purpose of process research is to validate these alternative hypotheses by pinning down conclusively the conditions under which psychotherapy is effective. For the moment, there is sufficient equivocality so that the choice of an hypothesis to support remains a matter of personal conviction. As Hersch (1968) points out, there is still no *convincing* proof that psychotherapy is effective, and in the meantime, "what we know with *certainty* about the effects of therapy is not heartwarming to the conscientious practitioner [italics mine]."

Despite the alternative hypotheses, there has been a noticeable dampening of enthusiasm for traditional psychotherapy in recent years. This has been manifested not so much by rejection of established techniques as by a willingness to consider new ones. Several recently developed approaches are currently receiving favorable consideration by the mental health professions. These newer techniques share certain common characteristics. Each places emphasis on current behavior patterns. Anamnestic appraisal is deemphasized. Conceptions like insight and the unconscious are unnecessary. Diagnostic categories are considered to have scant practical significance; little or no time is spent in formulating diagnoses. The significance of learning in the patient's life, rather than motivation, is stressed. It is anticipated that the duration of treatment will be measured in months, or even weeks, rather than years. Finally, there is a tendency toward the use of nonprofessional therapists, individuals other than the psychiatrist, clinical psychologist, and psychiatric social worker.

The emphases in these methods appear to render them most appropriate for the young and, indeed, we find that they have been used primarily with child and adolescent patients. They seem also to be most suited for dealing with behavioral symptoms rather than emotional states and thinking disorders. Again, the available reports suggest that those therapists who are using the techniques would agree.

Behavior Therapy

The technique that most clearly fits the descriptions in the previous paragraphs is called behavior modification or behavior therapy. In essence, it is a translation of learning theory, beginning with the Law of Effect, directly into therapy procedures. The symptom or "critical target behavior" is conceptualized as the consequence of disordered or maladaptive learning. The purpose of the therapy is to extinguish this behavior according to learning principles and, in some instances, to substitute a new, adaptive behavior.

Behavior therapy is actually a series of techniques using either operant or classical conditioning or desensitization, and varying along such dimensions as requisite skill of the therapist, requisite characteristics of the patient, and degree of control over reinforcements by the therapist, as well as the learning model (Kanfer and Phillips, 1966).

Since behavior therapy is extensively treated in other chapters of this volume, it will not be accorded any further consideration here. It is included only because it could not conceivably be omitted from any discussion of the newer approaches to psychological treatment.

Project Re-ED

The rationale and structure of this inpatient agency for children in the elementary school age range are described in two recent publications (Hobbs, 1966; Project Re-ED, 1967). The approach is clearly educative. The institutional setting itself is like a combination school and camp rather than a hospital or other conventional treatment center. The primary "therapist" is the *educateur* or teacher-counselor. As Hobbs (1966) notes, the teacher-counselors are the core of Re-ED, and a great deal of attention is devoted to selecting and training them. The training course requires nine months and covers a wide variety of subjects ranging from specialized teaching methods and use of professional consultants to arts, crafts, and games.

An evaluation of the effects of Re-ED on its first 250 inmates included such variables as social maturity and behavioral-emotional adjustment (Weinstein, in press). Surprisingly, all of the personality and emotional status variables reveal significant differences between preadmission and discharge or follow-up ratings, while changes in "academic adequacy" were statistically significant only for one of the two Re-ED schools. Six months after discharge, about 50 percent of all the cases were reported as substantially improved on behavioral-emotional ratings made by the Re-ED staff, using information provided by the child's regular school teacher. Parents and referring agencies were somewhat more impressed. Eighty-two percent of the mothers, 78 percent of the fathers, and 81 percent of the referring agencies viewed the ex-patients as moderately or greatly improved. The correlation between parent ratings was .67. Mothers and fathers are obviously not independent judges, and the coefficient cannot be used as a reliability estimate. Nonetheless, it can at least be stated that the parents are relatively in agreement, a circumstance which would exist if their respective ratings were indeed reliable.

Evidently, Re-ED has had a more pronounced effect on the child's behavior in the home than in the school. Perhaps it should be inferred that the teacher-counselors were more effective as counselors than as teachers, but it is nevertheless probable that they have succeeded in both roles to an unknown extent beyond the traditional residential treatment center. A best guess is that Re-ED's effectiveness is primarily a function of the careful selection and special training of the teacher-counselors, and secondarily of the school-camp, "unhospital" milieu.

Reality Therapy

Reality Therapy (Glasser, 1965) departs from traditional one-to-one and group treatment techniques along two theoretical lines. First, it places an announced premium on conventionally moral and responsible behavior on the part of the patient. The therapist is thus in the definite position of an advocate of social norms and mores, a purveyor of middle-class values. The assumption of this Mowrerian thinking is that the individual is capable of controlling his own behavior, analogous in a fashion to the Re-ED principle that "cognitive control can be taught" (Hobbs, 1966).

Second, the therapist seeks to exercise his influence on behalf of the moral and responsible by stepping out of the traditional, impersonal doctor role and deliberately seeking to involve himself with the patient. One is reminded of humanistic psychotherapy as espoused by Steinzor (1967) and the practical counselor-friend of Massimo and Shore (1967).

These two features of Reality Therapy suggest that it was tailored for use with adolescent delinquents and, in fact, the only published evaluation of its use to date reports on group therapy with institutionalized delinquent girls (Glasser, 1965). The outcome data are sketchy. Only 43 of a total of 370 treated inmates have been returned to the institution. Glasser states that his approach has been successful with 80 percent of the girls, but the basis of this contention is unclear.

Some Diagnostic Classifications: Juvenile Delinquency and School Phobia

Juvenile delinquency and school phobia are singled out for special attention in this chapter for several reasons. Both are characterized by clearly identifiable, manifest behavior and are thus diagnosed with relative facility. Both are viewed as a social problem by the community at large, and each has legal ramifications.

The differences between them are also striking. Delinquency has a comparatively high incidence, and a relatively low remission rate with treatment. School phobia has a low incidence and a high treatment remission rate. Perhaps the difference in remission rates accounts for the fact that there have been relatively few published, objective reports of evaluation of treatment of delinquency—especially considering the abundance of treatment programs—while evaluations of outcome with school phobia are relatively common, especially in light of the low incidence.

Delinquency

The diagnostic label "juvenile delinquent" is traditionally pinned to the nonadult whose primary symptoms include aggressive, hostile, destructive, or antisocial acting-out behaviors. The prevalence of delinquency is at an all-time high; nearly 700,000 cases were processed through the country's juvenile courts in 1965 (Task Force Report, 1967).

Delinquency is a special challenge for child guidance, not only because of its growing prevalence, but also because it carries over into adult life with a much greater frequency than other emotional disorders of childhood. Robins (1966), summarizing the findings of a 30-year follow-up of child guidance clinic patients, remarks:

> The neurotic children as adults resembled the control subjects. But the antisocial children produced a high proportion with arrests, alcoholism, divorce, poor job histories, child neglect, dependency on social agencies, and psychiatric hospitalization (p. v).

The report of the Task Force on Juvenile Delinquency and Crime of the President's Commission on Law Enforcement and Administration of Justice (1967) literally constitutes a volume in which sociological knowledge in these areas is summarized and synthesized.[5] Among more than 400 pages of text, only a single page is devoted to treatment. The authors of the relevant chapter (Rodman and Grams, 1967) explain as follows:

> A tremendous amount of effort and expenditure is going into a variety of delinquency prevention and rehabilitation programs involving psychotherapy and environmental therapy. As yet there is but a molehill of evaluation to confront the mountain of services that has developed ... moreover, the few careful evaluative studies carried out have shown treatment efforts to be largely unsuccessful. The only projects that seem able to report success are those that have not been independently evaluated (p. 212).

Conventional psychotherapy methods appear to be least effective with delinquents. The reported improvement rate is more than a standard deviation below the mean for all treated cases (Table 1). Hersch (1968) suggests that failure to respond to conventional psychotherapy is characteristic of patients from lower socioeconomic class milieus, which includes the bulk of delinquents. This may be the result of greater conflict between professional practice and expectations of the nature and structure of the therapy situation by lower-class patients. It has been hypothesized that such disharmony leads to poor therapy outcome (Levitt, 1966).

Gottesfeld's (1965) questionnaire survey of therapy concepts of professional workers and of male delinquents furnishes an objective account of the conflict. The traditional talking-listening-reflecting-nonjudgmental-impersonal role of the clinician is rejected by the delinquents in favor of an active, father-educator-counselor figure with heavy emphasis on the pragmatics of living. These discrepancies, Gottesfeld contends, suggest a need for new therapeutic strategies.

An innovative approach along the lines suggested by the Gottesfeld survey was carried out by Massimo and Shore with lower-class delinquent, adoles-

---

[5]For some unknown reason, the research staff and professional consultants of the Task Force seem to have been unaware of the recent work on treatment of delinquents which has appeared in the psychological literature.

cent boys. The therapist served as vocational counselor, remedial educator, and consultant on personal affairs, as well as psychotherapist in the usual sense (Massimo and Shore, 1967). Emphasis was placed on learning practical skills and dealing with various ordinary situations. The therapist went on shopping trips with his patient, helped him to get a driver's license, accompanied him when he went for an initial job interview, and so on. Place and time of session were informal.

The program ran for ten months and was effective in bringing about significant changes in a group of ten patients (Massimo and Shore, 1963). A two- to three-year follow-up (Shore and Massimo, 1966) indicated that the gains in therapy had been translated into successful community adjustment. Nine of the ten treated boys were employed, five had had additional education, five were married, and no one in the group had been arrested for a felony. In contrast, only six of the control patients were employed at the time of follow-up, and six had been convicted of felonies. These concrete, highly meaningful outcome measures make the Massimo-Shore study impressive even though the sample is small.

A report by Levinson and Kitchener (1966) from the National Training School for Boys suggests an analog in the treatment of delinquents with the Johns Hopkins findings concerning the relationship between personalities of patient and therapist (Whitehorn and Betz, 1954, 1960). Inmates at NTS live in cottages each having three counselors. The report concerns the method of assigning inmates to counselors within each cottage. In one cottage, the assignment was random. In another, the counselors selected the inmates whom they wanted, and in the third, selection was indirectly controlled by inmates themselves. The fourth type was a matching of counselor and inmate based on a Q sort of statements from the Edwards Personal Preference Schedule. The best-adjusted inmates in this cottage were assigned to a counselor to whom they were most similar in personality, while the poorly adjusted boys in this cottage were assigned to counselors who were dissimilar in personality. Over a period of five months, the matched counselor-inmate cottage ranked highest on six of eight objective indices of desirable behavior, and had a mean rank of 1.5 on all eight indices.

The conventional approach to therapy is represented by the studies of Persons (1966, 1967) and Truax et al. (1966). The former is a straightforward outcome evaluation of the effects of 80 hours of individual and group therapy on a group of institutionalized delinquent boys over a 20-week period. A one-year follow-up after discharge (Persons, 1967) disclosed that more of the treated boys, compared to a control group, were successfully employed, and fewer of them had committed parole violations or had had to be recommitted. Evidently, traditional methods can be effective, perhaps as a function of differences among therapists.

The concept of the "good therapist" personality (Truax and Carkhuff, 1967) led to a study of the effect of group therapy on institutionalized female delinquents (Truax et al., 1966). Moderately positive findings in favor of the treated group as compared to an untreated control were obtained on the Conformity Scale of the Minnesota Counseling Inventory and on a (more significant) objective index, the amount of time spent out of the institution during a one year follow-up period. However, since appropriate controls were not used, it cannot be inferred that these effects were due to the high levels of "accurate empathic understanding" and "nonpossessive warmth" of the two therapists rather than to group therapy itself.

School Phobia

The child who refuses to attend school is analogous to an adult who prefers not to be gainfully employed, and to whom the community applies terms of opprobrium like vagrant, tramp, bum, and idler. Each declines to carry out the primary function assigned to him by society and is therefore viewed with alarm by those forces responsible for maintaining social order.

Parents rarely fail to perceive school refusal as a problem that must be dealt with immediately by an agency outside the home. The decision to select a treatment or a correctional agency appears to depend upon whether anxiety is involved as a motivation for the child's behavior. When anxiety is not involved in school refusal, we ordinarily speak of *truancy*. When anxiety is a motivation, we refer to *school phobia.*[6]

Most comparisons of truants and school phobics (such as Leventhal and Sills, 1964; Hersov, 1960b) show clearly that unlike truants, the school phobic is of above average intelligence, doing at least fairly well in school, comes from an intact home, and manifests psychosomatic but not sociopathic symptoms. School phobia may appear at any age during the school years, but is most common in the 9- to 12-year-old group. Most studies report no sex difference in incidence.

Truants are seldom referred for psychotherapy, but referral for school phobia is not rare. School phobics constitute between one and two percent of child guidance clinic cases (Eisenberg, 1958), and as much as 14 percent of cases viewed as psychiatric emergencies (Morrison and Smith, 1967). Only suicide attempts or threats have a greater incidence among the emergency cases seen in clinics.

Table 3 summarizes findings of eight recent reports of the treatment of school phobia. The standard of success is invariably a complete remission of the symptom, that is, return to school. The outcome data in Table 3 indicate that school phobia is more amenable to therapy than the general run of emotional illnesses. Almost 83 percent of the cases were successfully treated. If the reports that include hospitalized cases (Weiss, 1967; Hersov, 1960a) are removed, the rate of cure is more than 86 percent. Follow-ups indicate that almost 89 percent of those cases that could be located showed no recurrence of symptoms.

A variety of different treatment approaches has been reported. Multidis-

---

[6]Adelaide Johnson is usually regarded as the originator of the term "school phobia" (Johnson, et al., 1941). It has been used consistently ever since, at least in this country, though it has become plain that in a number of instances, school phobia may not be a fear of school at all. The British seem to prefer the more behavioral, less dynamic expression, "school refusal."

TABLE 3. TREATMENT OF SCHOOL PHOBIA

Report	N	x̄ Age	x̄ IQ	Percentage Remission at Close	Percentage Remission at Follow-up
Weiss and Burke (1967)	14	13	—	—	79
Adams (1966)	21	10.2	above average	90	—
Kennedy (1965)	50	9.5	—	100	100
Coolidge et al. (1964)	49	7	113	—	96
Chazan (1962)	33	10.5	106	88	88
Davidson (1961)	27	11	hi average	93	—
Hersov (1960*)	50	11.8	106	68	100
Eisenberg (1959)	67	9.4*	110*	72	71*
Composite	311	9.9	108.9†	82.7	88.8

*Data from Rodriguez et al. (1959). The age and IQ data describe the 41 cases located on follow-up.
†Mean IQ is based on 173 cases for whom a numerical estimate was available.

ciplinary, many-faceted approaches are not uncommon (Kahn and Nursten, 1964; Davidson, 1961), but intensity and scope of treatment does not seem to be related to outcome. One of the most successful reports (Kennedy, 1965) had a maximum treatment course of only three days.

A factor that appears to be related to outcome is type of school phobia, a distinction first suggested by Coolidge et al. (1957) and exploited most clearly by Kennedy (1965). According to Coolidge, there are two primary types of school phobic. The "neurotic-crisis" phobic, called Type 1 by Kennedy, is essentially an overprotected, anxiety-prone child. The "way-of-life," or Type 2, phobic is a severely disturbed, possibly psychotic or incipiently psychotic child whose school refusal is only one facet of a deeply-seated disorder.

Using return to school as the sole criterion of outcome—the usual procedure—the prognosis for the "neurotic," Type 1 child is excellent with any form of therapy, but is poor for the more disturbed, Type 2 child. Some of the outcome reports in Table 3 note that a proportion of the sample was discarded because the cases were not true school phobics, that is, showed evidence of more extensive disorder (for example, Coolidge et al., 1964; Weiss and Burke, 1967). The discards were very probably Type 2 cases. Kennedy (1965) deliberately discarded six cases diagnosed as Type 2 so that he could report on a homogeneous sample. Hersov's (1960a) outcome report is the poorest listed in Table 3. Notably, his sample included 29 inpatients, many of whom were probably Type 2 phobics.

It is possible that Type 2 cases are customarily discarded, or perhaps not diagnosed as school phobias even though school refusal is the paramount, manifest symptom. This would be one factor accounting for the high success rate in the treatment of school phobia.

One might argue that school refusal in the Type 2 case is only one symptom—perhaps even a minor one—among many, that it is incidental to more serious problems, and that, thus, the Type 2 case is rightfully excluded from the category of school phobia. The cogency of the contention is questionable. School phobia is, in *every* instance, a symptom rather than a diagnosis in the usual sense. Most school phobics, regardless of type, have other psychological symptoms.

Another factor that seems to be related to treatment success is age. Most clinicians believe that therapy is more successful with younger school phobics. Eisenberg (1959) reports a 90 percent remission rate with children under 11 years old, compared to only 45 percent success with children older than 11 years.

A relationship between age and outcome can be crudely estimated from the reports in Table 3. The rank-order correlation between mean age of the sample and percentage of remitted cases at close (or follow-up if data at close are not given) is –.48. This coefficient falls short of conventional statistical significance, but is at least suggestive.

Age and type of phobia may be correlated, thus confounding the relationship between age and outcome. It is generally believed by clinicians that Type 2 cases tend to be older. It is notable that among the reports in Table 3, those that include inpatients have the highest mean ages (Hersov, 1960a; Weiss and Burke, 1967). A cautious, tentative inference would be that phobia type, rather than age per se, is the correlative factor.

School phobia as a symptom responds more frequently to therapy than other forms of maladjustment in children, often quickly and easily. Symptomatic treatment, though its usefulness is acknowledged, may very well leave an etiological core untouched. Some of the follow-ups of treated cases show little or no recurrence of the phobia among treated cases over periods of time ranging up to ten years (Chazan, 1962; Coolidge et al., 1964). Others report less favorable findings. The recurrence rate in the follow-up by Rodriguez et al. (1959) could be as high as 25 percent (the method of presentation of results does not permit a definite statement). Levenson (1961) reports on his treatment of ten school phobics in the 16- to 20-year-old range, all of whom had a history of the symptom in early childhood. Later behavior may suggest a continuing, underlying, causal factor, even though actual school refusal is not manifested. Coolidge et al. (1964) conducted one of the more careful, painstaking follow-up studies with a mean interval of nine years after close.

> In our study, 47 of the 49 subjects have returned to school and have either graduated or are still attending high school. . . . Fifty per cent of our subjects are, however, manifesting symptoms which, on investigation, can be traced back to the original phobia. This may be a continued chronic apprehension in relation to attending school, or an exaggerated and unwarranted concern regarding studies and exams. It may be expressed as Monday morning anergia, vague aches or pains or absences due to feigned illnesses. . . . Even the children who appear to be doing quite well and would be considered "normal adolescents" express more than the ordinary concerns about leaving home and in general show a cautious approach to new situations (Coolidge et al., 1964, pp. 676–677).

Do the encouraging reports of the treatment of school phobia reflect simply symptomatic improvement in many cases, without a true curative action? Are we being deceived by developmental symptom substitution? Is school phobia easily driven underground only to emerge later as test anxiety? As usual, there is a healthy suspicion, but no conclusive answer.

Some Miscellaneous Process Reports

Focus of Treatment

As previously noted, a unique aspect of child psychotherapy is that it is common for persons other than the child patient himself to enter into treatment. The argument holds that the therapist's influence on the child will be vitiated or negated unless therapeutic influence is exerted on the influential adults whose impacts have brought about psychopathology in the child. The mother, presumably the primary influence on the child, has always been a treatment focus. Some child guidance clinics insist on seeing every mother of every child in therapy. When the child is very young, sometimes only the mother will be treated. The father, as his influence is gradually being recognized, is also becoming a focus. In some cases, the entire family constellation will be involved in treatment.

The argument has rarely been subjected to objective examination, possibly because its logic appears to be overwhelming. Matarazzo's review (1965) of familial therapy does not include a single study directly relevant to assessment of effectiveness of treatment as a function of focus.

Several recent outpatient studies shed some provocative, though hardly definitive, light on the question. The patients came from a clinic in suburban Pittsburgh (Gluck et al., 1964), a large clinic in metropolitan Chicago (Lessing and Schilling, 1966), and from the Negro poverty community in New York City (D'Angelo and Walsh, 1967). The latter reports data in terms of mean change scores rather than percent of improvement as in the other two studies.

The pertinent data are summarized in Table 4. With a single exception, the three studies are in agreement that the order of effectiveness of treatment in terms of focus, from least to most, is (1) child alone, (2) mother alone, (3) mother and child, and (4) mother and father, or mother, father, and child.

TABLE 4. OUTCOME AS A FUNCTION OF TREATMENT FOCUS

	Study		
	Gluck et al. (1964)*	Lessing and Schilling (1966)*	D'Angelo and Walsh (1967)
Focus			
Child only	—	—	Worse
Mother only	55	62	—
Mother and child	67	71	No change
Mother and father	85	—	Improvement
Mother, father, and child	85	—	No change

*Data in percentage of improved cases.

The algebra of the Gluck study is clear; the critical factor in treatment success is a participating father. The D'Angelo and Walsh data suggest that there are two critical factors: a participating father and a nonparticipating child.

The hypothesis that treating parents has greater impact on the child than treating the child himself is regarded favorably by the child guidance movement. Acceptance by the mother of her responsibility for the child's symptoms is usually regarded as a positive prognostic sign. Frequently, treatment is not offered to children whose mothers do not verbalize such acceptance. It is tempting to conclude that the data in Table 4 support this position. There are several reasons why this conclusion would be premature.

First, there are alternative explanations for the data. It is conceivable that the improved prognosis when the father participates is due to the presence of a father interested and concerned enough to involve himself in the therapy process, not to the impact of the father's therapist.

Second, results from agencies other than conventional outpatient clinics are not necessarily in accord. For example, Hartmann et al. (1968) found that conjunctive parental treatment, either by a social worker or in group therapy, was unrelated to outcome with hospitalized adolescents. Seeman et al. (1964) report on a successful play therapy program with a group of second and third graders. Only the children were treated. Contact with the parents was deliberately kept to a bare minimum. Patients and controls were selected as the most poorly adjusted children after a screening of all second and third grades using peer and teacher ratings. This atypical procedure—actually an exercise in prevention—did not *require* participation of the parent. It would be impossible in the conventional outpatient setting, in which it is necessary for a parent to bring the child and usually to be involved in the diagnostic process.

It is conceivable that in some way, the importance of therapy for parents is a consequence of the child's awareness of parental responsibility for initiating the therapeutic contact. When the child does not perceive this responsibility, for whatever reason, the significance of parental involvement in therapy is diminished.

A study of remainers and terminators in child treatment by Cole and Magnussen (1967) suggests that terminating cases were more often ones in which only the mother participated, while the remainers more often included both mother and father. The authors infer support for the position that it is important to involve both parents in treatment. However, the data also suggest that whether the father becomes actively involved may depend partly upon the severity of the child's symptoms rather than on paternal motivation. Unfortunately, the data are not reported in sufficient detail to make a definitive inference concerning remaining in treatment and father participation.

The IJR Study

An attempt to relate treatment outcome to a number of patient, therapist, and process variables was carried out on cases treated at the Institute of Juvenile Research in Chicago during the period 1951–1960 (Lessing and

Schilling, 1966). In 505 cases, only the child had been treated; in 332 other cases, both mother and child had been seen. Outcome was rated by therapists at close on a scale essentially corresponding to Improved, Partly Improved, and Unimproved or Worse.

Relationships with 29 variables were computed. Among those that were *not* related to outcome in either group were frequency and number of treatment interviews and total time in treatment; profession and experience of therapist; and similarity of sex, race, and religion of therapist to that of the patient. These findings are parallel to those of Hartmann et al. (1968) in that five measures of treatment, including number of hours, length of sessions, and therapy for parents, were unrelated to outcome in institutionalized adolescents. Similar findings of a lack of correlation between outcome and number of treatment hours have been reported by Phillips (1960) and Shepherd et al. (1966), and are reflected in the reports of treatment of school phobia in Table 3. Parallel results have been found by investigators of psychotherapy with adults.

If psychotherapy were a generally effective treatment method, some positive correlation between outcome and number of treatment interviews would be expected. The absence of a relationship supports the conclusions derived from Table 1, and underscores the need for fresh conceptualizations of the psychotherapy process.

Six variables in the IJR study were found to differentiate the outcome groups for cases in which the mother alone had been treated. Three of the relationships are clear. Improvement is more likely to occur if the patient's siblings are of the same sex, and if the mother accepts her involvement in the patient's problems and does not unconsciously encourage the child's pathology. Relationships for the remaining three variables are not linear, and thus not subject to a clear interpretation. (The percentage of cases in the Unimproved category falls between those of the two categories of improvement.)

Only three variables differentiated the outcome groups for cases in which mother and child were treated. Improvement tended to be inversely related to degree of disturbance, which was more often rated as moderate in the Improved categories and less often as severe. Relationships for the other two variables—presence of a learning problem or of a somatic problem—were not linear.

The IJR study attempts to utilize routinely gathered clinical data in psychotherapy research. The effort is praiseworthy, but like all "fishing expeditions," runs afoul of an unfortunate mathematical contingency. Whenever a large number of nonindependent statistical analyses are computed in a single study, there is no known method of estimating the number of analyses that are statistically significant by chance alone. An appeal to the binomial theorem is futile; it applies only to independent events. The best solution lies in the use of a model or closed theoretical structure that predicts expected correlations. Unfortunately, such systems are not yet available.

Another problem with the fishing expedition approach is that the predictor variables are not always independent of the criterion variables. Some of the predictor variables will be employed, wittingly or unwittingly, in assessing severity of illness, outcome, or prognosis. In the Hartmann et al. (1968) study, a predictor variable like "discharged to hospital or home" is likely to be related to status at close. The presence of regression as a primary defense suggests a more serious illness, while "normal" handling of aggression indicates a milder one. It is not surprising to find that these two factors were related to outcome in the Hartmann study.

When a predictor and a criterion variable are nonindependent, a statistically significant correlation is an unavoidable artifact. It merely testifies to the successful employment of a predictor variable in measuring the criterion. No further inference is warranted.

Race

College and urban crises in recent years have, for the first time, brought some attention to the question of race as a factor in psychotherapy with children. There has yet been no quantitative investigation of this variable, and empirical data are not available. Two impressive clinical papers are noteworthy. Chethik et al. (1967) report on the first two Negro adolescents to be admitted to an inpatient treatment center that happens to have a high proportion of Negro workers. Lawrence (1968) forthrightly discusses his personal experiences as a Negro therapist working primarily with white children.

Some Indications for the Practicing Child Psychotherapist

Child guidance has its full share of standard rules of procedure, few of which have ever rested on a firm empirical basis. Many are now being directly challenged by recent research. These include such well-worn inheritances from psychoanalysis as:

1. The mother must invariably be a treatment focus if a school-aged child is to be treated successfully.

2. Involvement of the father is less significant in treating the child than is involvement of the mother.

3. Treatment outcome is positively related to intensity of treatment.

4. Permissiveness and encouragement to express negative feelings invariably constitute a desirable treatment procedure; punishment of undesirable behavior is never a desirable procedure.

5. Any home or family existence is likely to be more therapeutic than institutionalization.

6. Successful therapists are drawn exclusively from the ranks of psychiatry, clinical psychology, and psychiatric social work.

About a third of the children referred to child guidance clinics receive any kind of formal treatment.[7] There is an enormous investment of clinic time in the process—sometimes very elaborate—of identifying the fortunate third. Favorable prognosis is usually the paramount, determining factor. In turn, it is based on such variables as motivation of the mother for treatment, willingness of the parents to accept their responsibility for the child's symptoms, ego strength of the child, and the like. The outcome data suggest that we may have been treating the wrong children, that the establishment of a favorable prognosis means that the child will improve *with or without* formal intervention. It may be time for child guidance to give serious consideration to the possibility of revising prognostic criteria. For example, a high anxiety level in the mother may be an indication that developmental remission of symptoms is likely to occur and that formal treatment of the child is unnecessary.

Few conditions have been definitely established as requisite or even advisable for the treatment of the child patient. Innovation in therapy is the order of the day; rigid orthodoxies find scant empirical support. Finally, there seems to be no substitute for the *long-range,* follow-up study as the procedure for investigating either therapy outcome or therapy process when the patients are children.

References

Adams, P. L., McDonald, N. F., and Huey, W. P. School phobia and bisexual conflict: A report of 21 cases. *Amer. J. Psychiat.,* 1966, **123,** 541–547.

Beckett, P. G. S., Lennox, K., and Grisell, J. L. Responsibility and reward in treatment. *J. Nerv. & Ment. Dis.,* 1968, **146,** 257–263.

Bergin, A. E. Some implications of psychotherapy research for therapeutic practice. *Inter. J. Psychiat.,* 1967, **3,** 136–153.

Beskind, H. Psychiatric inpatient treatment of adolescents: A review of the clinical experience. *Comprehen. Psychiat.,* 1962, **3,** 354–369.

Betz, B. J., and Whitehorn, J. C. Relationship of the therapist to the outcome of therapy in schizophrenia. *Psychiatric Research Reports,* 1956, **5,** 89–140.

Chazan, M. School phobia. *Brit. J. Educ. Psychol.,* 1962, **32,** 209–217.

Chethik, M., Fleming, E., and Mayer, M. F. A quest for identity: Treatment of disturbed Negro children in a predominantly white treatment center. *Amer. J. Orthopsychiat.,* 1967, **37,** 71–77.

Cole, J. K., and Magnussen, M. G. Family situation factors related to remainers and terminators of treatment. *Psychother.,* 1967, **4,** 107–109.

Coolidge, J. C., Brodie, R. D., and Feeney, B. A ten-year follow-up study of sixty-six school-phobic children. *Amer. J. Orthopsychiat.,* 1964, **34,** 675–684.

Coolidge, J. C., Hahn, P. B., and Peck, A. L. School phobia: Neurotic crisis or way of life. *Amer. J. Orthopsychiat.,* 1957, **27,** 296–306.

D'Angelo, R., and Walsh, J. F. An evaluation of various therapy approaches with lower socio-economic group children. *J. Psychol.,* 1967, **67,** 59–64.

Davidson, S. School phobia as a manifestation of family disturbance: Its structure and treatment. *J. Ch. Psychol. & Psychiat.,* 1961, **1,** 270–287.

---

[7]Twenty-eight percent of the cases seen at the St. Louis Municipal Psychiatric Clinic between 1922 and 1944, and 21 percent of admissions to Maryland child clinics in 1958–59, were offered treatment (Robins, 1966). Nationally, the treatment rate was 34.9 percent for cases closed during 1966 (OPC Report, 1966).

DeFries, Z., Jenkins, S., and Williams, E. C. Foster family care—a non-sentimental view. *Child Welfare,* 1965, **44,** 73–84.

DeFries, Z., Jenkins, S., and Williams, E. C. Treatment of disturbed children in foster care. *Amer. J. Orthopsychiat.,* 1964, **34,** 615–624.

Eisenberg, L. The pediatric management of school phobia. *J. Pediat.,* 1959, **55,** 758–766.

Eisenberg, L. School phobia: A study in the communication of anxiety. *Amer. J. Psychiat.,* 1958, **114,** 712–718.

Eisenberg, L. The sins of the fathers: Urban decay and social pathology. *Amer. J. Orthopsychiat.,* 1962, **32,** 5–17.

Eisenberg, L., and Gruenberg, E. M. The current status of secondary prevention in child psychiatry. *Amer. J. Orthopsychiat.,* 1961, **31,** 355–367.

Eisenberg, L., Marlowe, B., and Hastings, M. Diagnostic services for maladjusted foster children: An orientation toward an acute need. *Amer. J. Orthopsychiat.,* 1958, **28,** 750–763.

Gardner, G. G. The relationship between childhood neurotic symptomatology and later schizophrenia in males and females. *J. Nerv. & Ment. Dis.,* 1967, **144,** 97–100.

Ginott, H. G., and Lebo, D. Most and least used play therapy limits. *J. Genet. Psychol.,* 1963, **103,** 153–159.

Ginott, H. G., and Lebo, D. Play therapy limits and theoretical orientation. *J. Consult. Psychol.,* 1961, **26,** 337–340.

Glasser, W. *Reality Therapy: A new approach to psychiatry.* New York: Harper & Row, 1965.

Gluck, M. R., Tanner, M. M., Sullivan, D. F., and Erickson, P. A. Follow-up evaluation of 55 child guidance cases. *Behav. Res. & Ther.,* 1964, **2,** 131–134.

Gottesfeld, H. Professionals and delinquents evaluate professional methods with delinquents. *Soc. Probs.,* 1965, **13,** 45–59.

Guerney, B. J., Jr. Filial therapy: Description and rationale. *J. Consult. Psychol.,* 1964, **28,** 304–310.

Haring, N. G., and Phillips, E. L. *Educating emotionally disturbed children.* New York: McGraw-Hill, 1962.

Hartmann, E., Glasser, B. A., Greenblatt, M., Solomon, M. H., and Levinson, D. J. *Adolescents in a mental hospital.* New York: Grune & Stratton, 1968.

Hawkins, R. P., Peterson, R. F., Schweid, E., and Bijou, S. W. Behavior therapy in the home: Amelioration of problem parent–child relations with the parent in a therapeutic role. *J. Exp. Ch. Psychol.,* 1966, **4,** 99–107.

Healy, W., and Bronner, A. F. The child guidance clinic: Birth and growth of an idea. In Lowrey, L. G., and Sloane, V. (Eds.), *Orthopsychiatry, 1923–1948: Retrospect and prospect.* American Orthopsychiatric Assoc., 1948.

Heinicke, C. M., and Goldman, A. Research on psychotherapy with children: A review and suggestions for further study. *Amer. J. Orthopsychiat.,* 1960, **30,** 483–493.

Hersch, C. The discontent explosion in mental health. *Amer. Psychol.,* 1968, **23,** 497–506.

Hersov, L. A. Refusal to go to school. *J. Ch. Psychol. & Psychiat.,* 1960, **1,** 137–145. (a)

Hersov, L. A. Persistent non-attendance at school. *J. Ch. Psychol. & Psychiat.,* 1960, **1,** 130–136. (b)

Hobbs, N. Helping disturbed children: Psychological and ecological strategies. *Amer. Psychol.,* 1966, **21,** 1105–1115.

Hood-Williams, J. The results of psychotherapy with children: A revaluation. *J. Consult. Psychol.,* 1960, **24,** 84–88.

Hunt, R. C. Ingredients of a rehabilitation program. *Proc. Ann. Conf. Milbank Memorial Fund, 1957.* 1958.

Johnson, A. M., Falstein, E. I., Szurek, S. A., and Svendsen, M. School phobia. *Amer. J. Orthopsychiat.,* 1941, **11,** 702–711.

Kahn, J. H., and Nursten, J. P. *Unwillingly to school.* New York: Macmillan, 1964.

Kanfer, F. H., and Phillips, J. S. Behavior therapy: A panacea for all ills or a passing fancy? *Arch. Gen. Psychiat.,* 1966, **15,** 114–128.

Kanner, L. History of child psychiatry. In Freedman, A. M., and Kaplan, H. I. (Eds.), *Comprehensive textbook of psychiatry.* Baltimore: Williams & Wilkins, 1967.

Kennedy, W. A. School phobia: Rapid treatment of fifty cases. *Abnorm. Psychol.,* 1965, **70,** 285–289.

Lapouse, R., and Monk, M. A. Fears and worries in a representative sample of children. *Amer. J. Orthopsychiat.,* 1959, **29,** 803–818.

La Vietes, R., Cohen, R., Reens, R., and Ronall, R. Day treatment center and school: Seven years experience. *Amer. J. Orthopsychiat.,* 1965, **35,** 160–169.

La Vietes, R., Hulse, W. C., and Blau, A. A psychiatric day treatment center and school for young children and their parents. *Amer. J. Orthopsychiat.,* 1960, **30,** 468–482.

Lawrence, L. E. The necessity for early confrontation concerning obvious racial characteristics. Paper read at the annual meeting of the American Association of Psychiatric Clinics for Children, 1968.

Lessing, E. E., and Schilling, F. H. Relationship between treatment selection variables and treatment outcome in a child guidance clinic: An application of data-processing methods. *J. Amer. Acad. Child Psychiat.,* 1966, **5,** 313–348.

Levenson, E. A. The treatment of school phobias in the young adult. *Amer. J. Psychother.,* 1961, **15,** 539–552.

Leventhal, T., and Sills, M. Self-image in school phobia. *Amer. J. Orthopsychiat.,* 1964, **34,** 685–695.

Levinson, R. B., and Kitchener, H. L. Treatment of delinquents: Comparison of four methods for assigning inmates to counselors. *J. Consult. Psychol.,* 1966, **30,** 364.

Levitt, E. E. The results of psychotherapy with children: An evaluation. *J. Consult. Psychol.,* 1957, **21,** 189–196. (a)

Levitt, E. E. A follow-up study of cases treated at the Illinois Institute for Juvenile Research: An evaluation of psychotherapy with children. Report of Mental Health Project No. 5503, Dept. of Public Welfare, State of Illinois, 1957. (b)

Levitt, E. E. A comparison of "remainers" and "defectors" among child clinic patients. *J. Consult. Psychol.,* 1957, **21,** 316. (c)

Levitt, E. E. A comparative judgmental study of "defection" from treatment at a child guidance clinic. *J. Clin. Psychol.,* 1958, **14,** 429–432.

Levitt, E. E. Psychotherapy with children: A further evaluation. *Behav. Res. & Ther.,* 1963, **60,** 326–329.

Levitt, E. E. Psychotherapy research and the expectation-reality discrepancy. *Psychother.,* 1966, **3,** 163–166.

Levitt, E. E., Beiser, H. R., and Robertson, R. E. A follow-up evaluation of cases treated at a community child guidance clinic. *Amer. J. Orthopsychiat.,* 1959, **29,** 337–347.

Lewis, W. W. Continuity and intervention in emotional disturbance: A review. *Exceptional Children,* 1965, **31,** 465–475.

Maas, H. S., and Engler, R. E. *Children in need of parents.* New York: Columbia Univ. Press, 1959.

Macfarlane, J. W., Allen, L., and Honzik, M. *A developmental study of the behavior problems of normal children between 21 months and 14 years.* Berkeley, Calif.: Univ. of California Press, 1954.

Massimo, J. L., and Shore, M. F. Comprehensive vocationally oriented psychotherapy: A new treatment technique for lower class adolescent delinquent boys. *Psychiat.,* 1967, **30,** 229–236.

Massimo, J. L., and Shore, M. F. The effectiveness of a comprehensive vocationally oriented psychotherapeutic program for adolescent delinquent boys. *Amer. J. Orthopsychiat.,* 1963, **33,** 634–642.

Matarazzo, J. D. Psychotherapeutic processes. In *Ann. Rev. Psychol.* Palo Alto, Calif.: Annual Reviews, Inc. 1965.

Morrison, G. C., and Smith, W. R. Emergencies in child psychiatry: A definition and comparison of two groups. Paper read at American Orthopsychiatric Assoc. meeting, 1967.

Persons, R. W. Psychological and behavioral change in delinquents following psychotherapy. *J. Clin. Psychol.,* 1966, **22,** 337–340.

Persons, R. W. Relationship between psychotherapy with institutionalized delinquent boys and subsequent community adjustment. *J. Consult. Psychol.,* 1967, **31**, 137–141.

Phillips, E. L. Parent–child psychotherapy: A follow-up study comparing two techniques. *J. Psychol.,* 1960, **49**, 195–202.

Reens, R. Intelligence quotients of children before and after intensive psychotherapeutic intervention. Unpublished paper, 1965.

Rioch, M. J. Elkes, C., Flint, A. A, et al. Pilot project in training mental health counselors. *U.S.P.H.S. Publ. No. 1254*, 1965.

Robins, L. N. *Deviant children grown up.* Baltimore: Williams & Wilkins, 1966.

Rodman, H., and Grams, P. Juvenile delinquency and the family: A review and discussion. In *Report of the Task Force on Juvenile Delinquency and Youth Crime of the President's Commission on Law Enforcement and Administration of Justice.* Washington, D.C.: U.S. Government Printing Office, 1967. Pp. 188–221.

Rodriguez, A., Rodriguez, M., and Eisenberg, L. The outcome of school phobia: A follow-up study based on 41 cases. *Amer. J. Psychiat.,* 1959, **116**, 540–544.

Schofield, W. *Psychotherapy: The purchase of friendship.* Englewood Cliffs, N.J.: Prentice-Hall, 1964.

Seeman, J., Barry, E., and Ellinwood, C. Interpersonal assessment of play therapy outcome. *Psychother.,* 1964, **1**, 64–66.

Shepherd, M., Oppenheim, A. N., and Mitchell, S. Childhood behavior disorders and the child guidance clinic: An epidemiological study. *J. Ch. Psychol. & Psychiat.,* 1966, **7**, 39–52.

Shore, M. F., Massimo, J. L., Kisielewski, B. A., and Moran, J. K. Object relations changes resulting from successful psychotherapy with adolescent delinquents and their relationship to academic performance. *J. Amer. Acad. Child Psychiat.,* 1966, **5**, 93–104.

Simmons, J. E. Are child guidance clinics becoming outmoded? Paper read at the Mideastern Regional meeting of the American Association of Psychiatric Clinics for Children, 1963.

Sonis, M. Implications for the child guidance clinic of current trends in mental health planning. *Amer. J. Orthopsychiat.,* 1968, **38**, 515–526.

Steinzor. B. *The healing partnership.* New York: Harper & Row, 1967.

Stover, L., and Guerney, B. G., Jr. The efficacy of training procedures for mothers in filial therapy. *Psychother.,* 1967, **4**, 110–115.

Strupp, H. H., and Bergin, A. E. Some empirical and conceptual bases for coordinated research in psychotherapy: A critical review of issues, trends, and evidence. *Inter. J. Psychiat.,* 1969, **5**, No. 2.

Truax, C. B. Effective ingredients in psychotherapy: An approach to unraveling the patient–therapist interaction. *J. Counsel. Psychol.,* 1963, **10**, 256–263.

Truax, C. B. Reinforcement and non-reinforcement in Rogerian psychotherapy. *J. Abnorm. Soc. Psychol.,* 1966, **71**, 1–9.

Truax, C. B. The use of trained practical counselors or therapists and the evolving understanding of counseling and psychotherapy. *Discussion Papers, Ark. Rehab. Res. & Trng. Ctr.,* 1968, **1**, No. 12.

Truax, C. B., and Carkhuff, R. R. *Toward effective counseling and psychotherapy: Training and practice.* Chicago: Aldine, 1967.

Truax, C. B., Wargo, D. G., and Silber, L. D. Effects of group psychotherapy with high accurate empathy and nonpossessive warmth upon female institutionalized delinquents. *J. Abnorm. Psychol.,* 1966, **71**, 267–274.

Wahler, R. G., Winkel, G. H., Peterson, R. F., and Morrison, D. C. Mothers as behavior therapists for their own children. *Behav. Res. & Ther.,* 1965, **3**, 113–124.

Warren, W. A study of adolescent psychiatric in-patients and the outcome six or more years later. I. Clinical histories and hospital findings. *J. Child Psychol. Psychiat.,* 1965, **6**, 1–17. (a)

Warren, W. A study of adolescent psychiatric in-patients and the outcome six or more years later. II. The follow-up study. *J. Child Psychol. Psychiat.,* 1965, **6**, 141–160. (b)

Weinstein, L. The Project Re-ED Schools for emotionally disturbed children: Effectiveness as viewed by referring agencies, parents and teachers. *Exceptional Children,* 1969, **35,** 703–711.

Weiss, M., and Burke, A. A five to ten-year follow-up study of hospitalized school phobic children and adolescents. Paper read at the annual meeting of the American Orthopsychiatric Association, 1967.

Whitehorn, J. C., and Betz, B. J. A study of psychotherapeutic relationships between physicians and schizophrenic patients. *American Journal of Psychiatry,* 1954, **111,** 321–331.

Whitehorn, J. C., and Betz, B. J. Further studies of the doctor as a crucial variable in the outcome of treatment with schizophrenic patients. *American Journal of Psychiatry,* 1960, **117,** 215–223.

Williams, R., and Pollack, R. H. Some non-psychological variables in therapy defection in a child-guidance clinic. *J. Psychol.,* 1964, **58,** 145–155.

Zeilberger, J., Sampen, S. E., and Sloane, H. N. Modification of a child's problem behaviors in the home with the mother as therapist. *J. Appl. Behav. Anal.,* 1968, **1,** 47–53.

Outpatient Psychiatric Clinics Annual Statistical Report, 1966. Biometry Branch, National Institute of Mental Health, 1966, PHS Publication 1854.

Project Re-ED: A demonstration project for the reeducation of emotionally disturbed children (revised). Nashville: George Peabody College for Teachers, 1967.

Report of the Task Force on Juvenile Delinquency and Youth Crime of the President's Commission on Law Enforcement and Administration of Justice. Washington, D.C.: U.S. Government Printing Office, 1967.

26. Individualized Therapy—A Summary

James O. Palmer

In the previous sections of this chapter, the question has been asked: Do the problems and needs of this child fit the goals and criteria of this form of treatment? However, only occasionally do the child's needs correspond to the stated goals and criteria of any one therapeutic approach. There are often as many contraindications as indications. Rather than ask whether the child fits any particular therapeutic mold, it would seem much more reasonable to use the data from the assessment to design an individualized program to fit the needs of the child. In this section, an attempt will be made to outline the ways in which therapy might be so programmed to the child.

To design such individualized treatment requires a careful and thorough assessment and thoughtful planning. Individualized therapy does not consist merely of a random sampling of therapeutic techniques, nor is it simply

From *The Psychological Assessment of Children* by James O. Palmer. Copyright © 1970 by John Wiley and Sons, Inc. Reproduced by permission.

an eclectic approach. The design should systematically take into account the following factors.

1. The needs and problems of the child.
2. The basic principles common to all forms of therapy.
3. The variations in techniques needed for the individual needs of the child.
4. The time sequence of the therapy.
5. The economic aspects of the therapy.
6. Some difficulties in implementing a plan for therapy.

1. . . . The overall need of every child is growth, that is, the development of a unique identity with an ego which is capable of independent need-gratification. The raison d'etre of any therapy is to promote such growth. Therapy, of course, does not create the urge to grow; this drive is a central aspect of the biological and social nature of the child. Rather, therapy is aimed at eliminating the obstacles and limitations to the child's growth, and thus deals with those specific behavioral stresses and conflicts which impede the child's development.

If therapy is to be planned to meet these impediments, then the first step is a comprehensive assessment. The assessment should not be limited to the questions asked by the referrant, but should explore in depth all ramifications of the child's ego development, and should contain a list of the various problems, that is, the manifest disturbing behaviors. Next, it should specify the different ways in which development is being impeded, the stresses and conflicts which underlie the disturbances. There should follow some reasonable hypotheses about the possible interrelationships of these factors, the dynamics or interacting forces. To plan therapy, an assessment should uncover and delineate the leitmotiv of the child's development, the core patterns of events and conflicts. These dynamics should be stated in terms of the child's stage of development. In particular, the assessment should specify the degree and nature of the child's dependency on others, and the process of internalization. The kinds of therapy to be used depend in part on the stage of development of the child's experience balance. The assessment should also contain a summary estimate of the overall ego strength of the child, again in terms of development, for the kinds of therapy and their implementation depend on the ability of the child to absorb and use the treatment.

2. As was repeatedly pointed out in the previous sections of this chapter, there are certain aspects of psychotherapy which all forms have in common and which appear to be fundamental to behavioral change. The therapeutic "couch" need not be a Proscrustean bed, but even though it comes in various shapes and sizes and designs, there are some basic elements. Any therapy must include to some degree and fashion, the following.

a. *A reflection or recognition of the child's affective states* or feelings. In behavior modification, which focuses on the environment, this recognition consists of the affective elements of the behavior of others in the environment and the affective responses of the child.

b. *The relationships between these affects and the environment.*

c. *The relationships between these affective states and the internal operations of the child.* In both client-centered therapy and behavior modification, this element of therapy is admittedly underestimated, since it is regarded as a constant.

d. *The relationship of these affective states to the motivations of the child* and of his parents and other authorities. All therapies are concerned with what the child is trying to do, learn, achieve, or obtain. His affective states reflect the frustration of these goals.

e. *The relationship between the child and the therapist.* In this relationship, the child both acts out the frustrations of his everyday life onto the therapist, and uses the therapist as a model.

f. *All therapists repeatedly reinforce* various aspects of the child's behaviors, in a working-through process, sometimes using simple operant rewards and punishments, sometimes using very complex verbal and behavioral situations.

g. Based chiefly on the therapeutic relationship, *all therapies use the therapeutic situation as a microcosm of everyday life.*

3. To design a therapeutic "couch" to fit the child, it is necessary to specify the variations needed in these basic dimensions of therapy. First, one needs to determine from the assessment which affective states need to be recognized and reflected. Which affective responses should be stressed? Which, possibly, ignored? Which are closest to the child's consciousness and are thus most available for reflection? Which feelings does he hide at all costs? How much spontaneity and lability does he demonstrate? How much does he limit his affective awareness and expression? How sensitive is he? All these questions can and should be answered as best as possible if the reflection of affect is to planned.

Second, the assessment should specify the relationships between these affects and observable environmental stresses. Are these affects a response to the environment, and to what degree? What stimuli set off these affective reactions? What stimuli inhibit them? Third, the assessment should specify the degree to which these affective responses reflect the internal state of the child. What memories, fantasies, impulses, and drives trigger off these feelings? Are these generalized affective states, or are they specific to certain external or internal stimuli? Assessment of these factors is basic to planning the degree to which the external and internal facts of behaviors are to be manipulated. Fourth, the therapist needs to be advised of the specific motivational patterns which drive the child to act and feel as he does. Where and why is the child frustrated in meeting his need-gratifications? How does he react to deprivation of needs? With knowledge of these motivational patterns, the therapist can make plans to help the child cope with his frustrations and to find effective means of gaining need-satisfactions. Usually the behaviors which require altering are these coping mechanisms. In other instances, the child may be very adept at coping, but needs to redirect his efforts.

The kinds of interactions that the therapist may initially expect from the child are those which the child currently conducts with other adults. These interactions appear during assessment, directly with the assessor and indirectly in the child's responses to various techniques, and parents may openly or inadvertently mention them. From assessment of these patterns, the therapist may be able to predict how the child may react to him and his behavior. Finally, on the basis of the assessment, it is possible to plan out the kinds of reinforcements which may need to be used for the child under consideration. One may also estimate the frequency of these reinforcements and how they should be varied. With these variables in mind, the therapeutic situations or microcosms may be selected.

4. In all therapies, the timing and sequence of reinforcements are a major factor. Some learning has to be spaced; some consists of a rapid repetition of rewards and punishments. The question facing all therapists is: What is to be done first? Most often, therapy proceeds step by step from one element to the next, in the order listed above in paragraph 2: the therapist initially reflects the child's feelings, relating them to his environment and then to his own internal stresses. At the same time, the therapist begins to explore the child's motivations and their relationships to these affects. As these patterns of behavior are demonstrated in the therapy hour, the therapist uses his relationship with the child as a reinforcement. These and other reinforcements are repeated to obtain specific modifications of the child's behavior, externally and internally.

However, it is not possible to conduct all therapy in this exact order. Sometimes a program of operant conditioning has to be instituted before the child will respond to anything as, for example, in the case of so-called autistic children. With other children, for example, delinquent adolescents, a direct confrontation of motivations may be necessary, even before very much affect is dealt with. The planning of therapeutic strategy is made possible by the assessment of the child's modes of operation. If all of the child's functioning is overwhelmed by a habit, it may be necessary to begin with a program of behavior modification; thereafter, the feelings and motivations underlying the habit may be attacked. If the child has retreated to his daydream world, an exploration of that world may have to precede any alteration of his social environment, which then might be attacked through some form of group treatment. In other instances, it may be necessary to focus on the family and its interactions if that is where the child is operating, before turning to treatment of internal conflicts and affects.

5. The cost of the treatment in time and money also should be estimated. Unfortunately, there is no known basis for budgeting the cost of treatment. This important facet of treatment planning has yet to be studied. At best, one can make rough estimates of the number of sessions, the number of months over which these sessions will be spread, and the consequent cost in therapist's fees or salary. However, if the other aspects of treatment are systematically planned according to the assessment, and if these plans are effectively implemented, then it may be possible subsequently to determine the time and cost of various plans, much as the construction of buildings or highways are budgeted. The cost in terms of dropouts from treatment should decrease, and planned treatment should motivate more patients to remain. Conversely, the average length of treatment for those who do continue should also decrease. The number of wasted hours and misdirected

efforts should be decreased by planning. The overall cost in terms of money spent on treatment may increase, but so should the number of successful outcomes.

6. *Difficulties and Objections.* If therapy is planned to meet the needs of the child, then there are no contraindications in the usual sense of the word. Each separate therapeutic endeavor is designed to be the indicated treatment of choice. However, this is not to deny that planning of therapy, in the present state of the scientific development, is often very difficult, if not nearly impossible. Admittedly, the above concepts of individually designed treatment are in many ways quite idealistic and only roughly outlined. Certainly, they are less specific than those proposed by advocates of other set plans, which do not take the variations of the individual into account. The only answer to this objection is that plans are necessary if treatment is not to be a hit-and-miss affair. Moreover, every expert in any kind of treatment does attempt to plan his therapy to fit the exigencies of the individual child. This proposal is intended to broaden such planning, so that by using the assessment, these individual variations may be made more definite and the opportunities for varying treatment may thus also be widened.

A second objection is that such individually designed treatment is, in effect, no treatment at all, but a potpourri of therapies. It does not seem to allow any one therapeutic technique to be completed. Admittedly, any plan must run its course to be effective. One might hesitate to cut a course of behavior modification short to begin a peer group or drop an individual psychoanalytic treatment in midstream to begin a conjoint family treatment. Any planned treatment has to allow for a completion of any component approach. However, these approaches may be considerably shortened by the very fact that more than one is being employed. Very often, any one approach is prolonged by the fact that there are other problems which cannot be easily handled by this single one. Moreover, it is often possible to conduct several therapeutic approaches at once—especially if a program is planned in advance. Reductio ad absurdum, a child might come daily for a therapeutic hour, but instead of receiving psychoanalytic treatment only, he might have such treatment only on Mondays; Tuesdays, he and his mother might be engaged in a behavior modification session; Wednesdays, he might meet in a peer group; Thursdays might be parents' day, for separate or joint sessions; and on Fridays, the whole family might gather for exploration of the family interactions. Unlikely as it is that any child should need such a mixture of treatments all at once, there is no reason that several approaches might not be used at once or in overlapping sequence. Moreover, through such a multiplex of treatment, the total time needed might well be reduced.

Although some therapists are skilled at several different approaches, it is rare that any one therapist can treat all the problems of a child. When a therapist is practicing by himself, he usually uses the methods which he knows best, hoping they will make sufficient changes in the child's behavior. If the child needs other forms of treatment, he may refer him elsewhere. Sometimes a child may be receiving a psychoanalytic treatment plus a conjoint family therapy from one therapist, but be attending some school or institute for learning difficulties where some form of operant conditioning is used. Unfortunately, in private practice, these forms of treatment are rarely coordinated. As a result, both in private practice and in public agencies there is an increasing trend toward the use of multiple therapies. Private practice is now being conducted by groups of several therapists of diverse training. The private school attempts to have several kinds of therapy available or the individual practitioner is associated with several colleagues or a private clinic. The implementation of a plan of therapy calls not only for a variety of therapists, but for a continuous administration of supervision and direction. Any such five-ring circus needs some kind of ringmaster. On the hospital ward, where such multiple treatment programs have long been used, the administrative director, usually a psychiatrist, is responsible for coordination of these treatment programs. However, the coordination of the treatment program for the individual child, within this milieu of treatments, is usually delegated to the individual therapist, the person who is working individually with the child. It is he who determines, in consultation with the staff, which treatments the child needs. Outpatient clinics seldom coordinate their treatment programs quite as closely, and more responsibility is placed on the individual therapist. Far too often, even in the best of clinics, one therapist has only a slight idea of what is going on in other treatments of the child. Such miscellaneous uncoordinated treatment can be avoided if there is careful planning by the whole staff prior to instituting any therapy. The assessment should be available to the whole staff and be used by all in a coordinated plan.

Finally, it may be objected that no plan of treatment can possibly meet the many exigencies that arise. Even if one could detail all the current stresses and conflicts which the child is enduring, it can be predicted with a high level of certainty that other stresses will occur. For example, the therapist may leave the clinic; the groups will change in membership; the child may be expelled from school; one of his parents may leave the home; the child may fall ill or be injured. Often these emergencies call for a rapid change in plans. In many instances, such emergencies are visibly imminent and it may seem that no planning is possible. In fact, some families present one crisis after another for the therapist to solve, playing a long-range game of family uproar, which in effect prevents therapy from ever beginning. However, treatment needs to be planned if only to prevent the therapy from being overwhelmed by crises. In a carefully outlined plan of treatment, it is possible to include these events as natural experiences to be worked through in treatment. Such treatment plans have to be flexible enough to allow for emergencies. Moreover, when the treatment is interrupted or disrupted by a crisis, there is no reason that the child's situation should not be reassessed. . . . If a family operates by creating one crisis after another, this fact usually is revealed in the assessment and plans can be made for approaching this mode of operations.

These modes of treatment do not exhaust all the possibilities of changing children's behaviors. Often it is necessary to make changes in the child's environment as well as in his actions and attitudes. . . .

Chapter Ten

Behavior Therapy

We have seen that traditional psychotherapy and play therapy have led to equivocal results, with some clinicians maintaining the virtues of these procedures and other investigators amassing considerable evidence suggesting that they lack adequate validity. Now let us consider another approach to treatment of personal and social maladjustment known as behavior modification, or behavior therapy.

Foundations for Behavior Therapy

Many years ago, the work of J. B. Watson (1925) and his collaborators laid the foundations for this currently popular form of treatment. Watson, founder of the school of psychology known as behaviorism, taught that all behavior is learned through the process of conditioning. His formulations were based on earlier work by Pavlov (1906, 1927), who demonstrated the process of "classical conditioning" in dogs. This Russian physician was interested in the physiology of digestion and designed a laboratory procedure whereby the biochemical secretions of dogs could be studied in the process of eating food. He noted that hungry experimental animals would salivate at the sight of food, and digestive processes would start before the food was actually in the dog's mouth.

Even more important for psychology was the observation that after a number of these laboratory sessions, the dog would salivate at the sight of other objects in the situation that had been associated with the presentation of food. To study this procedure systematically, Pavlov paired food (unconditioned stimulus) with a tone (conditioned stimulus) and recorded the dog's salivary response. After a number of trials, the dog would dependably salivate whenever he was presented with the tone alone. Drawing on Pavlov's experimental findings, Watson stated that through proper application of conditioning principles one could largely determine the capabilities and future attainments of the growing child.

The specific study from this early period in the history of behaviorism that is most pertinent to our present concerns is the experiment by Watson and Rayner (1920) in which little Albert was conditioned to fear a white rat.

This little boy showed no fear of the animal until the experimenters accompanied its presentation with a loud noise that startled Albert. Through this process of classical conditioning, pairing the rat (conditioned stimulus) with the loud noise (unconditioned stimulus), Albert learned to make the conditioned response of crying whenever he saw the white rat. Certain other basic facts of conditioning were evidenced in this study.

When Albert learned to fear the rat, he soon showed the same fear reaction to other white furry objects, such as a rabbit or a piece of terrycloth, which demonstrates a process known as "stimulus generalization." On the other hand, if the object he had learned to fear was presented on several occasions without being accompanied by the unconditioned stimulus, Albert no longer appeared frightened, thus demonstrating a process known as "experimental extinction." However, sometimes the conditioned response reappeared following a period in which it had apparently been extinguished, a phenomenon known as "spontaneous recovery." Another important observation from these early studies (Jones, 1924a, 1924b) was that it was much more efficient to pair the feared object with something pleasant (such as eating some favorite food) than merely waiting for the learned fear response to extinguish. This latter observation is related to a currently popular procedure in behavior therapy known as reciprocal inhibition or counterconditioning, in which the person is first encouraged to become very relaxed and then to think about anxiety-provoking material. The incompatibility of relaxation and tension are supposed to lead to elimination of the learned fear response (anxiety) in the subject.

Mowrer's Treatment of Enuresis

Another pioneer researcher in this field that later became known as behavior modification was O. H. Mowrer, who applied conditioning principles in treating the problem of enuresis (bed-wetting) in children. Using principles derived from earlier studies with animals, Mowrer and Mowrer (1938) designed a procedure in which a pad connected to a loud buzzer was placed over the mattress in the child's bed. Whenever water got on this pad it triggered an electrical current that sounded the buzzer, causing the child to awaken. Thus, the procedure followed the paradigm of a full bladder leading to urination, while still asleep, which caused the buzzer to sound and awaken the child. Through the conditioning process the child gradually learned to wake up in response to the bladder tension which preceded the buzzer, thus avoiding the undesirable behavior of bed-wetting.

Dollard and Miller's Contributions

Another milestone in the development of behavior therapy was the classic work by Dollard and Miller (1950) demonstrating the usefulness of stimulus-response learning theory in the treatment of psychological disorders. These investigators were heavily influenced by the theoretical contributions and animal experiments developed under Clark Hull at Yale University. The four fundamental concepts from this theory, which is meant to explain the acquisition of behavior, are drive, cue, response, and reward. That is, in order to learn a behavior, the organism must be motivated (drive) and guided by a stimulus (cue) to behave in a certain way (response) in order to obtain something it wants (reward). Through manipulation of these four conditions it is possible for the organism to acquire new behaviors and also to eliminate old behaviors.

This procedure is known as "instrumental conditioning" in that the organism's response is instrumental in obtaining the reward. While in classical (or "respondent") conditioning the conditioned response is elicited from the organism (that is, the organism has no control over it), in instrumental conditioning the response is emitted from the organism (the organism decides whether it will make the learned response). For example, in classical conditioning, a puff of air that causes an eye-blink can be paired with a tone, and following a few trials of presentation the tone alone will elicit an eye-blink. The conditioned response and the unconditioned response are just about identical (both are eye-blinks), and the organism has no voluntary control over the reflexive responses that are elicited through the experimental procedure.

On the other hand, in instrumental conditioning the hungry animal is placed into a box containing a lever that can be pressed to deliver a food pellet that can then be eaten. In this situation hunger serves as the drive, the lever is the conditioned stimulus, or cue, pressing the lever is the conditioned response, and eating the food is the unconditioned response that constitutes the reinforcement, or reward, making it possible for the organism to learn this behavior pattern. Note that while the conditioned and unconditioned response are the same in classical conditioning, they are usually very different from each other in instrumental conditioning.

These two types of conditioning are believed capable of accounting for large portions of behavior evidenced by organisms throughout the animal kingdom, including much that is regarded as uniquely human behavior. Dollard and Miller, a sociologist and psychologist who are well-versed in psychoanalytic theory, showed that many features of abnormal personality and much of what transpires in psychotherapy could be accounted for in terms of stimulus-response learning theory.

Escape and Avoidance Learning

Much of the original research on instrumental learning focused on approach learning. That is, studies were concerned with understanding the process by which the animal learns to make certain responses in order to obtain something he seeks (positive reward). Miller (1944) became interested in avoidance learning and designed studies in which rats learned to make certain responses in order to avoid something that was painful to them (negative reward). Just as one could study the process by which the rat learned to press a bar in order to obtain a food pellet, one could also observe the process by which the rat learned to press a bar in order to avoid an electric shock.

A typical study here might involve putting a rat into a box with a grid floor and containing a light and a lever. Whenever the light comes on it is followed shortly by the floor becoming electrified, delivering a shock, which can be terminated by pressing the lever, to the rat's feet. The animal soon learns to press the lever when the light comes on. This is known as escape learning. In a slightly modified form of this procedure, there is a time interval (perhaps 5 seconds) between the light coming on and the floor becoming electrified; if the animal presses the lever during this interval the shock is not administered. This is known as avoidance learning.

In one experimental design the animal receives the negative reinforcement (shock) and can terminate it by making the correct response (escape learning). In an extension of this design, if the animal makes the correct response (avoidance learning) he does not receive the negative reinforcement. Miller (1944) conducted what are now viewed as classic studies on approach-avoidance conflicts. He used a procedure in which the animal learned to make a certain response in order to obtain something he wanted and also learned to make a response in order to avoid something painful or unpleasant. Miller carefully studied and developed theories predicting the behavior of animals placed in situations where they were motivated to display both types of conflicting responses. Much of this research on conflict behavior is fundamental to understanding the kinds of learning situations that have been encountered by neurotic human beings in the course of their psychosocial development.

Experimental Neurosis in Animals

A related line of investigation has been concerned with "experimental neurosis" in laboratory animals. By placing animals in conflict situations it has been demonstrated that they often become abnormal and show strange and maladaptive behaviors that appear similar to those evidenced by neurotic and psychotic humans. The following example shows the kind of laboratory conditions that have been used to make animals "neurotic."

Masserman (1943) placed hungry cats in a cage containing a box with a lid that could be lifted to obtain food. Cats readily learned that when the light came on in the cage they could lift the cover and obtain a tasty piece of fish from the box. This is another example of what we have described as instrumental approach-learning. At a certain point in the experiment, however, when the light came on and the cat lifted the cover, to his surprise and dismay, he encountered a strong blast of air in his face. The cat soon learned to stay away from the box whenever the light came on, providing an example of instrumental avoidance-learning.

The conflict arose when the cat was sufficiently hungry that he was willing to approach the box and lift the cover and again encountered the frightening air blast. From this procedure most cats become "neurotic," defecating and urinating all over the cage, crying, howling, and crouching in the corner. Some refused to eat in the cage even when the air blast no longer was part of the experimental procedure. Various "therapies" were used, including petting and comforting the animals while in the cage, forcing them to approach the box by sliding them toward it with a movable partition, and feeding them alcohol to help them "relax." It was found that considerable therapeutic effort was required in order to get the cats to overcome their avoidance response and to learn once again to experiment with the box and its contents. This, then, is an example of one type of investigation that has been used to study experimental neurosis resulting from approach-avoidance conflicts.

Traumatic Avoidance Learning

Solomon and his collaborators for many years have been conducting a program of research on traumatic avoidance learning in dogs (Solomon, 1964; Solomon, Kamin, & Wynne, 1953; Solomon & Wynne, 1954). These experiments use a shuttle-box consisting of two compartments separated by a barrier and a movable gate atop the barrier. The floors of these compartments are made of steel bars that can be electrified to provide a very strong electric current to the animal's paws. A dog is placed into the darkened compartment, a light comes on and the gate is raised, and 10 seconds later the floor becomes electrified. The strength of the shock is just short of tetanizing the animal, causing the animal to howl, urinate, defecate, and thrash about the cage until he somehow scrambles over the barrier. After a brief interval the procedure is repeated. Again the dog manages to scramble over the barrier, thus escaping from the shock. It does not take many trials before the dog learns to jump over the barrier as soon as the light comes on and the gate goes up, thereby not waiting around to receive the shock but showing what is known as traumatic avoidance learning.

More interesting than the acquisition of the avoidance response are the findings from attempts at extinguishing this learned behavior. Literally hundreds of trials were run with shock no longer a part of the experimental procedure, yet not a single animal ever learned to stop jumping when the light came on. In other words, when it was no longer necessary to make the avoidance response, the animal never discovered this fact because the avoidance learning was so rigidly established and resistant to extinction.

This type of avoidance behavior is believed to be analogous to much of the maladaptive behavior shown by human beings. That is, behavior learned under traumatic or threatening conditions tends to be perpetuated in a rigid, unchanging fashion long after it serves any adaptive function. Because it originally engendered anxiety and distress, the individual avoids any further attempts at mastering the situation, and new learning is blocked in a neurotic fashion. Many therapeutic efforts involve procedures designed to encourage the person to reconsider an originally threatening situation and to attempt new learning that might be more adaptive than the defensive behavior being perpetuated.

Learned Helplessness

In more recent experiments, Solomon's students (Seligman, Maier, & Geer, 1968) have extended this research to include what they term "learned helplessness." With this procedure, a dog is placed in a hammock-like sling, suspended above the ground with his legs protruding through openings in the canvas. The animal is then submitted to a series of trials in which a signal is followed by strong electric shock applied to his paws. In this experimental procedure, the animal can do nothing to escape or avoid the shock. The signal comes on, followed by several seconds of very painful stimulation to his paws, and the dog is completely helpless to do anything about this traumatic experience.

At first glance, there is nothing enlightening about this procedure, and many people might view it merely as an horrendous example of psychologists torturing helpless animals. What is scientifically interesting, however, is that when dogs are first given this kind of traumatic experience and then placed in the shuttle-box situation they do not learn to make the escape response. In other words, when the light comes on and the gate goes up, dogs who have originally learned that they were helpless continue to act as though they are helpless in this new learning situation and never learn to jump the barrier to escape or avoid the shock. It takes special types of handling and training to get the animals to overcome their abnormal behavioral tendencies, and these corrective efforts can be viewed as forms of behavior therapy.

Skinner's Contributions

Having discussed several prominent investigators whose work is highly relevant to behavior therapy, let us now consider the contributions of B. F. Skinner, who is probably the most influential behavioral scientist behind this therapeutic movement. In 1938 Skinner published his classic work, *The Behavior of Organisms*, and then devoted many years to conducting painstaking and ingenious research on rats and pigeons that served to establish firmly a variant of instrumental conditioning known as "operant conditioning." Skinner's experiments usually involve placing an animal in an experimental situation in which it is free to make a certain response whenever it chooses. When it makes the correct response, it receives a reinforcement; thus, the conditioned response operates to reward the organism with something it wants from the environment.

Skinner and his students have conducted detailed studies of the effects of reinforcement, since Skinner believes that the main factor in any learning situation is that the organism receive reinforcement for its behavior. Characteristically, Skinnerians measure the rate of responding as a function of different schedules of reinforcement. While many of these laboratory studies of rats making literally thousands of responses as a function of varying reinforcement schedules are not particularly fascinating to non-scientists, some of his more unusual experiments have received wide public notice. For example, using his conditioning techniques, Skinner taught pigeons to play Ping-Pong and, during World War II, to peck on signal in the nose-cones of guided missiles, thereby steering them to their targets.

At the human level, Skinner's contributions have provided the basis for programmed instruction and the use of teaching machines in school systems. That is, applying principles of operant conditioning and using knowledge of reinforcement schedules, students are more efficiently taught to master conventional academic subject matter. Not only have Skinner's experiments contributed to the field of education, but some years ago he and one of his students initiated a program of applied research that served as the forerunner of much of what is now known as behavior therapy.

Development of Behavior Therapy

At this point, we will briefly review various avenues of clinical work that led to development of this field. Actually, the behavior therapy movement got its start on three relatively independent fronts in America, England, and South Africa. Odgen Lindsley, a psychology student of Skinner's at Harvard University, established an experimental program for behavior modification with chronic psychotic patients at Metropolitan State Hospital in Massachusetts. Adapting many of the procedures that Skinner had used successfully in studying the behavior of rats and pigeons, Lindsley and Skinner (1954; Lindsley, 1956) showed that seemingly bizarre behaviors of psychotic patients could be understood and controlled in a laboratory setting. Patients who had been given up as hopeless and believed to be completely unmotivated to conform to conventional standards of behavior were found to respond in a meaningful, predictable manner when placed in an operant-conditioning situation.

Shortly after the initiation of this behavior modification program for psychotic patients, Eysenck (1959, 1960) published reports of behavior therapy with neurotic patients in England. As mentioned previously in Chapter Nine, Eysenck, who was a psychologist at Maudsley Hospital, had earlier published critiques of conventional psychotherapy. He now attempted to show how much better behavior therapy fared in comparison with psychotherapy.

At about this time, Wolpe, a psychiatrist working in South Africa, published his influential book on psychotherapy by reciprocal inhibition in which he described techniques that have become cornerstones in behavior therapy as now practiced throughout America (1958). These, then, are the beginnings from which this currently popular treatment method developed. For a more comprehensive review of these historical developments, as well as scholarly discussion of all aspects of behavior therapy, see the recent book by Yates (1970).

Bandura's Modeling and Observational Learning

While not falling into the camp conventionally known as behavior therapy, Bandura and his collaborators have made important contributions to this field through their research on social learning and personality development (Bandura & Walters, 1963; Bandura, 1969). Highly significant aspects of this theory and research have been concerned with the demonstration of the importance of modeling and observational learning in the behavior of children. In varied situations, they have shown how greatly children are influenced by observing the performance of adults and how prone they are to imitate the behaviors they have seen rewarded in others. Bandura (1969) has summarized the evidence and shown that principles of behavior modification can be used effectively in socialization, education, and therapy with children.

Use of Non-Professional Behavior Therapists

One major advantage of behavior therapy is that it does not require highly trained, professionally educated personnel to conduct the treatment successfully. While the treatment programs should be designed and supervised by professionals with proper academic background of theory and expertise, the actual behavior therapy can be efficiently conducted by technicians who apply the behavioral principles in working with patients. In some settings, high school graduates and college undergraduates are employed as behavior modifiers, and there have been experimental programs in which patients serve as behavior therapists for other patients. A related development is the emphasis on training parents to apply behavior modification techniques in handling their own abnormal children. That is, in many treatment centers for severely disturbed children, there are training programs in which parents are taught the principles and procedures of behavior therapy and are then expected to serve as therapists for the child when he returns to the home situation.

This de-emphasis of professionalism and the belief that principles and procedures are more important than academic degrees or personal qualities has encouraged some investigators to consider the possibility of using machines to serve in place of human behavior therapists. Eysenck (1967) has discussed the feasibility of "treatment machines" and cites some evidence indicating that they have already proven useful in certain cases. However, another recent discussion of behavior therapy maintains that "... the personal qualities of a good psychotherapist are just as essential in a good behavior therapist. He should be warm and understanding, and he should be able to communicate these attributes to his client ... .Although the behavioral techniques are typically quite different from most traditional psychotherapeutic methods, clients present themselves and their nebulous, but hurting, problems in the same way to all therapists [*Abnormal Psychology*, 1972, p. 443]." Thus, there is some disagreement on the role of personal qualities of behavior therapists. It seems likely, however, that programs of research may well provide empirical evidence that will help decide these matters in the future.

Comparisons of Behavior Therapy and Psychotherapy

There have been several attempts to compare the relative effectiveness of behavior therapy and psychotherapy, but most of them have been with adult patients. In general, the outcomes suggest that behavior therapy is a more effective therapeutic approach. It had been argued that behavior therapy, focusing only on symptoms and ignoring the underlying causes of abnormal behavior, could lead only to symptom substitution. That is, the behavior therapy might well serve to eliminate the specific abnormal behavior it focused on, but since it would not remove the "unconscious" basic conflict behind the abnormality, other signs or symptoms would appear to take its place. In fact, however, this has not been found. The elimination of symptoms and behavioral abnormalities has not led to symptom substitution, and there appear to be general personal and social benefits that accompany the removal of disturbing symptoms.

A recent study comparing the relative effectiveness of operant conditioning and play therapy in schizophrenic children (Ney, Palvesky, & Markely, 1971) has found greater improvement following operant conditioning. These authors, however, state that this study generated more questions than it answered, including the question of whether some combination of psychodynamic therapy and behavioral therapy might be more effective than either approach used alone.

Recently, an exceptionally well-designed study has been described; it compares the effectiveness of behavior therapy (reciprocal inhibition), conventional child psychotherapy, and being placed on a waiting list as methods of treating phobic children (Miller, Barrett, Hampe, & Noble, 1972). For the overall sample of 67 children, each of the three methods proved to be effective in improving symptomatic behavior. When the sample was broken down into a younger and older sub-group of phobic children, it was found that none of the treatments were effective with the older children (11 to 15 years of age). However, with the younger children (6 to 10 years of age) therapy was highly effective (96 percent showing improvement) and was superior to being placed on the waiting list for treatment. The findings further demonstrated that neither the therapist's experience nor the type of therapy (behavioral versus psychotherapy) differentially affected the outcomes. In other words, with the younger phobic children, either treatment approach—whether conducted by experienced or inexperienced therapists—proved highly effective in "curing" the phobic behavior.

The Issues

The paper by Donna M. Gelfand and Donald P. Hartmann reprinted in this chapter presents a scholarly, comprehensive review of behavior therapy with children showing varied types of problem behaviors. Next, I discuss the therapeutic work of Lovaas and his colleagues with autistic children. In the area of behavior therapy with psychotic children, Lovaas is probably the most influential recent worker. His films demonstrating the procedure and outcomes of reinforcement therapy have been shown nation-wide to college students in psychology courses, and his published papers have made major contributions to the professional literature. The description of Lovaas' research and findings presented here reveals the great effort required in conducting behavior modification programs and the relatively small amount of lasting success that results from these therapeutic endeavors. It may turn out, however, that the behavioral and the psychodynamic approaches to treatment have much more in common than has been recognized to date, and that greater therapeutic gains will come from future application of "psychodynamic behavior therapy."

References

Abnormal psychology: Current perspectives. Del Mar, Calif.: CRM Books, 1972.

Bandura, A. *Principles of behavior modification*. New York: Holt, Rinehart & Winston, 1969.

Bandura, A., & Walters, R. H. *Social learning and personality development*. New York: Holt, Rinehart & Winston, 1963.

Dollard, J., & Miller, N. E. *Personality and psychotherapy: An analysis in terms of learning, thinking, and culture*. New York: McGraw-Hill, 1950.

Eysenck, H. J. Learning theory and behavior therapy. *The Journal of Mental Science*, 1959, **105**, 61–75.

Eysenck, H. J. (Ed.) *Behavior therapy and the neuroses*. London: Pergamon Press, 1960.

Eysenck, H. J. New ways in psychotherapy. *Psychology Today*, 1967, **1**, 39–47.

Jones, M. C. The elimination of children's fears. *Journal of Experimental Psychology*, 1924, **7**, 382–390. (a)

Jones, M. C. A laboratory study of fear: The case of Peter. *Pedagogical Seminar*, 1924, **31**, 308–315. (b)

Lindsley, O. R. Operant conditioning methods applied to research in chronic schizophrenia. *Psychiatric Research Reports*, 1956, **5**, 118–139.

Lindsley, O. R., & Skinner, B. F. A method for the experimental analysis of the behavior of psychotic patients. *American Psychologist*, 1954, **9**, 419–420.

Masserman, J. H. *Behavior and neurosis*. Chicago: University of Chicago Press, 1943.

Miller, L. C., Barrett, C. L., Hampe, E., & Noble, H. Comparison of reciprocal inhibition, psychotherapy, and waiting list control for phobic children. *Journal of Abnormal Psychology*, 1972, **79**, 269–279.

Miller, N. E. Experimental studies of conflict. In J. McV. Hunt (Ed.), *Personality and the behavior disorders*. Vol. 1. New York: Ronald Press, 1944.

Mowrer, O. H., & Mowrer, W. M. Enuresis: A method for its study and treatment. *American Journal of Orthopsychiatry*, 1938, **8**, 359–436.

Ney, P. G., Palvesky, A., & Markely, J. Relative effectiveness of operant conditioning and play therapy in childhood schizophrenia. *Journal of Autism and Childhood Schizophrenia*, 1971, **1**, 337–349.

Pavlov, I. P. The scientific investigation of the psychical faculties or processes in the higher animals. *Science*, 1906, **24**, 613–619.

Pavlov, I. P. *Conditioned reflexes*. G. V. Anrep (Trans.) London: Oxford University Press, 1927.

Seligman, M. E. P., Maier, S. F., & Geer, J. H. Alleviation of learned helplessness in the dog. *Journal of Abnormal Psychology*, 1968, **73**, 256–262.

Skinner, B. F. *The behavior of organisms*. New York: Appleton-Century-Crofts, 1938.

Solomon, R. L. Punishment. *American Psychologist*, 1964, **9**, 239–253.

Solomon, R. L., Kamin, L., & Wynne, L. C. Traumatic avoidance learning: The outcome of several extinction procedures with dogs. *Journal of Abnormal and Social Psychology, 1953, 48,* 291–302.

Solomon, R. L., & Wynne, L. C. Traumatic avoidance learning: The principle of anxiety conservation and partial irreversibility. *Psychological Review,* 1954, **81,** 353–385.

Watson, J. B. *Behaviorism*. New York: Norton, 1925.

Watson, J. B., & Rayner, R. Conditioned emotional reactions. *Journal of Experimental Psychology*, 1920, **3**, 1–14.

Wolpe, J. *Psychotherapy by reciprocal inhibition*. Stanford, Calif.: Stanford University Press, 1958.

Wolpe, J., & Lazarus, A. A. *Behavior therapy techniques*. London: Pergamon Press, 1966.

Yates, A. J. *Behavior therapy*. New York: Wiley, 1970.

27. Behavior Therapy with Children: A Review and Evaluation of Research Methodology

Donna M. Gelfand
Donald P. Hartmann

As compared to adults, children have become an increasingly popular client population for behavioristically oriented therapists. Some reasons for the widespread use of learning-theory-based therapy for children's problems may be the comparative brevity of the treatment, the relative ease with which children's social environments can be controlled, and the types of maladaptive behaviors for which children are often referred for treatment. An important element of most behavioristic treatment interventions is the manipulation of the client's environment so that undesirable behavior patterns are eliminated and prosocial responses are positively reinforced (Ullmann & Krasner, 1965, Ch. 1). The requisite environmental control is often easier to achieve for children in their homes and schools than in the typically more complex and varied social interactions of noninstitutionalized adults. Since the young child spends the major part of his time either among his family or at school, the therapist can effectively manipulate the child's social experiences by instructing a fairly small group of people, the teacher and parents. Moreover, these people have considerable control over the child, and are specifically responsible for the child's welfare and for teaching him appropriate behavior patterns. When treating adults, it is usually more difficult to find and solicit the cooperation of persons who can serve as equally powerful reinforcement-dispensing or controlling agents, and it is highly unlikely that they would have the degree of authority over the adult client that adults typically possess with respect to children.

In addition, children are often referred for professional help for maladaptive behaviors which have proved among the most amenable to behavior-therapy techniques. When parents or school personnel refer children for treatment, the presenting complaint is often a well-defined behavior such as bedwetting, a phobia, or temper tantrums, the types of problems which, as Grossberg (1964) has pointed out, behavior therapy most successfully treats. It has also been suggested (Krasner & Ullmann, 1965, p. 57) that the type of specific and detailed instructions parents receive from behavior therapists more nearly meet the parents' initial treatment expectations than do the more general and vague directions, for example, to be demonstrative and accepting, traditionally given by children's therapists.

From *Psychological Bulletin*, 1968, **69**, 204–215. Copyright 1968 by the American Psychological Association and reproduced by permission.

As a consequence, parents may be more likely to aid than to interfere with the therapeutic effort. Parental sabotage is thought to occur notoriously often in the more traditional play-therapy interventions, and it is not uncommon to hear a therapist state his belief that the parents do not sincerely want their child's adjustment to improve. To date, the same charge has not been made with any frequency by behavioristically oriented therapists who, by and large, report parents to be cooperative and interested in aiding in the treatment process.

As used here, the term behavior therapy refers to treatment techniques derived from theories of learning and aimed at the direct modification of one or more problem behaviors rather than at effecting more general and less observable personality or adjustment changes. Because behavior therapists assume that both desirable and deviant social responses are learned, their treatment interventions consist of laboratory-derived learning procedures, for example, modeling and operant and classical conditioning.

Results of behavior therapy with a variety of subject samples have previously been reviewed (Bandura, 1961, 1967; Grossberg, 1964; Rachman, 1962; Werry & Wollersheim, 1967) and critically evaluated (Breger & McGaugh, 1965; Weitzman, 1967). It is the purpose of this paper to survey the behavior-therapy literature for subjects between infancy and 18 years of age, examine the range of problems treated, the methods used, and to critically review the adequacy of the therapy-evaluation attempts. This literature review is limited to reports of the clinical application of behavior-modification techniques.

Behavior-therapy studies can conveniently be classified in terms of the desired effect on rates of children's emission of both undesirable and prosocial behaviors.[1] Some treatment interventions aim to decrease the production of problem behaviors, others attempt to enhance the variety and likelihood of occurrence of desirable responses such as adequate language and motor skills, while a third approach combines acceleration of rates of prosocial behaviors with elimination of problem behaviors. This classification schema may have an advantage in clarity over those more commonly employed (e.g., Bandura, 1961; Rachman, 1962) in which learning mechanisms have often been confounded with treatment procedures, for example, extinction and negative practice (Grossberg, 1964). Moreover, a confusing variety of terms has been used to describe essentially identical manipulations; for example, desensitization, reciprocal inhibition, counterconditioning, deconditioning, and unconditioning have all been used to describe a single technique for the treatment of phobias. And finally, the sheer number of categories required by the use of previously employed descriptive terms plus the addition of new terms required by the increased use of operant techniques would be unwieldy.

It is recognized that in the case of some therapy reports the categories used in this paper do not include mutually exclusive techniques. A therapist who intends chiefly to use a deceleration technique may also informally include some social reinforcement of his client's prosocial behaviors. In such

---

[1]This classification scheme was suggested by O. R. Lindsley in a workshop presentation, University of Utah, November 30, 1965.

cases, the study will be categorized according to the therapist's stated intentions. Any classification system is somewhat arbitrary, and the schema used is designed simply to allow adequate description of a wide range of problems and treatment techniques.

Deceleration of Maladaptive Behaviors

Phobias

A large group of therapeutic interventions have as their aim a decrease in the magnitude and frequency of a variety of problem behaviors. Jones' (1924a, 1924b) elegant and long-neglected treatment of a child's fear of animals falls within this treatment classification. The technique used by Jones and others in the behavioristic treatment of phobias involves pairing incompatible experiences of relaxation and enjoyment with the presentation of anxiety-evoking stimuli so the previously fear-provoking stimuli become associated with pleasurable feelings (Bandura, 1961). Modifications of techniques developed for use with adults by Wolpe and his colleagues (Wolpe, 1958; Wolpe & Lazarus, 1966) are most often used in the treatment of children's phobias. Briefly, the procedure involves inducing feelings of relaxation in the child by the therapist through suggestion, hypnosis, or drugs. An anxiety hierarchy is constructed with items ranging from least to most fear-provoking situations, and the child is helped to imagine progressively stronger fear items under uninterrupted relaxation. This treatment technique has been used to combat irrational fear of water (Bentler, 1962), fear of hospitals and ambulances (Lazarus & Rachman, 1957), school phobia (Garvey & Hegrenes, 1966; Lazarus & Abramovitz, 1962), and dog phobia (Lazarus, 1959). Patterson (1965b) has also treated school phobia with a shaping procedure, direct praise and candy reinforcement given to a child for tolerating separation from his mother and for making statements about a boy doll's bravery in a structured doll-play situation. An interesting and methodologically sophisticated variation in the treatment of dog phobia has been described by Bandura, Grusec, and Menlove (1967) who demonstrated that exposure to a fearless peer model displaying approach responses produces stable and generalized reduction in children's avoidance behavior. The Bandura et al. study was particularly impressive because the authors: (a) precisely identified the active therapeutic ingredient through the inclusion of several matched treatment and control groups, (b) developed a specialized performance scale to measure the strength of avoidance responses, and (c) included pretests and posttests as well as follow-up measures.

Antisocial and Immature Behavior

Behavior therapists have also reported considerable success in the treatment of aggressive, antisocial, and immature behaviors. In a relatively early study, Williams (1959) controlled temper tantrums in a 21-month-old child through extinction. The customary reinforcement the parents had accorded the child for his refusal to sleep was abruptly discontinued, and his crying was effectively controlled at the tenth extinction trial. Periods of time out from positive reinforcement have been used to decrease rates of thumbsucking (Baer, 1962), vomiting (Wolf, Birnbrauer, Williams, & Lawler, 1965), and stealing (Wetzel, 1966). A combination of mild punishment and time-out techniques was successfully used to control the generalized negativism of a 5-year-old child truly gifted as a trouble maker (Boardman, 1962), while aggression in a nursery school class was controlled by instructing the teachers not to attend to either physical or verbal aggression and instead to reward cooperative behavior (Brown & Elliott, 1965).

Hyperactivity

The hyperactivity often associated with neurological deficit has long been thought unamenable to psychological manipulation and has been treated chiefly by administration of a variety of tranquilizing drugs. Patterson (1965a) and Patterson, Jones, Whittier, and Wright (1965), however, have used positive reinforcement in a classroom setting to control hyperactivity in 9- and 10-year-old boys diagnosed as brain damaged. Observing that the boys' inappropriate activities frequently earned them the acclaim of their classmates, Patterson reinforced the entire class for the subjects' desirable responses with a consequent increase in their attending behaviors. Doubros and Daniels (1966) also reported success in controlling children's overactive behavior through positively reinforcing low-magnitude responses in a playroom setting, while another group of investigators (Homme, deBaca, Devine, Steinhorst, & Rickert, 1963) imaginatively used the opportunity to engage in noisy play as a reinforcer for children's sitting quietly and attending to their nursery school teacher. James (1963) reported dramatic changes in a group of five hyperactive children by programming the teacher's behavior so that social reinforcers were made contingent upon the occurrence of socially acceptable behavior.

Tics

A popular technique for the control of tics is massed practice of the problem behavior voluntarily engaged in by the tiqueur. Massed practice has been used successfully with adults (Jones, 1960; Yates, 1958), and Yates predicted that it would be even more effective with child subjects because in their briefer learning histories the tic would not be over-learned so that, according to Hullian learning theory, massed practice would contribute more to growth of reactive inhibition than to habit strength. This expectation has, by and large, not been confirmed in the child-therapy literature. Although Walton (1961) effectively controlled multiple facial, arm, leg, and vocalization tics in an 11-year-old boy in only 36 treatment sessions and Ernest (1960) reported eliminating a girl's inspiratory tic, two recent studies have reported massed practice to be ineffective in controlling bizarre, repetitive rocking at night (Evans, 1961) and head-jerk and eyeblink tics (Feldman & Werry, 1966). In the latter study, both tics actually increased in frequency over base-line levels as a result of massed practice of the head jerk. A third tic which had previously disappeared also recurred concurrent with the treatment attempt. Feldman and Werry (1966) attributed their negative results to a probable buildup in the child's anxiety level which was thought to be responsible for the tics.

The conditions under which a massed-practice technique will be successful have not yet been well established, and consequently descriptions of therapeutic failures can provide valuable information regarding crucial controlling variables. Unsuccessful outcome may be related to difficulty in policing the massed-practice trials in that the experience is probably very fatiguing and aversive for the child who will attempt to avoid the practice session whenever possible, thereby defeating the treatment attempt. The therapist must also be careful not to inadvertently reinforce the tics, for example, by writing or marking a record sheet each time the tic occurs, thus increasing the rate.

Self-Destructive Behavior

Lovaas and his colleagues (Lovaas, Berberich, Perloff, & Schaeffer, 1966; Lovaas, Freitag, Gold, & Kassorla, 1965; Lovaas, Freitag, Kinder, Rubenstein, Schaeffer, & Simmons, 1964; Lovaas, Schaeffer, & Simmons, 1965) have treated self-injurious behaviors in schizophrenic children through administration of punishment via electric shock, critical comments, and slapping. Having in this manner focused the children's attention upon relevant social stimuli, their appropriate behaviors could then be more effectively positively reinforced. Both time out from reinforcement and electric-shock punishment were used to control a variety of self-destructive responses in a 9-year-old psychotic boy (Tate & Baroff, 1966). Not surprisingly, the shock procedure was the more powerful modification technique. In the course of the avoidance conditioning, the buzzing sound produced by the stock prod used to administer shock acquired secondary reinforcing properties and was used to promote the child's eating and to control his holding a lake of saliva in his mouth and his persistent clinging to people. Although the main techniques used by Tate and Baroff (1966) were time-out and punishment, praise was also given the child for his prosocial responses.

Acceleration of Prosocial Behaviors

In some instances, therapists are faced not with the prospect of minimizing undesirable responses, but with increasing the extent of the child's behavior repertoire, which may be inadequate and restricted for his age group (Quay, Werry, McQueen, & Sprague, 1966). For example, Johnston,

Kelley, Harris, and Wolf (1966) enhanced the development of motor skills of a generally awkward and inhibited nursery school boy by making his teachers' attention and approval contingent upon his using a play-yard climbing frame. The same group of investigators also eliminated regressed crawling in a 3-year-old girl through differential social reinforcement of her walking rather than crawling (Harris, Johnston, Kelley, & Wolf, 1964) and increased the frequency of peer as opposed to teacher interaction in a socially isolated nursery school girl (Allen, Hart, Buell, Harris, & Wolf, 1964). In an attempt to maximize the extratherapeutic maintenance of new behaviors, Ferster and Simons (1966) have emphasized the importance of capitalizing on natural reinforcers in dealing with behavioral deficits in disturbed children.

Toilet Training

Toilet training is another developmental task apparently facilitated through judicious use of positive reinforcement (Madsen, 1965; Pumroy & Pumroy, 1965). To increase training efficiency, Van Wagenen and Murdock (1966) have developed a transistorized device which is placed in training pants and automatically activates a tone signal when the child has urinated or defecated, thus allowing parents to shape appropriate toilet use through the method of successive approximations. On successive trials the infant is positively reinforced for elimination closer and closer to the proper location.

The Mowrer electric-alarm method (Mowrer & Mowrer, 1938) and later modifications have seen considerable recent use in the treatment of enuresis (Coote, 1965; Jones, 1960; Lovibond, 1963, 1964; Werry, 1966; Wickes, 1958). Well-controlled studies by De Leon and Mandell (1966) and Werry and Cohrssen (1965) have demonstrated the comparative superiority of the bed-buzzer method over unspecified psychotherapy-counseling techniques and no-treatment controls.

Making positive reinforcement contingent upon bowel movements has been reported to be an effective procedure in cases of encopresis with mental retardates (Dayan, 1964; Hundziak, Mauer, & Watson, 1965), psychotics (Keehn, 1965; Neale, 1963), and children with no other reported problems (Gelber & Meyer, 1965; Peterson & London, 1965). Peterson and London also used hypnotic-like suggestion and reasoning with the child to help promote behavior change.

Retardation

The instatement and acceleration of prosocial behavior have also been accomplished in children displaying severe retardation in the learning of necessary social and motor skills. As a dramatic example, Fuller (1949) trained a bedridden 18-year-old vegetative idiot to move his arm to earn a food reinforcer. Rice and McDaniel (1966) provided useful methodological suggestions for manipulating the motor behavior of profoundly retarded children. Psychotic and mentally retarded children have been successfully treated for poverty in generalized imitation tendencies (Metz, 1965), self-help behavior (Bensberg, Colwell, & Cassel, 1965), and speech deficiency (Commons, Paul, & Fargo, 1966; Cook & Adams, 1966; Kerr, Meyerson, & Michael, 1965; Salzinger, Feldman, Cowan, & Salzinger, 1965; Straughan, Potter, & Hamilton, 1965). The treatment techniques used in the latter group of studies were combinations of modeling procedures and positive reinforcement for imitation or correct responding.

Multiple Treatment Techniques

The studies discussed in this section have combined manipulations designed to promote adaptive behaviors with attempts to decrease the occurrence of problematic behavior. The use of such technique combinations with individual clients appears to be growing in popularity among behavior therapists possibly because the child who displays a particular maladaptive behavior is likely also to have learned relatively few socially desirable means of acquiring the reinforcement which his deviant responses were intended to secure. Under such circumstances, it is possible that apparent "symptom substitution" will occur, with another problem behavior emerging after a treated deviant response has been successfully eliminated, simply because the child's response hierarchies include few prosocial behavior patterns (Bandura & Walters, 1963, p. 32). Thus the therapist can help prevent the appearance of additional problems through teaching the child alternative desirable responses which are likely to be maintained through positive reinforcement available in the child's social situation.

Delinquents

Delinquents typify a group exhibiting a number of undesirable response patterns (e.g., stealing, fighting, lying) in combination with a deficiency in prosocial responses such as cooperation with authorities, regular work habits, and sufficient self-control. Not surprisingly, behavior-therapy interventions with delinquents have frequently involved use of combined acceleration-deceleration techniques. For example, Burchard and Tyler (1965) used time out in an isolation room to control an institutionalized delinquent boy's antisocial behaviors, and at the same time positively reinforced his adaptive behaviors. He was awarded tokens which could be turned in for a number of reinforcing events for each hour he managed to remain out of isolation. Tyler (1965) has also reported successful use of time out in an isolation room for delinquents' misbehavior while playing pool. In the same paper, Tyler described promising pilot-study data indicating that reinforcing an adolescent delinquent's approximations to satisfactory academic performance will produce improvement in his school grades. Schwitzgebel

(1967) has also demonstrated a significant increase in adolescent delinquents' cooperative and constructive behaviors when this class of responses was followed by positive consequences such as verbal praise or a gift. In a matched delinquent group, attempted punishment of hostile, antisocial statements through the therapist's disagreement or inattention failed to produce a corresponding decrease in deviant responding. Since Schwitzgebel's subjects were not institutionalized and engaged in the interview sessions on a purely voluntary basis, the experimenters were reluctant to jeopardize the boys' willingness to participate by exposing them to powerful aversive stimuli. Consequently, it is probable that the aversive consequences for deviant responses were simply too mild to have any effect, as Schwitzgebel himself hypothesized. In an earlier study (Schwitzgebel & Kolb, 1964), prosocial behavior was increased in adolescent delinquents through administration of positive reinforcers (small change and cigarettes) on a variable-interval schedule. The boys received reinforcement for keeping appointments, appropriately discussing and analyzing their feelings, and performing job-training tasks. Three years after termination of treatment, these subjects showed a significant reduction in frequency and severity of criminal offenses as compared to a matched-pair control group.

Autistic Behaviors

Simultaneous use of acceleration and deceleration modification techniques has proved to be a powerful approach to the treatment of particularly maladaptive and resistant behavior patterns, such as those often observed in psychotic children (Lovaas, Freitag, Gold, & Kassorla, 1965). For example, working with a severely autistic 3-year-old boy, Wolf, Risley, and Mees (1964) produced considerable positive behavior change through a combination of positive reinforcement (food) and a procedure described as "mild punishment and extinction" which involved isolating the boy in his bedroom contingent upon his having had a temper tantrum. Other investigators have described similar brief isolation sessions as time out from positive reinforcement (Hawkins, Peterson, Schweid, & Bijou, 1966). Similarly, Zimmerman and Zimmerman (1962) have combined extinction of bizarre and tantrum behaviors with social reinforcement for appropriate responses in a special classroom situation, and Marshall (1966) has successfully used food reinforcement and mild punishment (slaps on the buttocks, extinguishing room lights) to toilet train an 8-year-old autistic child. Davison (1964) reported extinction of fear and aggressive responses as well as increased responsiveness to adult requests in a 9-year-old autistic girl through contingent application of candy, attention, and opportunities to look into a mirror and withdrawal of social reinforcement for undesirable behavior. Treatment of nonpsychotic children's aggression (Gittelman, 1965; Sloane, Johnston, & Bijou, 1966), storm phobia and anorexia nervosa (Hallsten, 1965; White, 1959), school phobia (Lazarus, Davison, & Polefka, 1965), and operant crying (Hart, Allen, Buell, Harris, & Wolf, 1964) seems also to be facilitated through simultaneous use of acceleration and deceleration techniques.

Parental Training

A new treatment technique which seems to have considerable promise is the training of parents to become appropriate reinforcement-dispensing agents. In some instances, parents are invited to observe reinforcement-treatment sessions, first, to see that the reinforcement contingency actually does control their child's problem behavior, and second, to learn how and when to dispense reinforcers, both tangible and social. Thus far, parents have been reported to have been successfully trained as behavior therapists for their children's antisocial behavior (Hawkins et al., 1966; Russo, 1964; Straughan, 1964; Whaler, Winkel, Peterson, & Morrison, 1965; Zeilberger, Sampen, & Sloane, 1966), excessive scratching and self-mutilation (Allen & Harris, 1966), and psychotic temper tantrums (Wetzel, Baker, Roney, & Martin, 1966). Patterson and Brodsky (1966) have recently ambitiously attempted the treatment of a child's multiple problem behaviors through the concurrent use of several conditioning programs including training the parents. The child's temper tantrums were modified through the use of an extinction-counterconditioning procedure, his separation-anxiety reactions were treated through another extinction-counterconditioning program, positive reinforcement was used to increase his positive interactions with peers, while his parents were trained to extinguish his negativistic and immature behaviors and to reward any evidences of cooperation and independence. Since there is some evidence that the environmental reinforcement contingencies to which delinquents (Buehler, Patterson, & Furniss, 1966) and adult psychotics (Gelfand, Gelfand, & Dobson, 1967) are exposed probably maintain their deviant behaviors, it is likely that the best hope for permanent positive behavior change rests in modifying the client's social environment. In the case of children, it may well prove more efficacious to modify the parents' child-rearing practices than to bring the child to the laboratory or clinic for direct interaction with the therapist. Parental education of this type may well have important preventive aspects also in that parents who are aware of the nature of their control of their children's behavior may be better able to prevent the occurrence of future problems and to promote appropriate interpersonal behavior.

Research Methodology

Paradigms for psychotherapy research using the more traditional treatment versus control groups designs have recently been discussed in detail by other writers (Bergin, 1966; Goldstein, Heller, & Sechrest, 1966; Kiesler, 1966) so this paper will deal only with evaluation of treatment with single subjects. As is the case with traditional play-therapy evaluation reports, the vast majority (96%) of the child-behavior-therapy papers reviewed here are case studies which describe modification of the behavior of individual subjects or of small groups of children displaying similar problem behaviors. Some writers have concluded that demonstrations of therapeutic efficacy with single cases represent no scientifically acceptable evidence at all. For example, Breger and McGaugh (1965) have argued that the behavior therapists' reliance upon single-subject therapy evaluations necessarily creates doubts about their claims of therapeutic success, and that, therefore, most of the reported successes "must be regarded as no better substantiated than those of any other enthusiastic school of psychotherapy . . . [p. 351]." This criticism has application only insofar as the methods used by therapy researchers studying individual subjects fail to meet the criteria usually applied to laboratory "free operant" studies. The "single organism, within-subject design" (Dinsmoor, 1966) has been extensively described elsewhere (Bachrach, 1964; Honig, 1966; Sidman, 1960, 1962), so this paper will discuss only a few of the major features. The contention here is that use of this method in therapy evaluation can powerfully demonstrate behavior control if certain specified procedures are followed. For instance, adequate base-line measures of the occurrence of the problem behavior (and, when applicable, frequency of prosocial responses) should be collected over a period of time long enough to provide reliable rate information. Obviously, these data should be collected in a rigorous, planned manner and not retrospectively recounted by the child's parents or teachers, as is frequently done in both traditional and behavior-therapy case studies. The therapist-experimenter should also provide a specific and detailed description of the treatment procedures, which should include sufficient data to permit replication by other investigators. Included should be information on the total number of treatment sessions, the length of each session, description of their spacing over time, and the total time span of the therapeutic intervention. The nature and extent of contacts with parents, teachers, and other involved individuals also ought to be provided. This body of information allows the reader to make comparisons regarding the efficiency and power of various treatment techniques. The work of Paul (1966), Lang and Lazovik (1963), and Lang, Lazovik, and Reynolds (1965) provides a high standard regarding adequate description of treatment procedures. The former author also presented a useful analysis of problems and alternative strategies in the design of therapy-evaluation studies.

Therapy-process data on the rate of occurrence of the behavior under investigation should be collected during every treatment session. Continuous data collection during therapy aids both in precise identification of the variables controlling the child's behavior and in the evaluation of treatment efficacy (Reyna, 1964).

A technique refinement not often observed is the systematic variation of the treatment reinforcement contingencies. After substantial and apparently reliable behavior modification has taken place, the reinforcement contingencies should be altered temporarily, for example, reversed, so the problem behavior is once again reinforced, or a prosocial response, instated through positive reinforcement, is extinguished. Correlated changes in the observed response rate provide a convincing demonstration that the target behavior is unmistakably under the therapist's control and not due to adventitious, extratherapeutic factors. This design feature is extremely important, if not essential, when $N = 1$, as Sidman (1960) and Dinsmoor (1966) have pointed out. The problem of the feasibility of such reinforcement-contingency reversals in clinical research is a knotty one, but this procedure should have high priority when the report is presented as a research study and the method described is to be taken seriously as an effective treatment technique. If the problem behavior precludes the reinstatement of natural contingencies, a number of substitute techniques might be considered. Use of a yoked control treated identically to the treatment subject with the exception that the active therapeutic ingredient is not systematically administered should prove useful in desensitization studies where contingency reversal is not feasible. Demonstration of behavioral control also might be accomplished by breaking the target behavior into subunits, for example, on the basis of response magnitude or object, and independently manipulating the separate units.[2] Less desirable substitutes for complete contingency reversal include the following control techniques: contingency changes that have predictable effects on response emission, for example, schedule changes; contingency reversal for a limited aspect of the target behavior and/or for the target behavior under limited, discriminable conditions.

Unfortunately, all of the previously discussed experimental control procedures are undermined if the accuracy of the rate measures is open to question. As in all psychotherapy research, extreme care must be taken to assure that truly objective behavior observations and measures are used. Since therapists are notoriously unobjective observers when the validity of their favorite treatment technique is in question, the best procedure would require either automatic recording of the target behaviors or the use of observers who are naive regarding the treatment procedure. Two additional refinements used by Brackbill (1958) in her study of the extinction of the smiling response in infants seem highly desirable for use in therapy evaluation also. First, sound-film recordings should be made at several points in the treatment process to permit independent and, if necessary, repeated observer reliability checks. Such a film record would also be useful to therapists wishing to learn the techniques which are often not adequately described in the published report. Another impressive design feature used by Brackbill was the establishment of high interobserver reliability prior to the inception of the study proper, a procedure rarely, if ever, followed in the child-therapy research literature where observer reliability is typically shaped while the behavior modification is proceeding. A possible result is that the observations made early in therapy lack reliability.

Lest the state of affairs in the reliability department look too black, it should be pointed out that the types of behaviors usually dealt with by behavior therapists are well defined, easily observed, and difficult to mistake, for example, the incidence of temper tantrums, enuresis, or speech deficit. Therefore, observer bias should less seriously affect the results than would be the case where the variables under investigation are less rigorously defined, such as lack of positive self-regard, covert hostility, and high anxiety.

---

[2]This technique was suggested by Florence R. Harris in a workshop presentation, University of Utah, April 28, 1967.

Nevertheless, investigators should not ignore Rosenthal's (1963, 1964) convincing demonstrations that experimenter bias can distort results even when seemingly very unmistakable response classes are under study.

One further therapy-evaluation procedure which should be undertaken in single-case as well as in treatment versus control group designs is a follow-up analysis of the stability of the behavior modification. A series of follow-up evaluations over a period of time, perhaps several years, would provide much-needed information concerning "symptom substitution" and generalization effects and would be a highly desirable design feature. Naturally, it is proposed that any follow-up data collection be made in a form more rigorous than the all too typical therapist's phone call to the child's parents or teacher, a procedure very likely to be subject to the Hello-Goodbye effect (Hathaway, 1948), according to which the persons contacted for information feel it is only polite to assure the therapist that he had helped the child, whether or not any change in behavior is actually observable.

Unfortunately, many of the behavior-therapy studies reviewed in this paper fail to meet most of the assessment standards suggested in the evaluation paradigm and thus represent no improvement over the traditional clinical case study in terms of experimental rigor. Nevertheless, in contrast to the play-therapy case-study literature, there are a small but growing number of carefully designed behavior-therapy case studies which meet most, if not all, of the suggested evaluation criteria and which convincingly demonstrate the power and efficiency of behavioristic treatment approaches (Allen et al., 1964; Doubros & Daniels, 1966; Harris et al., 1964; Whaler et al., 1965). While it is still possible to argue the merits of the theoretical bases for behavior-therapy techniques, careful application of the "single organism, within-subject design" should leave little question about the method's effectiveness.

References

Allen, K. E., & Harris, F. R. Elimination of a child's excessive scratching by training the mother in reinforcement procedures. *Behaviour Research and Therapy*, 1966, **4**, 79–84.

Allen, K. E., Hart, B., Buell, J. S., Harris, F. R., & Wolf, M. M. Effects of social reinforcement on isolate behavior of a nursery school child. *Child Development*, 1964, **35**, 511–518.

Bachrach, A. J. Some applications of operant conditioning to behavior therapy. In J. Wolpe, A. Salter, & L. J. Reyna (Eds.), *The conditioning therapies: The challenge in psychotherapy.* New York: Holt, Rinehart & Winston, 1964.

Baer, D. M. Laboratory control of thumbsucking by withdrawal and representation of reinforcement. *Journal of the Experimental Analysis of Behavior*, 1962, **5**, 525–528.

Bandura, A. Psychotherapy as a learning process. *Psychological Bulletin*, 1961, **58**, 143–159.

Bandura, A. Behavioral psychotherapy. *Scientific American*, 1967, **216**, 78–86.

Bandura, A., Grusec, J. E., & Menlove, F. L. Vicarious extinction of avoidance behavior. *Journal of Personality and Social Psychology*, 1967, **5**, 16–23.

Bandura, A., & Walters, R. H. *Social learning and personality development.* New York: Holt, Rinehart & Winston, 1963.

Bensberg, G. J., Colwell, C. N., & Cassel, R. H. Teaching the profoundly retarded self-help activities by shaping behavior techniques. *American Journal of Mental Deficiency,* 1965, **69,** 674–679.

Bentler, P. M. An infant's phobia treated with reciprocal inhibition therapy. *Journal of Child Psychology and Psychiatry,* 1962, **3,** 185–189.

Bergin, A. E. Some implications of psychotherapy research for therapeutic practice. *Journal of Abnormal Psychology,* 1966, **71,** 235–246.

Boardman, W. K. Rusty: A brief behavior disorder. *Journal of Consulting Psychology,* 1962, **26,** 293–297.

Brackbill, Y. Extinction of the smiling response in infants as a function of reinforcement schedule. *Child Development,* 1958, **29,** 115–124.

Breger, L., & McGaugh, J. L. Critique and reformulation of "learning-theory" approaches to psychotherapy and neurosis. *Psychological Bulletin,* 1965, **63,** 338–358.

Brown, P., & Elliott, R. Control of aggression in nursery school class. *Journal of Experimental Child Psychology,* 1965, **3,** 102–107.

Buehler, R. E., Patterson, G. R., & Furniss, J. M. The reinforcement of behavior in institutional settings. *Behaviour Research and Therapy,* 1966, **4,** 157–167.

Burchard, J. D., & Tyler, V. O., Jr. The modification of delinquent behavior through operant conditioning. *Behaviour Research and Therapy,* 1965, **2,** 245–250.

Commons, M. L., Paul, S. M., & Fargo, G. A. Developing speech in an autistic boy using operant techniques to increase his rate of vocal-verbal responding. Paper presented at the meeting of the Western Psychological Association, Long Beach, California, April 1966.

Cook, C., & Adams, H. E. Modification of verbal behavior in speech deficient children. *Behaviour Research and Therapy,* 1966, **4,** 265–271.

Coote, M. A. Apparatus for conditioning treatment of enuresis. *Behaviour Research and Therapy,* 1965, **2,** 233–238.

Davison, G. C. A social learning theory programme with an autistic child. *Behaviour Research and Therapy,* 1964, **2,** 149–159.

Dayan, M. Toilet training retarded children in the state residential institution. *Mental Retardation,* 1964, **2,** 116–117.

De Leon, G., & Mandell, W. A comparison of conditioning and psychotherapy in the treatment of functional enuresis. *Journal of Clinical Psychology,* 1966, **22,** 326–330.

Dinsmoor, J. A. Comments on Wetzel's treatment of a case of compulsive stealing. *Journal of Consulting Psychology,* 1966, **30,** 378–380.

Doubros, S. G., & Daniels, G. J. An experimental approach to the reduction of overactive behavior. *Behaviour Research and Therapy,* 1966, **4,** 251–258.

Ernest, E. (Personal communication.) Cited by H. G. Jones, Continuation of Yates' treatment of a tiqueur. In H. J. Eysenck (Ed.), *Behavior therapy and the neuroses.* Oxford: Pergamon Press, 1960. P. 257.

Evans, J. Rocking at night. *Journal of Child Psychology and Psychiatry,* 1961, **2,** 71–85.

Feldman, R. B., & Werry, J. S. An unsuccessful attempt to treat a tiqueur by massed practice. *Behaviour Research and Therapy,* 1966, **4,** 111–117.

Ferster, C. B., & Simons, J. Behavior therapy with children. *Psychological Record,* 1966, **16,** 65–71.

Fuller, P. R. Operant conditioning of a vegetative human organism. *American Journal of Psychology,* 1949, **62,** 587–590.

Garvey, W. P., & Hegrenes, J. R. Desensitization techniques in the treatment of school phobia. *American Journal of Orthopsychiatry,* 1966, **36,** 147–152.

Gelber, H., & Meyer, B. Behavior therapy and encopresis: Complexities involved in treatment. *Behaviour Research and Therapy,* 1965, **2,** 227–231.

Gelfand, D. M., Gelfand, S., & Dobson, W. R. Unprogrammed reinforcement of patients' behavior in a mental hospital. *Behaviour Research and Therapy,* 1967, **5,** 201–207.

Gittelman, M. Behavior rehearsal as a technique in child treatment. *Journal of Child Psychology and Psychiatry,* 1965, **6,** 251–255.

Goldstein, A. P., Heller, K., & Sechrest, L. B. *Psychotherapy and the psychology of behavior change.* New York: Wiley, 1966.

Grossberg, J. M. Behavior therapy: A review. *Psychological Bulletin,* 1964, **62,** 73–88.

Hallsten, E. A., Jr. Adolescent anorexia nervosa treated by desensitization. *Behaviour Research and Therapy,* 1965, **3,** 87–91.

Harris, F. R., Johnston, M. K., Kelley, C. S., & Wolf, M. M. Effects of positive social reinforcement on regressed crawling of a nursery school child. *Journal of Educational Psychology,* 1964, **55,** 35–41.

Hart, B. M., Allen, K. E., Buell, J. S., Harris, F. R., & Wolf, M. M. Effects of social reinforcement on operant crying. *Journal of Experimental Child Psychology,* 1964, **1,** 145–153.

Hathaway, S. R. Some considerations relative to nondirective counseling as therapy. *Journal of Clinical Psychology,* 1948, **4,** 226–231.

Hawkins, R. P., Peterson, R. F., Schweid, E., & Bijou, S. W. Behavior therapy in the home: Amelioration of problem parent-child relations with the parent in a therapeutic role. *Journal of Experimental Child Psychology,* 1966, **4,** 99–107.

Homme, L. E., deBaca, P. C., Devine, J. V., Steinhorst, R., & Rickert, E. J. Use of the Premack principle in controlling the behavior of nursery school children. *Journal of the Experimental Analysis of Behavior,* 1963, **6,** 544.

Honig, W. K. (Ed.) *Operant behavior: Areas of research and application.* New York: Appleton-Century-Crofts, 1966.

Hundziak, M., Mauer, R. A., & Watson, L. S., Jr. Operant conditioning and toilet training of severely mentally retarded boys. *American Journal of Mental Deficiency,* 1965, **70,** 120–124.

James, C. E. Operant conditioning in the management and behavior of hyperactive children: Five case studies. Unpublished manuscript, Orange State College, 1963. Cited by G. R. Patterson, R. Jones, J. Whittier, & M. A. Wright, A behaviour modification technique for the hyperactive child. *Behaviour Research and Therapy,* 1965, **2,** 218.

Johnston, M. K., Kelley, C. S., Harris, F. R., & Wolf, M. M. An application of reinforcement principles to development of motor skills of a young child. *Child Development,* 1966, **37,** 379–387.

Jones, H. G. The behavioral treatment of enuresis nocturna. In H. J. Eysenck (Ed.), *Behaviour therapy and the neuroses.* London: Pergamon Press, 1960.

Jones, M. C. The elimination of children's fears. *Journal of Experimental Psychology,* 1924, **7,** 382–390. (a)

Jones, M. C. A laboratory study of fear: The case of Peter. *Pedagogical Seminar,* 1924, **31,** 308–315. (b)

Keehn, J. D. Brief case-report: Reinforcement therapy of incontinence. *Behaviour Research and Therapy,* 1965, **2,** 239.

Kerr, N., Meyerson, L., & Michael, J. A procedure for shaping vocalization in a mute child. In L. P. Ullmann & L. Krasner (Eds.), *Case studies in behavior modification.* New York: Holt, Rinehart & Winston, 1965.

Kiesler, D. J. Some myths of psychotherapy research and the search for a paradigm. *Psychological Bulletin,* 1966, **65,** 110–136.

Krasner, L., & Ullmann, L. P. (Eds.) *Research in behavior modification.* New York: Holt, Rinehart & Winston, 1965.

Lang, P. J., & Lazovik, A. D. Experimental desensitization of a phobia. *Journal of Abnormal and Social Psychology,* 1963, **66,** 519–525.

Lang, P. J., Lazovik, A. D., & Reynolds, D. J. Desensitization, suggestibility, and pseudotherapy. *Journal of Abnormal Psychology,* 1965, **70,** 395–402.

Lazarus, A. A. The elimination of children's phobias by deconditioning. *Medical Proceedings,* South Africa, 1959, **5,** 261–265.

Lazarus, A. A., & Abramovitz, A. The use of "emotive imagery" in the treatment of children's phobias. *Journal of Mental Science,* 1962, **108,** 191–195.

Lazarus, A. A., Davison, D. C., & Polefka, B. A. Classical and operant factors in the treatment of school phobia. *Journal of Abnormal Psychology,* 1965, **70,** 225–229.

Lazarus, A., & Rachman, S. The use of systematic desensitization in psychotherapy. *South African Medical Journal,* 1957, **31,** 934–937.

Lovaas, O. I., Berberich, J. P., Perloff, B. F., & Schaeffer, B. Acquisition of imitative speech by schizophrenic children. *Science,* 1966, **161,** 705–707.

Lovaas, O. I., Freitag, G., Gold, V. J., & Kassorla, I. C. Experimental studies in childhood schizophrenia: Analysis of self-destructive behavior. *Journal of Experimental Child Psychology,* 1965, **2**, 67–84.

Lovaas, O. I., Freitag, G., Kinder, M. I., Rubenstein, D. B., Schaeffer, B., & Simmons, J. B. Experimental studies in childhood schizophrenia: Developing social behavior using electric shock. Paper presented at the meeting of the American Psychological Association, Los Angeles, September 1964.

Lovaas, O. I., Schaeffer, B., & Simmons, J. B. Building social behavior in autistic children by use of electric shock. *Journal of Experimental Research in Personality,* 1965, **1**, 99–109.

Lovibond, S. H. The mechanism of conditioned treatment of enuresis. *Behaviour Research and Therapy,* 1963, **1**, 17–21.

Lovibond, S. H. *Conditioning and enuresis.* Oxford: Pergamon Press, 1964.

Madsen, C. H., Jr. Positive reinforcement in the toilet training of a normal child: A case report. In L. P. Ullmann & L. Krasner (Eds.), *Case studies in behavior modification.* New York: Holt, Rinehart & Winston, 1965.

Marshall, G. R. Toilet training of an autistic eight-year-old through conditioning therapy: A case report. *Behaviour Research and Therapy,* 1966, **4**, 242–245.

Metz, J. R. Conditioning generalized imitation in autistic children. *Journal of Experimental Child Psychology,* 1965, **2**, 389–399.

Mowrer, O. H., & Mowrer, W. M. Enuresis: A method for its study and treatment. *American Journal of Orthopsychiatry,* 1938, **8**, 436–459.

Neale, D. H. Behavior therapy and encopresis in children. *Behaviour Research and Therapy,* 1963, **1**, 139–150.

Patterson, G. R. An application of conditioning techniques to the control of a hyperactive child. In L. P. Ullmann & L. Krasner (Eds.), *Case studies in behavior modification.* New York: Holt, Rinehart & Winston, 1965. (a)

Patterson, G. R. A learning theory approach to the treatment of the school phobic child. In L. P. Ullmann & L. Krasner (Eds.), *Case studies in behavior modification.* New York: Holt, Rinehart & Winston, 1965. (b)

Patterson, G. R., & Brodsky, G. A behavior modification programme for a child with multiple problem behaviors. *Journal of Child Psychology and Psychiatry,* 1966, **7**, 277–296.

Patterson, G. R., Jones, R., Whittier, J., & Wright, M. A. A behaviour modification technique for the hyperactive child. *Behaviour Research and Therapy,* 1965, **2**, 217–226.

Paul, G. L. *Insight versus desensitization in psychotherapy.* Stanford: Stanford University Press, 1966.

Peterson, D. R., & London, P. A role for cognition in the behavioral treatment of a child's eliminative disturbance. In L. P. Ullmann & L. Krasner (Eds.), *Case studies in behavior modification.* New York: Holt, Rinehart & Winston, 1965.

Pumroy, D. K., & Pumroy, S. S. Reinforcement in toilet training. *Psychological Reports,* 1965, **16**, 467–471.

Quay, H. C., Werry, J. S., McQueen, M., & Sprague, R. L. Remediation of the conduct problem child in the special class setting. *Exceptional Child,* 1966, **32**, 509–515.

Rachman, S. Learning theory and child psychology: Therapeutic possibilities. *Journal of Child Psychology and Psychiatry,* 1962, **3**, 149–163.

Reyna, L. J. Conditioning therapies, learning theory, and research. In J. Wolpe, A. Salter, & L. J. Reyna (Eds.), *The conditioning therapies.* New York: Holt, Rinehart & Winston, 1964.

Rice, H. K., & McDaniel, M. W. Operant behavior in vegetative patients. *Psychological Record,* 1966, **16**, 279–281.

Rosenthal, R. On the social psychology of the psychological experiment. *American Scientist,* 1963, **51**, 268–283.

Rosenthal, R. Experimenter outcome orientation and the results of the psychological experiment. *Psychological Bulletin,* 1964, **61**, 405–412.

Russo, S. Adaptations in behavioral therapy with children. *Behaviour Research and Therapy,* 1964, **2**, 43–47.

Salzinger, K., Feldman, R. S., Cowan, J. E., & Salzinger, S. Operant conditioning of verbal behavior of two young speech-deficient boys. In L. Krasner & L. P. Ullmann (Eds.) *Research in behavior modification.* New York: Holt, Rinehart & Winston, 1965.

Schwitzgebel, R., Short-term operant conditioning of adolescent offenders on socially relevant variables. *Journal of Abnormal Psychology,* 1967, **72,** 134–142.

Schwitzgebel, R., & Kolb, D. A. Inducing behavior change in adolescent delinquents. *Behaviour Research and Therapy,* 1964, **1,** 297–304.

Sidman, M. *Tactics of scientific research.* New York: Basic Books, 1960.

Sidman, M. Operant techniques. In A. L. Bachrach (Ed.), *Experimental foundations of clinical psychology.* New York: Basic Books, 1962.

Sloane, H. N., Jr., Johnston, M. K., & Bijou, S. W. Successive modification of aggressive behavior and aggressive fantasy play by management of contingencies. Unpublished manuscript, University of Utah, 1966.

Straughan, J. H. Treatment with child and mother in the playroom. *Behaviour Research and Therapy,* 1964, **2,** 37–41.

Straughan, J. H., Potter, W. K., & Hamilton, S. H. The behavioral treatment of an elective mute. *Journal of Child Psychology and Psychiatry,* 1965, **6,** 125–130.

Tate, B. G., & Baroff, G. S. Aversive control of self-injurious behavior in a psychotic boy, *Behaviour Research and Therapy,* 1966, **4,** 281–287.

Tyler, V. O. Exploring the use of operant techniques in the rehabilitation of delinquent boys. Paper presented at the meeting of the American Psychological Association, Chicago, September 1965.

Ullmann, L. P., & Krasner, L. (Eds.) *Case studies in behavior modification.* New York: Holt, Rinehart & Winston, 1965.

Van Wagenen, R. K., & Murdock, E. E. A transistorized signal-package for toilet training of infants. *Journal of Experimental Child Psychology,* 1966, **3,** 312–314.

Walton, D. Experimental psychology and the treatment of a tiqueur. *Journal of Child Psychology and Psychiatry,* 1961, **2,** 148–155.

Weitzman, B. Behavior therapy and psychotherapy. *Psychological Review,* 1967, **74,** 300–317.

Werry, J. S. The conditioning treatment of enuresis. *American Journal of Psychiatry,* 1966, **123,** 226–229.

Werry, J. S., & Cohrssen, J. Enuresis: An etiologic and therapeutic study. *Journal of Pediatrics,* 1965, **67,** 423–431.

Werry, J. S., & Wollersheim, J. P. Behavior therapy with children: A broad overview. *American Academy of Child Psychiatry Journal,* 1967, **6,** 346–370.

Wetzel, R. Use of behavioral techniques in a case of compulsive stealing. *Journal of Consulting Psychology,* 1966, **30,** 367–374.

Wetzel, R. J., Baker, J., Roney, M., & Martin, M. Outpatient treatment of autistic behavior. *Behaviour Research and Therapy,* 1966, **4,** 169–177.

Whaler, R. G., Winkel, G. H., Peterson, R. F., & Morrison, D. C. Mothers as behavior therapists for their own children. *Behaviour Research and Therapy,* 1965, **3,** 113–124.

White, J. G. The use of learning theory in the psychological treatment of children. *Journal of Clinical Psychology,* 1959, **16,** 227–229.

Wickes, I. G. Treatment of persistent enuresis with the electric buzzer. *Archives of Disease in Childhood,* 1958, **33,** 160–164.

Williams, C. D. The elimination of tantrum behavior by extinction procedures. *Journal of Abnormal and Social Psychology,* 1959, **59,** 269.

Wolf, M. M., Birnbrauer, J. S., Williams, R., & Lawler, J. A note on apparent extinction of the vomiting behavior of a retarded child. In L. P. Ullmann & L. Krasner (Eds.), *Case studies in behavior modification.* New York: Holt, Rinehart & Winston, 1965.

Wolf, M. M., Risley, T., & Mees, H. Application of operant conditioning procedures to the behavior problems of an autistic child. *Behaviour Research and Therapy,* 1964, **1,** 305–312.

Wolpe, J. *Psychotherapy by reciprocal inhibition.* Stanford: Stanford University Press, 1958.

Wolpe, J., & Lazarus, A. A. *Behavior therapy techniques.* Oxford: Pergamon Press, 1966.

Yates, A. J. The application of learning theory to the treatment of tics. *Journal of Abnormal and Social Psychology,* 1958, **56,** 175–182.

Zeilberger, J., Sampen, S. E., & Sloane, H. N., Jr. Modification of child problem behavior in the home with the mother as therapist. Unpublished manuscript, City College of New York, 1966.

Zimmerman, E. H., & Zimmerman, J. The alteration of behavior in a special classroom situation. *Journal of Experimental Analysis of Behavior,* 1962, **5,** 59–60.

28. On Lovaas' Behavior Therapy Program for Autistic Children

Anthony Davids

O. Ivar Lovaas and his collaborators have recently presented an extensive report of follow-up measures on autistic children treated with behavior therapy (Lovaas, Koegel, Simmons, & Stevens, in press). The findings were based on 20 autistic children who had received operant conditioning therapy in the course of a 5-year program at UCLA. This program was carried out with a heavy research orientation focusing on a limited set of behaviors, one of which was speech. As Lovaas mentions, when this experimental program was instituted in 1964, behavior therapy with psychotic children was new. Consequently, much of their work was exploratory and contained many shortcomings that were realized only as the program progressed. Moreover, the children selected for this experimental program were those with the poorest prognosis.

These children were described as showing the following characteristics: (1) apparent sensory deficit (abnormal vision or hearing); (2) severe affect isolation (indifference to people); (3) high rate of self-stimulatory behavior (rocking, spinning, arm flapping); (4) mutism (found in about half the children); (5) echolalia (echoing the speech of others); (6) minimal evidence of receptive speech; (7) minimal presence of social and self-help behaviors; and (8) self-mutilation in a minority of cases, but severe aggressive outbursts in all cases.

In general, the treatment program attempted to extinguish or suppress pathological behaviors and to establish socially desirable behaviors. In attempting to extinguish pathological behaviors (such as biting, scratching, and feces smearing), they used the techniques of (1) reinforcement withdrawal (leaving the child alone); (2) aversive stimuli (slapping or administering electric shock); or (3) reinforcement of incompatible behavior (rewarding for sitting quietly in a chair).

Simultaneously with suppressing undesirable behavior, the therapist attempted to establish a kind of primitive stimulus control. That is, he picked some simple behavior, such as the child looking at the therapist, and taught the child to make this response when requested to do so. Following these introductory steps, the main emphasis was on language training using operant procedures. Lovaas readily admits that this particular emphasis may not have been the best one for every child in the program, and some would perhaps have benefited more from other treatment emphases.

While attempting to build speech in these children, the investigators also initiated programs designed to facilitate social and self-help skills. The focus was on building the kinds of behaviors that would make the children easier to live with—dressing themselves, brushing their teeth, eating properly at the dining table, and showing signs of affection. The emphasis throughout the program was on making the children look as normal as possible, by rewarding them for desirable behavior and punishing them for psychotic behavior. In essence, the children were taught that adults were in control. In Lovaas' words, "... we attempted to teach these children what parents of the middle-class western world attempt to teach theirs. There are, of course, many questions which one may have about these values, but faced with primitive psychotic children, these seem rather secure and comforting as initial goals."

In establishing these behaviors, therapists used reinforcers that were functional for each particular child. Many children would work only for food, quieting down and paying attention only if given an occasional slap on the rear. For some children, symbolic approval and disapproval were sufficient reinforcers for obtaining the desired behaviors. In this regard, Lovaas mentions individual differences found among behavior modifiers. Based on his several years of intensive work in this field, Lovaas states "The degree of expertness of the behavior modifier will dictate his results, and the field is so new that it is difficult to specify the exact conditions under which one produces such an expert."

The main findings from this study can be summarized as follows. "Sick" behaviors (self-stimulation and echolalia) decreased during treatment, and "healthy" behaviors (appropriate speech, play and social behaviors) increased. Scores on IQ tests and on the Vineland Social Maturity Scale showed large gains during treatment. All children improved, but some improved more than others. Follow-up measures taken two years after treatment showed large differences depending on the environment the child returned to following treatment. Children whose parents were trained to carry out behavior therapy in the home continued to improve, while those who were institutionalized deteriorated. Brief reinstatement of behavior therapy served to reestablish the original therapeutic gains in the children who had been institutionalized.

Lovaas et al. concluded that despite its limitations, behavior therapy with autistic children is helpful. It proved especially effective in suppressing self-destruction in children who had mutilated themselves for years. In many cases, if the child was not mute, the operant conditioning techniques were able to produce noteworthy improvements in language and intellectual behavior. The treatment was found to result in some stimulus generalization and response generalization, although not to the extent the investigators had hoped. However, they believe that teaching parents to treat their own children by these techniques will lead to even better results in the future.

These investigators also discuss the many disappointments encountered in the course of their treatment program and follow-up assessments. Most significant was the failure to isolate a pivotal response, or one key behavior that could be modified and thus result in profound personality change. In this regard, they state most emphatically, "Our treatment was not a cure for autism." They also point out that the underlying pathology in autism may ultimately be discovered to be biochemical and, if so, the proper treatment may require correction of a biochemical imbalance.

One indisputable finding from this research is the importance of including parents in the treatment program. However, they found that not all parents are equally effective behavior modifiers; they listed the qualities found in the parents who were successful. Among these were a willingness to: (1) use strong consequences (deprivation of food, spanking) and to become angry as well as very loving; (2) deny that the child is "ill" and to give him some responsibility; and (3) commit a major part of their lives to managing the child.

In closing, Lovaas et al. emphasize that the principles and procedures they use are not new. For, as they state, "Reinforcement, like gravity, is everywhere, and has been around for a long time." What is new about behavior therapy is the fact that it involves systematic evaluation of how its principles and procedures affect the individual. Thus, it is not the content of behavior therapy that is new, but its utilization of research methodology. In the hands of investigators as skilled and dedicated as Lovaas and his collaborators, this methodology should make major contributions to the understanding and application of psychological treatment.

Reference

Lovaas, O. I., Koegel, R., Simmons, J. Q., & Stevens, J. Some generalization and follow-up measures on autistic children in behavior therapy. *Journal of Applied Behavior Analysis,* in press.

Part IV

Ethical Considerations and General Conclusions

Chapter Eleven

Aversive Control

Perhaps one of the most significant issues in the field of abnormal child psychology is the use of aversive stimuli in attempting to modify the behaviors of abnormal children. This issue is closely related to certain ethical considerations in the general use of behavior modification techniques, but this chapter will focus on application of various forms of aversive control in working with disturbed children.

From our study of behavior therapy we have seen that positive and negative reinforcements constitute fundamental ingredients in the therapeutic process. There has been little expressed concern over the application of positive reinforcements, although recently the use of tangible reinforcers such as prizes, candy, and cigarettes has been criticized because these forms of positive reward can easily be used as bribes (O'Leary, Poulos, & Devine, 1972); investigators have been urged to be on the alert for possible misuses of tangible rewards. This, however, is not the kind of misuse and abuse with which we are concerned here. Our focus is on various kinds of negative experiences that are imposed on defenseless children in the course of their supposedly therapeutic treatment.

Time-Out Procedures

A commonly used technique in behavior modification is "time-out," a short form of what was originally called "time-out from positive reinforcement." The original term referred to the fact that when the child became uncooperative and disruptive he would be removed from the situation in which he could obtain positive reinforcement (Bijou & Baer, 1967). In other words, if the child were in a learning situation in which he could earn positive reinforcements and he became uncontrollable, he was sent away from the situation ("time-out from the positive reinforcement") until he was again in a condition to work for the positive rewards. This procedure soon became applied to control unmanageable behavior. For example, if a child had a tantrum he could be sent to his room until he calmed down.

As the behavior modification movement gained momentum and enjoyed wider currency throughout the psychological community, it became recognized that merely going to one's room could actually entail many positive aspects. The practice then became to make the "time-out" unpleasant and something that the child would want to avoid. Thus, rather than merely being excluded from some positive ongoing activity or being sent to a comfortable room, the child would be placed in a small, barren room or even a closet. "Time-out" then becomes highly discomforting, with the child being sentenced to a form of punishment. That is, he is placed alone in a small room just as prisoners are sentenced to solitary confinement.

Time-out can take other forms that do not necessitate placing the child in a room away from the remainder of a group of patients. The adult can merely order the child to stay fixed in a certain place or position. For example, one technique is to force the child to stand with his nose and knees touching the wall, with his arms outspread against the wall, and to maintain this position for a given period. In other words, when the child does not behave as the behavior therapist dictates, he is assigned a "time-out" period that could range from a matter of minutes to a half hour or even an hour sentence against the wall. If this description does not convey the discomfort involved, the reader should assume this position for 10 minutes.

Extreme Isolation

A therapeutic procedure making use of severe isolation, but not as a form of "time-out," has been described by Churchill (1969). Working with psychotic children, this particular method involves isolating the child in an 8 by 15-foot room, where he stays 24 hours a day, seven days a week, for three to five weeks. During this period the child hears or sees nothing other than what is provided by adults who work with him individually for a total of six hours a day. The room contains only a potty chair and a mattress on the floor. Food, water, and the social contact are used as reinforcers, and if the psychotic child does not show the behaviors that are being conditioned, he is deprived of these essential positive reinforcements. So here we see a process of relearning that uses a combination of long periods of total isolation and possible withholding of such essentials as food and water. While this procedure may appear blatantly cruel, it should be pointed out that noteworthy improvements in the behavior of some seriously disturbed children have resulted from this form of behavior therapy.

Many of these techniques may seem unduly harsh, but they do not include any form of actual physical punishment or purposeful infliction of pain. That is, the aversive procedures described so far require the child to endure something that is only uncomfortable, frightening, exhausting, or frustrating. Now let us consider the application of painful stimuli in attempting to modify or control abnormal behavior in children.

Application of Painful Stimuli

The most commonly used technique, and the one that has led to much public concern, is the use of a cattle-prod to administer electric shock to child patients. The following excerpt from a published paper will serve to describe the kind of apparatus used for the purpose of manipulating the self-destructive behavior of a retarded boy.

> Punishment, in the form of a 1-sec. electric shock, was delivered by a hand-held inductorium ("Hot-shot," by Hot-shot Products Company, Inc., Savage, Minnesota). The inductorium was a 1-ft. long rod with two electrodes 0.75 in. apart protruding from its end. The shock, delivered from five 1.5-v. flashlight batteries, had spikes as high as 1400 v. at 50,000 ohms resistance. It was definitely painful to the experimenter, like a dentist drilling on an unanesthetized tooth, but the pain terminated when the shock ended. As soon as (within 1 sec.) the child hit himself, the experimenter, holding the inductorium, reached over and applied it to the child's leg [Lovaas & Simmons, 1969].

Before judging the appropriateness of using a technique such as this, we should understand the kind of self-abusive behavior that was being displayed by this child. John was an 8-year-old mentally retarded boy who had no speech, showed little understanding of language, and functioned on an exceptionally low level in all areas of psychosocial adjustment. The major disturbing problem, however, was that this boy beat himself unmercifully and was covered with self-inflicted bruises and contusions. Because of this, for six months before this attempt at behavior therapy, John had continuously worn restraints on both legs and arms. Whenever he was removed from these restraints he became extremely agitated, consequently requiring constant care and attention.

Before using the electric shock stimulus, the investigators studied John's self-destructive acts when he was placed alone in a small room, with restraints removed, for a 90-minute period. He was observed from an adjoining room through a one-way mirror, and exact counts were made of his self-destructive acts. This procedure was carried out for several days, and it was observed that John showed 2750 destructive acts on the first day, with gradual decrease on succeeding days, until he finally stopped hitting himself after a total of almost 9000 self-inflicted blows. While this extinction procedure finally produced a deceleration in the undesirable behavior, it was noted that John started to hit himself again whenever he was placed into another situation. Thus, the therapists attempted to control his abusive behavior by means of strong negative reinforcement in the form of electric shock. This procedure was very successful in getting John to stop hitting himself, and this inhibition generalized to situations beyond the experimental room. John's social awareness and overall level of functioning seemed somewhat improved as the self-abusive behavior was successfully eliminated by means of the electric shock, and he could be allowed to live without physical restraints.

Use of Positive Rewards

Attempts to inhibit self-destructive behavior by means of positive rein-forcements have met with little success. Davids (1972) describes an 8-year-old psychotic boy who persisted in beating himself throughout his two years of residential psychiatric treatment. Whenever his hands were free, Jeff beat his face until it bled, his eyes were blackened, and he became groggy from his own blows. Attempts to prevent this included requiring him to wear a football helmet or boxing gloves, placing restraints on his elbows, or tying his hands behind his back. An experiment in behavior modification was designed in which Jeff could have all sorts of positive reinforcements as long as he did not hit himself—candies and his favorite foods; soda, which he liked very much; listening to his favorite music played on a phonograph; playing with sand and water, which he enjoyed; and so forth.

In this experimental situation, whenever Jeff hit himself he was placed in a large, specially designed box. It was much like a steam-cabinet used in health studios, with the body encased in the box and only the head pro-truding through the top opening. This aspect of the experimental procedure could be viewed as a form of negative reinforcement, or punishment, but its intended purpose was merely to give Jeff a "time-out" from positive rein-forcement and to prevent him from hitting himself without having to be held by a person (which might be rewarding to him).

Many weeks of an entire summer were devoted to this attempted behavior modification, but with no success. Jeff enjoyed the positive reinforcements, but did not seem to mind being placed in the box, and he continued to hit himself with great frequency. He was discharged from the residential treatment center with his hands still tied behind his back, just as he had come in two years before. One wonders if the application of aversive stimuli in the form of electric shocks administered each time he hit himself might have served to decelerate his self-destructive behavior. Unfortunately, we will never know, although several reports published since that time suggest that this technique might well have been effective.

Treating Chronic Ruminative Vomiting

The application of electric shock has been used to treat serious childhood abnormalities other than self-abuse. An excellent example is provided by Lang and Melamed's (1969) use of avoidance conditioning therapy in treating chronic ruminative vomiting. This study was conducted with a 9-month-old male infant whose life was seriously endangered by persistent vomiting and chronic rumination (rechewing of the vomitus). This child was literally wast-ing away (down to a weight of 12 pounds) and, according to the attending physician, was likely to die if he continued this behavior, which had been unaffected by various forms of medical therapy attempted during the child's hospitalization.

It was therefore decided to institute a program of behavior therapy in which electrodes were attached to the child's leg and an electromyograph (EMG) was used to record sucking, swallowing, and vomiting. The EMG recordings, together with a nurse's observations, provided accurate measures of the initiation of vomiting, and whenever this occurred electric shock could be applied immediately to the child's leg. After only two 1-hour conditioning sessions, the infant reacted to the shock by crying and cessation of vomiting. A few additional sessions led to complete elimination of this undesirable behavior, not only in the experimental set-up but also throughout the remainder of the day and night. Moreover, it was noted that the child's activity level increased, he became more interested in his environment, played more contentedly, smiled and reached out to be held by nurses and his mother. He was discharged from the hospital after only 5 days of treatment, and a follow-up assessment one month later found him to be a healthy looking, alert and active 21-pound child with no signs of problem behavior. This rapid recovery following brief aversive conditioning certainly provides vivid evidence of the effectiveness of behavior modification in treating this type of psychosomatic disorder.

Building Social Behavior

A quite different use of electric shock in building social behavior in autistic children was reported by Lovaas, Schaeffer, and Simmons (1965). These investigators designed an experimental procedure in which the child was placed in a room with grids across the floor that could be charged electrically. On either side of the room were human adults whom the child could approach if he so chose. These children, however, tended to avoid human contacts and engaged mainly in self-stimulation and tantrum-like behaviors. In this experimental procedure, the investigators turned on the current, which delivered a painful electric shock to the child's bare feet. The first phase of the experiment involved escape learning, with the child being able to terminate the shock by going to one of the adults. That is, the child was in the middle of the room, the floor became electrified, and he continued to be shocked until he approached one of the adults at either side of the room. Following this phase, the procedure was changed to an avoidance learning situation with the child being able to avoid receiving shock by complying with the adult's invitation for the child to approach him. If the child did not comply with this social request within a specified time interval, the current was turned on and he was shocked until he made the escape response.

This study involved twin boys as subjects, and they both learned to show the social behavior in order to avoid shock. Moreover, the shock was effective in eliminating pathological behaviors such as self-stimulation and tantrums. Interestingly, affectionate and other social behaviors toward the adults increased after these adults became associated with shock reduction. In other words, the children were conditioned to learn that these adults represented safety and comfort, and this learning appeared to improve their social adjustment.

The Issues

Thus we see that electric shock has been used in different ways. In one procedure, the shock is applied to suppress specific undesirable responses, and in the other procedure shock reduction is used as a way to establish social reinforcers (that is, to make adults more meaningful and rewarding to the child). In commenting on the use of electric shock to build social behavior in autistic children, Breger (1965) stated, "I think there is a real ethical problem here when pain is deliberately inflicted on subjects without their consent in an attempt to 'control' their behavior. The argument that nothing else has worked is really beside the point, though it has been evoked in the past to justify such ethically dubious practices as the widespread use of prefrontal lobotomies."

So here we are faced with a dilemma with ample ethical and practical implications. Among psychotic and retarded children there are those who show extreme forms of self-injurious behavior—pummeling their faces, banging their heads against hard objects, biting themselves or tearing off bits of flesh, cutting themselves with sharp objects, or repeatedly sticking damaging objects into various body orifices. In order to prevent serious injury, these children are often placed in complete restraints such as strait-jackets or are kept immobilized on a chair or a bed with their arms and legs firmly tied. Is this sort of treatment any more humane or socially accept-able than the administration of painful but brief electric shocks that might enable the child patient to move about more freely without injuring himself?

We will here present three papers that elaborate on this issue. In the first paper, George S. Baroff and Bobby G. Tate present a detailed description of the use of aversive stimulation (electric shock) in treating self-injurious behavior. The second paper, by William H. Shaw, demonstrates the applica-tion of a quite different form of aversive control (punishment by injections) in the treatment of a girl who refused to speak. In the third paper, Donald M. Baer concludes that punishment is a legitimate tool for modifying severely troublesome behavior.

The paper by Baer appeared as an appendix to Neuringer and Michael's *Behavior Modification in Clinical Psychology* (1970). It was written in re-sponse to a paper by Kushner (1970) on the use of electric shock as an aversive control in clinical practice. In this scholarly paper, Kushner reviews the research literature about aversive controls and discusses the advantages of electric shock as a form of aversive treatment. He then presents numerous case examples of the successful use of this procedure in treating a wide variety of patients seen in institutional as well as private practice settings. One of the cases described was a 17-year-old girl who had been vigorously and rapidly sneezing for six months with no relief. Another was a 7-year-old severely retarded boy who showed self-destructive behavior in the form of hand-biting. At the adult level, there was a 33-year-old man with the fetish of stealing women's panties, putting them on, and masturbating. In each of these cases, and in several others described by Kushner, conditioning procedures using electric shocks led to rapid elimination of the socially undesirable and disabling behavior. Stimulated by Kushner's chapter, Baer emphasizes that these abnormal behaviors are painful to the individual and that it is more humane to apply a momentarily painful treatment leading to an improved state of overall adjustment than it is to withhold such treatment. These papers may help the reader decide which is the lesser of the evils.

References

Bijou, S. W., & Baer, D. M. (Eds.) *Child development: Readings in experimental analysis.* New York: Appleton-Century-Crofts, 1967.

Breger, L. Comments on "Building social behavior in autistic children by use of electric shock." *Journal of Experimental Research in Personality*, 1965, **1**, 110–113.

Churchill, D. W. Psychotic children and behavior modification. *American Journal of Psychiatry*, 1969, **125**, 1585–1590.

Davids, A. *Abnormal children and youth: Therapy and research.* New York: Wiley-Interscience, 1972.

Kushner, M. Faradic aversive controls in clinical practice. In Neuringer, C., & Michaels, J. L. (Eds.), *Behavior modification in clinical psychology.* New York: Appleton-Century-Crofts, 1970.

Lang, P. J., & Melamed, B. G. Avoidance conditioning therapy of an infant with chronic ruminative vomiting. *Journal of Abnormal Psychology*, 1969, **74**, 1–8.

Lovaas, O. I., Schaeffer, B., & Simmons, J. Q. Building social behavior in autistic children by use of electric shock. *Journal of Experimental Research in Personality*, 1965, **1**, 99–109.

Lovaas, O. I., & Simmons, J. Q. Manipulation of self-destruction in three retarded children. *Journal of Applied Behavior Analysis*, 1969, **2**, 143–157.

Neuringer, C., & Michael, J. L. (Eds.) *Behavior modification in clinical psychology.* New York: Appleton-Century-Crofts, 1970.

O'Leary, K. D., Poulos, R. W., & Devine, V. T. Tangible reinforcers: Bonuses or bribes? *Journal of Consulting and Clinical Psychology*, 1972, **38**, 1–8.

29. The Use of Aversive Stimulation in the Treatment of Chronic Self-Injurious Behavior

George S. Baroff
Bobby G. Tate

Chronic self-injurious behavior is a dramatic form of psychopathology which is seen both in severely retarded and in psychotic children. It consists of relatively repetitive self-hitting which may occur in the absence of obvious environmental determinants giving it, thereby, the quality of stereotyped behavior. Examples of self-injurious activity are hard head banging, slapping and punching of face and head, and kicking, scrátching and biting one's self. A number of workers have sought to explain this bizarre manifestation which has been variously labeled as self-destructive behavior and as masochism, autoaggression, and self-aggression (Cain, 1961; Berkson, in press; Collins, 1965; Dizmang, 1966; Dollard et al., 1939; A. Freud, 1954; Goldfarb, 1945; Greenacre, 1954; Hartmann et al., 1949; Mahler et al., 1959; Sandler, 1964; Zuk, 1960). Our own preference is for the term "self-injurious behavior" (Tate and Baroff, 1966) because it is descriptive rather than interpretive. The term denotes behavior which *results* in physical injury and it does not imply an attempt to hurt the self.

Self-injurious behavior presents formidable management problems as it may prevent the therapist from providing the child with potentially growth-producing social, emotional, educational, and recreational experiences. Failure of adequate control of self-hitting may also lead to permanent injury as in the case reported here. Until recently, the management of such patients was achieved only through physical restraint or through heavy dosages of drugs. In 1964, however, Lovaas et al. reported that chronic self-injurious behavior in schizophrenic children was rapidly reduced by punishing[1] it with painful but physically noninjurious electric shock. The same result with a severely retarded girl has been reported by Ball (1965). The present paper is a description of similar work with a psychotic youngster whose eventual freedom from continuous self-hitting permitted his exposure to other therapeutic endeavors and the possibility of future noninstitutional living.

From *Journal of Child Psychiatry*, 1968, **7**, 454–470. Copyright 1968 by the American Academy of Child Psychiatry. Reproduced by permission.
[1]Punishment in Skinnerian theory as in common parlance refers either to the use of a negative reinforcer (aversive stimulus) or to the withdrawal of a positive reinforcer (rewarding stimulus).

Case Presentation

The Patient

Sam is a nine-year-old boy with a history of self-hitting since age four. His vision is severely impaired due to bilateral cataracts and to one fully and one partially detached retina. It is thought that the fully detached retina was actually caused by self-hitting. Sam is the only child of the mother's second marriage. The pregnancy was unwanted but eventually accepted and the mother states that she looked forward to his birth. His birth weight was seven pounds and periodic examinations by the family pediatrician during the first year revealed normal physical development. From the beginning, Sam's environment was stormy. The father who later was hospitalized with a paranoid psychosis was already quite disturbed and there were two periods when Sam lived with his maternal grandparents. The father is described as a bright but odd person who was extremely critical of the boy. He is characterized as "menacing" and "unpredictable" but not physically abusive. That the latter statement may not be accurate is suggested by Sam's later purportedly inappropriate fear of another adult male, the maternal grandfather. By age two Sam showed deviant reactions to stress; crying was followed by withdrawal and later by confusion and hyperactivity, and language of two-word phrase complexity which had developed gradually disappeared. Sam returned to his maternal grandparents for the second time at age two and a half when his father's condition worsened. The grandmother describes the boy at that time as a very frightened child who screamed in terror at the approach of an adult male. Sam is described as completely abnormal in behavior at the age of two years and eight months; he had no speech, emitted animal-like sounds, and the family pediatrician who had not seen him since age one reported that he was shocked at his appearance. At age four, the self-hitting began. He would punch his face or chest, but the grandmother was able temporarily to control the frequency of this behavior through the use of a football helmet and by placing towel padding on the chest. At this time, diagnosed as a case of infantile autism, he received his first psychiatric care. Sam is said to have benefited from treatment, but the psychiatrist left the hospital and the child rapidly worsened. He began hard head punching and head banging and at age five was admitted to a state hospital where he was described as overactive, agitated, negativistic and disorganized. He was too disturbed to respond to formal psychological testing, but his clinical behavior suggested organicity. With regard to intellectual functioning, a previous psychological examination in connection with his hospitalization at age four is said to have shown evidence of normal intelligence. At the state hospital Sam received extensive individual and group play therapy but without significant effect. Various drugs were tried but produced only temporary gains. The only dependable procedure for preventing self-hitting was physical restraint; the prognosis was considered very poor.

Description of Sam on Admission to Murdoch Center

Our involvement with Sam began with his admission to Murdoch Center, a state institution providing programs for mentally retarded and emotionally disturbed children with which the Department of Psychology of the University of North Carolina has a training affiliation. Sam was initially seen in Murdoch Center's diagnostic clinic where a comprehensive evaluation was conducted prior to our starting to work with him. During a week of study, observations were made by the ward nurse, a social worker, a psychiatrist, and a psychologist. The nurse reported that Sam constantly hit himself when not restrained, except when being fed, and that he occasionally screamed at night. He followed simple directions, used two-word phrases, was only partially toilet trained, sought physical closeness and enjoyed listening to music on the radio. The social worker also observed him on the ward and described him as withdrawn, rocking, moaning, screaming, and face-slapping. The psychiatrist reported that Sam's hitting seemed to increase with anxiety and that when Sam hit himself, it was difficult to avoid making an immediate response which would interfere with the hitting. With regard to Sam's desire for physical closeness, the speculation was offered that this might be due to the blindness itself, to the seeking of external restraint for self-hitting, and for maintaining a sense of self. The psychologist also noted variation in self-hitting according to the degree of anxiety and Sam's possible use of physical closeness as a means of protecting himself from his own self-hitting. The diagnostic impression was of childhood psychosis with autistic and symbiotic features.

Sam's Mother

Sam's mother was our primary informant, and most striking was her difficulty in giving any detailed information about the nature of her interaction with her son. Her description of what must have been a very harrowing existence was marked by detachment. Though she was clearly concerned, the expected affect was lacking. Her psychological evaluation by means of the Minnesota Multiphasic Personality Inventory yielded the picture of a hysterical character who seeks childlike dependency relationships. No psychotic elements were indicated; she showed the classic hysterical picture of *la belle indifférence*.

Preliminary Description of the Self-Injurious Behavior

Although it was difficult to obtain information from the mother, a special effort was made to secure as much material as possible about the self-injurious behavior. To add to the observation of the diagnostic clinic team, we were particularly interested in a description of the self-hitting, the conditions which appeared to elicit and suppress it, the youngster's reaction to presumably noxious stimulation, and apparent attempts at self-restraint. We were also interested in the natural history of the behavior and in those activities which the boy enjoyed. The latter would serve as potential positive reinforcers (rewards) in the work contemplated.

1. Description of symptom: by age nine, Sam's repertoire of self-injurious behavior consisted of face-slapping and punching, hard head banging, striking his shoulder with his chin, and kicking himself. He occasionally punched, bit, and scratched others.

2. Conditions of elicitation: he would hit himself when released from restraint, when angry, frightened, startled, when he desired attention, and when left alone.

3. Conditions of temporary suppression: for at least brief periods hitting was reduced through padding, by actually holding him, and by distracting his attention. It was also noted that hitting was reduced when he was riding in a car. Except for padding and automobile riding, suppression appeared to be associated with some kind of direct adult attention.

4. Response to noxious stimulation: it has been suggested that self-injurious behavior may be associated with diminished pain sensitivity (Mahler et al., 1959), but our observations of Sam's response to pinching and to electric shock indicate that his pain response to external irritants is not grossly altered. In fact, it may well be that the self-hitting *is* experienced as unpleasant but that the intensity of the discomfort is reduced because it serves as a cue to positive reinforcement through attention. That an aversive stimulus can be deprived of its noxious potential when immediately followed by a rewarding one is clearly demonstrated in an experiment of Pavlov summarized by Melzack (1961). While dogs ordinarily respond violently to electric shock to the paw, Pavlov found that by presenting food after the shock, the dog's response to shock was radically altered. Instead of showing discomfort, the dog eventually responded to shock by salivating, wagging its tail, and turning toward the food dish. The dog's conditioned response to a painful stimulus persisted as the intensity of shock was increased and even when shock was supplemented by burning and wounding of the animal's skin. The effect of psychological processes on pain has been discussed by Beecher (1965) and Melzack (1961). The latter views pain as a complex perceptual rather than a purely sensory experience the quality and intensity of which are influenced by past history, by momentary state of mind, and by the *meaning* given to the pain-producing situation.

5. Behavior suggesting attempts at self-restraint: in work with an eighteen-year-old girl who also engages in self-hitting, behavior was often observed which suggested attempts at *self-restraint*. This interesting feature has not been noted in the reports of other investigators and we sought to determine whether it also occurred in Sam. The mother reported that, indeed, when Sam's restraints were accidentally lost, he would put his hands together and approach her holding his hands out as if he wanted the restraints restored. It will also be recalled that the psychiatrist and psycholo-

gist who evaluated Sam in the diagnostic study independently concluded that at least one dimension of the desire for physical closeness was to obtain external control for self-hitting.

We have now observed four individuals who practice self-hitting and three of them show apparent efforts at self-restraint. The eighteen-year-old girl reacts to hand and arm freedom by first striking her face and then either holding her arm rigid on the bed or placing it under her body. Another boy slaps his face and then quickly places his hands beneath his undershirt and against his body. These observations suggest that self-hitting is experienced as an unpleasant event over which the individual has inadequate control. Also consistent with this possibility is the acceptance of relatively long periods of complete physical restraint without apparent discomfort. Finally, we have often seen a rapid disappearance of agitation in Sam following the reinstatement of restraints.

6. Sources of pleasure: Sam is said to enjoy music, motoring, candy, ice cream, being rocked and sung to, and being held.

The Treatment Process

During the first month of Sam's admission, his behavior was observed in a variety of settings and situations. He had a private room in the infirmary and when unattended he was restrained in bed with leather wrist and ankle cuffs. This was necessary in order to prevent further eye injury through self-hitting. During this observation period Sam was cooperative at times and particularly enjoyed activity associated with close physical contact. He followed some verbal directions, but expressive language was quite meager and consisted mainly of unintelligible vocalizations. Two weeks after admission we began a systematic recording of the self-injurious behavior during daily mid-afternoon thirty-minute sessions. Sam's restraints were removed and a research assistant sat next to him on his bed. She placed her arm around him and talked and played with him. The second research assistant recorded all self-hits as well as vocalizations. Much self-injurious behavior occurred and consisted primarily of face-slapping and punching, of striking his shoulder with his chin (accompanied by a loud clucking noise), and, occasionally, hard head banging. Its severity seemed to be associated with his apparent state of agitation and during the first month his average rate of self-hitting was about two blows per minute.

In the second month of his admission, Sam's behavior worsened and the frequency of self-hitting, as recorded during our observation period, increased to an average rate of five blows per minute. There was occasional blooding of the mouth, screaming, and once he struck at a research assistant. The little communicative language that had been present essentially disappeared as his utterances were almost entirely gibberish. During periods of extreme agitation and self-hitting, he had to be restrained in bed and, as noted earlier, this generally resulted in a rapid diminution of distress. At this time a study was undertaken on the effects of presumably pleasurable stimulation (music and a vibrator) on self-hitting. At first these stimuli were presented on a noncontingent basis: that is, they were offered irrespective of his behavior. While some response was evoked, his hit rate was unaffected. Subsequently, an attempt was made to reduce self-hitting by interrupting stimulation as the consequence of a self-hit. This, too, proved ineffective. As the second month ended he began to be very insistent on going outside for walks and showed less interest in play and songs. If his desire for a walk was frustrated, he responded with screaming, self-hitting, and on one occasion he tried to scratch and bite the research assistant.

During the third month he became increasingly uncooperative and the first instance of catatoniclike behavior occurred. While being undressed following an unusually calm walk, he suddenly froze with his hands in the position of a begging dog, eyes wide open and smiling slightly. He remained in this position for many minutes and then suddenly dropped to the floor, banged his head against it and began hitting himself. At about this time he also began retaining spittle in his mouth for long periods.

As we worked with Sam it was evident that he had a great need to maintain close physical contact with people. Separation would result in screaming and self-hitting; it was decided, therefore, to try to employ this powerful reinforcer as a means of controlling his behavior.

Control by Withdrawal and Reinstatement of Physical Contact

A four-week experiment was devised which consisted of applying alternately two different responses to self-hitting that occurred during a twenty-minute walk. In the first and third weeks, the "control" periods, the research assistants made no response to any self-injurious behavior. Sam would walk between them holding their hands and when he hit himself it was ignored. The experimental (punishment) sessions consisted of introducing an aversive consequence to self-hitting by abruptly terminating physical contact with him as soon as he hit himself. Following any self-hit, the research assistants would jerk their hands free and keep them free for three seconds following the hit or for three seconds following the last hit if there were a series of them. Sam's typical response to the sudden loss of contact was to freeze and to remain motionless until his hands were grasped again. During these walks virtually all self-injurious responses were chin-to-shoulder hits. On a few occasions during the "punishment" periods he punched his head, but he rarely withdrew his hand from an assistant and struck himself. The concentration of self-hitting in the form of chin-to-shoulder blows and his reaction to sudden loss of physical contact were probably due to the experimental situation itself. Removed from the familiar surroundings of his room, even a blind child without prominent symbiotic features would be in jeopardy without the assistance of a guide.

The difference in frequency of self-injurious behavior between the two treatment procedures was striking, especially as between the first control and experimental sequences. In the first control sequence the daily rate varied from 5.8 to 8.0 hits per minute with a median rate of 6.6. The introduction of an aversive contingency during the first experimental sequence produced a dramatic and instantaneous reduction in self-hitting to a negligible 0.1 hits per minute, a 66-fold decrease. During the second control sequence the median daily rate was 3.3 hits per minute. The reinstatement of the aversive contingency during the second experimental sequence again resulted in a lowered rate of self-hitting—from 3.3 to 1.0 hits per minute, but the contrast is not as dramatic as between the first control and experimental sequences. Not only was the control rate down by half, but the experimental rate was twice as high. The former may be an extinction phenomenon (due to ignoring the self-hitting), while the latter may reflect some adaptation (loss of fear) to the aversive consequence. In any case the experiment demonstrated that the frequency of self-injurious behavior was a function of how the environment responded to it. Sam's reaction to the alternating conditions also revealed his sensitivity to the environment, his capacity quickly to grasp simple causality, and, most important, *some degree of control* over his self-injurious behavior.

Control by Electric Shock

Although the punishment procedure resulted in less self-hitting, we were concerned that *any* degree of future head banging or face-punching might result in the detachment of the one still possibly salvageable retina and produce irreversible blindness. It was decided, therefore, to try to eliminate the self-hitting as rapidly as possible. Parental and institutional permission were obtained for the use of painful but physically noninjurious electric shock. The shock apparatus is a cattle prod (Sears and Roebuck No. 325971) similar to the one used by Lovaas et al. (1964). Approximately 130 volts are delivered when the prod is touched to the skin. Prior to using this with Sam, the investigators shocked each other and were impressed with its aversive potential; it produced quite a jolt!

Two days after completing the experiment which revealed the effectiveness of punishment by withdrawal of physical contact, the more powerful negative reinforcer (shock) was first employed. Accompanied by a physician and with an assistant recording Sam's behavior, we entered his room. We chatted pleasantly with him and freed his hands but left his feet restrained. As soon as his hands were free he began punching himself in the face and the intensity of self-hitting rapidly increased. A temper tantrum developed during which he screamed, flailed his arms, and banged his head against the railing on the side of the bed. We placed our hands on the railing in order to cushion the blows and prevent real damage. No attempt was made to interfere with the tantrum as we wanted to have a period of free responding which could then be compared with effects of shock. During the six minutes of temper tantrum he hit himself at the rate of fourteen blows per minute,

but this subsided and during the eighteen minutes prior to the first administration of shock the rate was down to two per minute.

The first shock evoked neither cry nor scream but rather a startle which
was followed by whining. After two face hits the type of hitting changed
to chin-to-shoulder blows and each of these was also shocked. He also began
to wince as soon as he struck himself and to try to avoid the shock device,
but there was no vocal indication of extreme distress. As noted earlier, there
is no evidence of grossly altered pain sensitivity, yet while the shock was
clearly aversive to him his reaction to it was less extreme than anticipated.

In the first few minutes four shocks were administered and then there
was a complete cessation of self-hitting. With that, his limbs were freed and
we sat him up in bed, talked and tried to play with him. He was offered
the rocking chair, but he refused it. He was then placed in the rocker and,
in spite of some agitation, he hit himself only once. He was promptly shocked
again after which he settled down, smiled and seemed quite happy.
Quoting from notes of that day, "We stayed with him . . . and were ready
to shock him at any moment he hit himself. It is remarkable how quickly
the hits stopped." During the ninety minutes after the onset of shock there
were only five hits (average rate of 0.06 per minute) and there were none
at all for the last sixty minutes of that period.

We left Sam's room but kept him under observation via closed-circuit
television. During the next ninety-minute observation period only four hits
occurred and these were followed by shock. For the most part he lay quietly
in bed, but he did engage in some manneristic behavior with his hands.
At the end of ninety minutes Sam was offered dinner which he refused.
He was then restrained for the night.

On the next day Sam's restraints were removed at 9:00 A.M. and he was
left completely free but under continuous observation. He spent most of
this time in bed on which some toys were placed, but he was also out of
bed for one hour during which he was encouraged to use a rocker and
to walk around his room. In this five-and-a-half-hour period there were twenty
hits and all were of a light intensity. Each hit was shocked either immediately
or within thirty seconds. The average hit rate was 0.06 per minute which
was identical to that of the first shock day. On the third day Sam's period
of complete freedom from physical restraint was extended to eight and a
half hours (8:00 A.M. to 4:30 P.M.). There were only fifteen hits throughout
the day; an average rate of 0.03 per minute, and most of these occurred
during one period of agitation at noon. He was out of bed for three hours
during which he used the rocking chair, walked, and "played" with toys.

In the ensuing days Sam's freedom from restraint was gradually increased
until he was out of bed nine hours a day. Because of limited personnel
he was still restrained at night, but this did not seem to bother him. He
began attending a class for severely retarded children with major physical
handicaps where he was encouraged to play with a variety of toys. In fact,
he rarely used toys in a constructive manner and his chief interest was in
turning the pages of a magazine. He did, however, enjoy walks and using
swings in a playground area. Wherever Sam went, the person accompanying

him carried the shock stick, but its use became rare. In the nine months following shock, twenty-eight incidents of self-hitting have been reported. Twenty-three of these occurred during the first five months after shock (an average rate of one self-hit in every ten days), while only five have been seen in the last four months (an average rate of one hit in every twenty-four days). Considering that Sam was hitting himself at a rate of two blows per minute on admission to Murdoch Center, the self-injurious behavior can be viewed as essentially eliminated. Self-hitting is no longer a problem; it now occurs so rarely that those attending Sam have long since ceased carrying the shock stick. In short, a pattern of self-injurious behavior which had existed for more than five years, had resulted in blindness in one eye, and had been completely refractory to standard forms of treatment, was interrupted literally within minutes, reduced to a noninjurious minimum within days, and all but disappeared in five months.

Other Behavioral Changes

In addition to Sam's self-hitting, his eating habits and language were of special concern to us. His food and liquid intake had gradually decreased following admission and five days before shock his weight was lower by 14 pounds. On days when he ate nothing he often held large quantities of saliva in his mouth for hours, emptying his mouth only accidentally or under coercion. In the thirty-six hours preceding shock, Sam ate only a small portion of one meal and consumed 400 c.c. of liquids. He refused supper on the first shock day and on the next day consumed nothing except for a little milk and cereal at breakfast. He was again retaining saliva and was also posturing with his hands. On the third post-shock day he refused all food in the morning and appeared very apathetic. At 2:00 P.M. he was offered juice which he refused by turning his head away. He was then told firmly to drink, but he would not open his mouth. At that time, out of our concern for his weight loss and general physical condition, it was decided to threaten him with shock if he did not eat. Simultaneous with the delivery of shock, the shock stick produces a buzz and Sam had previously demonstrated a conditioned fear to that sound. It was decided to couple a firm command to drink with the shock stick buzz, and this resulted in his not averting his mouth, but he still refused to open it. Successive commands followed by the buzz resulted in his opening his mouth and accepting the juice, though he refused to swallow it. A command and a buzz produced the swallowing, and this was continued until he had consumed all of the juice. Verbal praise and affectionate pats followed each desired response. With each step, he was less resistive and by the time he came to his milk he was gulping down large quantities. He fed *himself* the ice cream! It was evident from his eventual "eager eating" that he had been very hungry but was caught in a kind of negativistic bind which the threat of shock had interrupted. This procedure had to be repeated at supper and also during the following day. On the third day, however, he began eating spontaneously. In similar fashion posturing and saliva-holding were quickly eliminated and were not replaced with other symptoms. Subsequently there has been only one other episode of prolonged fasting and this was similarly terminated. For the first seven months after shock, Sam's behavior at mealtimes was quite variable. Often he ate well, but on other occasions he was quite balky and much prompting was necessary. Meals became the one place where negativistic behavior was likely to occur. In the last two months, however, this has also largely disappeared apparently in conjunction with a generalized state of well-being.

With the cessation of hitting following shock, a program of language training was undertaken in which we were shortly joined by a speech therapist. Our initial attempts to evoke appropriate sounds and words on command (imitative speech) were notably unsuccessful and the speech therapist lost interest, observing that Sam's attention span was too limited.[Procedures for obtaining speech consisted primarily of positive reinforcement using as rewards sugar flakes, food at mealtimes, and attention, but some *ad hoc* use was also made of negative reinforcement.] Here the relief of distress was contingent on the use of words that were known to be in his repertoire. The effect was to increase the degree of vocalization but in the form of sounds and not words. Since Sam had, in the past, spontaneously used some two-word phrases, the possibility of willful refusal to emit speech was entertained. As the first period of intensive language work ended it was our impression that, in spite of some spontaneously used appropriate speech, he was unable to produce the same sounds and words imitatively. As pressure for speech was reduced, energies were redirected both toward reducing his negativism at meals and his clinging behavior.[Two months after the end of the first period of language training, an increase in the spontaneous use of new words was noted, e.g., "cookie, ice cream, more." This stimulated us to resume speech work and, with the exception of two episodes of obvious negativism, his response has been increasingly positive. Now appearing were two-word phrases which included an adjective or a verb as well as a noun, e.g., "more milk, more patty-cake, go outdoors, do nothing." Sam cooperated readily in giving words on demand; he appeared to enjoy these sessions and was very attentive. Intelligibility of his speech was also increasing. We were again using positive reinforcers and the sugar flakes were considered the most powerful of the incentives. Within another month Sam was repeating on command, "take me outside." Such sentences were *not* used spontaneously, but were more complex equivalents of two-word phrases. In the last two months talking has become a highly preferred activity. Sam requests the research assistants to initiate "talking" which he seems to view as a game.]

A review of Sam's language behavior sheds some light on our earlier perplexity over his failure to produce on command what he had uttered spontaneously. Sam had achieved a degree of verbal competence in two types of settings. Words were occasionally used spontaneously and appropriately to effect some need-reducing action on the part of others, and words were understood in the context of following verbal directions. Each of these conditions was unidirectional from a speech standpoint since words were reinforced by *actions* and not by other *words*. When Sam was asked to repeat words on command, a word-word sequence, we were asking him to use words in a context which differed from those in which he had previously achieved some competence. This highly particularized or contextual use of words suggests that Sam lacks the *concept* of words. This inference is not offered as an explanation of Sam's lack of imitative language since children can imitate speech before they have presumably attained the concept of words or of the speech process itself. The most parsimonious explanation offered here for the unevenness of Sam's language development is that speech in the service of need reduction was reinforced but that speech-speech sequences were not. This formulation has, of course, direct treatment implications.

Summary

Problems historically associated with the use of punishment have right-fully generated an accent on love, tenderness, and understanding in our child-rearing and treatment procedures. The results of the present study as well as those of other investigators (Lovaas et al., 1964; Ball, 1965) would suggest, however, that to this armamentarium can be added punishment as a potentially effective means of rapidly modifying unacceptable behavior in psychotic children. Our aversion to punishment stems, in part, from what Solomon (1964) has described as persisting legends concerning both the ineffectiveness of punishment as an agent of behavioral change as well as the inevitability of a neurotic outcome as a legacy of all punishment procedures.

In the present study, punishment dramatically reduced and essentially eliminated chronic self-injurious behavior in a blind psychotic boy. Relatively mild punishment associated with the withdrawal of physical contact contingent on self-hitting was more effective than ignoring the behavior while physically noninjurious but painful electric shock resulted in almost immediate cessation of behavior that had existed for more than five years. Behavioral control has been maintained for nine months and it has been possible for the boy to participate in therapeutic activities which were hitherto impossible because of the need for physical restraint. Punishment with electric shock also prevented accidental reinforcement of self-hitting. Before treatment began, self-hitting was often suppressed by sitting behind him and placing one's arms about him. While this was clearly reinforcing to him and may be a function of his symbiotic level of development, one would certainly hope that Sam could learn less destructive techniques for obtaining close physical contact.

Punishment not only rapidly eliminated self-hitting, but it was found that the threat of punishment signaled by the association of a buzz with shock could reinstate eating and terminate posturing and saliva-saving. Of special significance, except for the creation of a phobic response to buzzing sounds, no deleterious effects of shock have been observed.

Punishment did not produce a dog-in-the-manger attitude. Sam "understood" the bargain that was made; he apparently expected to be punished for behavior which punishment itself had revealed could be suppressed. Further, he had no way of judging the appropriateness of the punishment itself. If some of the hostility which may be engendered by punishment stems from failure to understand why one is being punished, this element was absent in the present situation.

Not only did punishment not evoke anger; on the contrary, we were struck by the rapid brightening of mood which frequently followed punishment. During experimental sequences when punishment was used, Sam was described as "bright-eyed and bushy-tailed" in contrast to a whining negativistic mood when self-hitting was ignored. Was this oft-observed association between fear-induced cessation of hitting (punishment) and mood change causal or are they concomitant effects? At this time no formulation is offered in which we have any conviction, but we hope to make this phenomenon the object of future investigation. One might posit "attention" as the key, because it was only under the punishment condition that Sam's caretakers responded promptly, albeit aversively, to his self-hitting. But if attention per se was rewarding, then the rate of hitting under punishment would have increased rather than decreased! One can also speculate that punishment resulted in the interruption (short-circuiting) of tension which Sam could not himself reduce and which, in nonpunishment situations (self-hitting ignored), was associated with increased frustration, irritability, and self-hitting. Here, cessation of hitting and mood change would be construed as concomitant effects. Punishment in this context could be conceived of as a high intensity stimulus of very brief duration which has the effect of breaking up an ongoing state of discomfort which the organism cannot itself reduce.

Reference

Ausubel, D. P. (1950), Negativism as a phase of ego development. *Amer. J. Orthopsychiat.*, 20:796–805.

Ball, T. S. (1965), Personal communication.

Beecher, H. K. (1965), Quantification of the subjective pain experience. In: *Psychopathology of Perception*, ed. P. H. Hoch & J. Zubin. New York: Grune & Stratton, pp. 111–128.

Berkson, G. (in press), Abnormal stereotyped motor acts. In: *Comparative Psychopathology*, ed. J. Zubin & H. Hunt. New York: Grune & Stratton.

Cain, A. C. (1961), The presuperego 'turning-inward' of aggression. *Psychoanal. Quart.*, 30:171–208.

Collins, D. T. (1965), Head-banging: its meaning and management in the severely retarded adult. *Bull. Menninger Clin.*, 29:205–211.

Dizmang, L. H. (1966), Ending the hopelessness surrounding "headbangers." [Roche Report] *Frontiers of Hosp. Psychiat.*, 3.

Dollard, J., Doob, L. W., Miller, N. E., Mowrer, O. H., & Sears, R. R. (1939), *Frustration and Aggression*. New Haven: Yale University Press.

Freud, A. (1954), In: Problems of infantile neurosis: a discussion. *The Psychoanalytic Study of the Child*, 9:16–71. New York: International Universities Press.

Goldfarb, W. (1945), Psychological privation in infancy and subsequent adjustment. *Amer. J. Orthopsychiat.,* 15:247–255.

Greenacre, P. (1954), In: Problems of infantile neurosis: a discussion. *The Psychoanalytic Study of the Child,* 9:16–71. New York: International Universities Press.

Hartmann, H., Kris, E., & Loewenstein, R. M. (1949), Notes on the theory of aggression. *The Psychoanalytic Study of the Child,* 3/4:9–36. New York: International Universities Press.

Lovaas, O. I., Freitag, G., Kinder, M. I., Rubenstein, D. B., Schaeffer, B., & Simmons, J. B. (1964), Experimental studies in childhood schizophrenia: developing social behavior using electric shock. Paper read at American Psychological Association, Annual Convention, Los Angeles, California.

Mahler, M. S., Furer, M., & Settlage, C. F. (1959), Severe emotional disturbances in childhood: psychosis. In: *American Handbook of Psychiatry,* ed. S. Arieti. New York: Basic Books, pp. 816–839.

Melzack, R. (1961), The perception of pain. *Sci. American,* 204 (2):41–49.

Sandler, J. (1964), Masochism: an empirical analysis. *Psychol. Bull.,* 62:197–204.

Solomon, R. L. (1964), Punishment. *Amer. Psychologist,* 19:239–253.

Tate, B. G. & Baroff, G. S. (1966), Aversive control of self-injurious behavior in a psychotic boy. *Behav. Res. & Ther.,*4:281–287.

Zuk, G. H. (1960), Psychodynamic implications of self-injury in defective children and adults. *J. Clin. Psychol.,* 16:58–60.

30. Aversive Control in the Treatment of Elective Mutism

William H. Shaw

Elective mutism is a relatively rare childhood behavior pattern for which a variety of explanations have been propounded and treatment methods tried (Pustrom and Speers, 1964; Elson et al., 1965). In recent years, learning theory principles have been applied in the treatment of some cases: these have mostly taken the forms of social reinforcement and nonreinforcement (Reed, 1963; Straughan et al., 1965). In the case to be presented, the systematic use of a noxious stimulus was the essential element in a successful treatment program. This method involved practical, theoretical, and ethical issues.

Case Report: Wilma

This girl was born in Holland, the fourth of six children, and the younger of two girls, to a family which valued emotional control and verbal reserve. Her mother was strong, stoical, and quietly authoritative; her father was

From *Journal of Child Psychiatry*, 1971, **10**, 572–581. Copyright 1971 by the American Academy of Child Psychiatry. Reproduced by permission.

inadequate, excitable, talkative, and dependent on his wife. Wilma was an attractive but self-contained child, whose speech development in Dutch was quite normal. When she was 2½ years old, the family moved to an English-speaking community in Canada. Her father's dreams of prospering failed repeatedly in the ensuing years, and he blamed this on his difficulty in learning the new language. Unlike her sister and brothers, Wilma did not begin to speak English, although she continued to use Dutch normally. When she was aged 3 to 5 her older sister had a period of elective mutism confined to the school setting; this behavior was forcibly terminated by corporal punishment at school. Wilma was aware of this at the time. She told her brothers that she intended never to speak English, and after starting school herself she made good this undertaking. She also began a progressive reduction in the number of Dutch-speaking people to whom she would use even that language. From age 8 onward, she spoke only to members of her immediate family, and exclusively in Dutch, although by now English was the language generally used in her home. She became increasingly rejecting of her father, while still apparently admiring and identifying with her mother and older sister. Her academic progress over the years was normal, apart from her persistent silence, for which she was physically punished at least twice by school staff members. At age 7 and again at age 9 she was referred to the local mental health clinic, but she and her parents failed to cooperate in outpatient treatment. At age 10½, following the third such referral, her parents consented to her admission to Thistletown Hospital (Rexdale, Ontario).

In the hospital her manner was self-possessed and reserved. Although rather rigid and independent-seeming, Wilma conformed smoothly to most hospital routines and presented no behavior problems. She came to be recognized as an intelligent, capable, self-sufficient girl, and although she was sometimes haughty with the other children, she gained unique prestige and influence among them. Although she refused to cooperate in formal psychological testing, she did do a Metropolitan Achievement Test, on which at age 11 she scored at the grades 9 and 10 level in English language skills. However, despite months of speech therapy, individual psychotherapy, and milieu therapy, Wilma's mutism stubbornly persisted.

Meanwhile, a number of tentative inferences had been made regarding intrafamilial factors contributing to the development of her elective mutism. These included: the "strong, silent" mother, the inadequate father blaming his failures on having to learn to speak English, and the example of her older sister's mutism. While these factors may have been causative originally, it seemed that Wilma's mutism had come to have an independent life of its own, now mainly related to other forces. It was hypothesized that a major current obstacle to her normal use of English speech was the fact that most of her repertoire of social behavior had been built up around the maladaptive practice of mutism, the abandonment of which would therefore be difficult and probably anxiety-provoking for her. More obviously (but ultimately less significantly) passive aggressiveness was also involved. There were on the other hand a number of indications that she had some desire to begin using speech appropriately—to deepen her relationships with a few preferred staff members, to get out of the hospital, and to live as a normal teen-ager in the years to come.

At the beginning of her second year in the hospital, Wilma was started on a series of twice-weekly intravenous injections of amobarbital sodium (7½ gr.) and methamphetamine hydrochloride (30 mg.) aimed at helping her overcome her presumably strong inhibitions regarding speech (Delay, 1949; Houston, 1952). After four weeks the amobarbital sodium was stopped, but she continued to receive twice-weekly injections of methamphetamine hydrochloride (20 mg. I.V.), and showed a consistently intense dislike of these. After three weeks of this treatment Wilma finally whispered her first word since admission. This occurred in a secluded site away from the hospital, when she was alone with her favorite staff member, who was putting great pressure on her to speak as a proof of their friendship; as Wilma spoke a single English word ("yes") in a whisper, her manner was very tense, self-conscious, and furtive.

During the next few months further progress was only minimal, confined to single words spoken in private to the same counselor on a few occasions. Even this output ceased entirely when injections were temporarily discontinued, but resumed when injections were resumed. Significantly, it began to appear not only that the small gains were indeed related to the methamphetamine hydrochloride injections, but also that this effect was based on her perceiving them as punishment for nonspeech—punishment which she was trying to avoid by producing this minimal speech.

It was decided to try exploiting more systematically this apparent effect of the injections. A formal program was set up in which her verbal output was to be expanded gradually toward normal. At the outset of this program her verbal behavior showed the following characteristics: whispered voice, single-word utterances, at a frequency much less than once daily, addressed to a single well-liked adult female without witnesses, in secluded locations. These characteristics represented the extreme ends of a number of continua through which she was expected to move toward the normal use of speech. The program involved specific daily expectations regarding her verbal behavior, with periodic upgradings related to these continua. Each day's minimal speech requirements were made explicit to her, as was the condition that if she did not meet these requirements by bedtime, she would receive an injection (methamphetamine hydrochloride, 20 mg. I.V.) on the following morning. This program was carefully explained to her at the outset. She was subsequently given explicit information regarding each successive expansion in requirements, and her progress was frequently reviewed with her.

This program lasted seven months. Wilma's early speech had a definite Dutch accent, which faded only gradually. She continued speaking in a whisper for several months, until a more normal voice was formally required from her. Although she continued to show a consistently strong dislike of the injections, her attitude to the program otherwise seemed more often positive than negative. On most days she spoke first (thereby satisfying the formal requirement of speech at least once daily) during the first half of her waking hours. When by thus speaking as required she won a day's reprieve from injection, her feeling of relief was usually apparent. With each successive expansion in her verbal behavior (whether use of more normal speech, or use of speech in more normal situations) she initially showed tension, hesitation, and self-consciousness. These reactions cleared on subsequent repetitions, and the gains were maintained spontaneously thereafter. The threat of injection could thereupon be related to yet a further expansion.

Although Wilma was not formally required to speak more than once daily (expansions being instead confined to how, where, and to whom she spoke), she exceeded this required minimal frequency increasingly often as the months passed. At the same time, she was increasingly able to avoid the potentially daily injections—eight injections being needed during the first month, six during the next three months, and only two in the last three months. As her conversation expanded and became more spontaneous, she began to give spoken confirmation of a number of the assumptions on which the program was based. She emphatically confirmed that she found the injections noxious, because they made her feel extremely "dizzy." She confirmed that avoidance of these injections was her main immediate motive for each expansion in her verbal behavior, and glumly acknowledged that she felt the injections were necessary for her progress. Regarding her difficulty in expanding her speech, she once exclaimed to her favorite counselor, "You expect too much of me! It's easy for you, but not for me!"

Normal social reinforcers appeared to play an increasingly important role in conditioning Wilma's speech as the months passed. Once they saw that she was really able to speak, staff members could more easily make mutism difficult for her by declining to respond to nonverbal communication. However, despite social pressures, her progress lapsed during two periods in which the threat of injections was removed (once on a trial basis, and once when the author was absent on vacation).

Wilma's progress in speech was accompanied by an increase in her spontaneous use of vivacious gestures and facial expressions, and by an increasingly outgoing and cooperative attitude. For example, after her previous persistent refusal, she now calmly permitted dental work to be done. She also agreed to a limited amount of psychometric testing, obtaining a full-scale score of 120 (Verbal 111, Performance 125) on the WISC, and scoring at the 97th percentile on the Raven Matrices. After seven months, it was possible to remove the threat of injections permanently, and ordinary social reinforcers now proved sufficient to continue shaping her verbal behavior toward normal. On the California Test of Personality, done at this time, the main findings were "a relatively high sense of personal worth and personal freedom." On a visit to her home community a few months later, she used English speech appropriately, and her discharge from the hospital followed soon after.

On follow-up one year after discharge Wilma was found to be maintaining normal adjustment in her home, community, and school. She was using speech appropriately in all settings, had closer relationships with other family members and normal relationships with peers, was making very good academic progress, had participated in a public spelling contest, and was captain of a baseball team.

Discussion

The anxiety Wilma clearly showed with each new expansion in her use of speech confirmed our working hypothesis that a major reason for the persistence of her mutism was that the experience of speech was anxiety-provoking for her. Removing this restraint would not alone have immediately enabled her to start using English speech appropriately. Her history indicated that she had no experience in speaking English, and her initially accented speech confirmed this. She also had to learn to use spoken English (and to rebuild much of her social repertoire accordingly).

[The formal treatment program consisted of a series of rising expectations in her use of English speech, with failures to meet daily requirements resulting in punishment by injections. What directly promoted her progress was not the injections, however, since these were relatively infrequent (only sixteen in seven months) and delayed so long (until the following morning) as not to have had a direct effect. The function of the injections was essentially an indirect one, that of sustaining the *threat* of injection. The periodic injections served to establish this threat situation as a conditioned aversive stimulus, and their decreasing frequency over the months presumably reflected at least in part the progressive strengthening of the conditioning. (Other factors contributing to this decreasing frequency probably included: increasing adaptation to the total situation of the program, increasing motivation, and increasing influence of social reinforcement.)]

This daily renewed threat situation became sufficiently aversive that on a large and increasing majority of days Wilma sought relief by speaking as required, usually early in the day. The anxiety-provoking experience of speaking was thus accompanied virtually daily by the relief associated with the termination of an aversive stimulus, and this event appeared to have two results: the operant of speech was reinforced, and the experience of speaking was paired with "aversion relief," a response incompatible with anxiety (Thorpe et al., 1964; Solyom and Miller, 1967). That operant conditioning occurred, with shaping of her speech in English through successive approximations to normal, is evidenced by the increasing frequency of speech (beyond formal requirements), and by its progressive changes from whispered to normal vocal tone, and from single-word utterances to normal sentences. That aversion relief was conditioned to the experience of speaking, progressively replacing anxiety (or in Wolpeian terms reciprocally inhibiting it), is indicated by the increasing spontaneity of her speech, and by her decreasing anxiety with subsequent exposures to each situation, starting with an audience of one favored female adult far from the hospital, and progressing up the stimulus-generalization gradient. In brief, Wilma's speech training involved both classical conditioning (threat situation becoming a conditioned aversive stimulus) and operant conditioning (speech being reinforced by termination of this conditioned aversive stimulus), and it thus exemplified Mowrer's (1950) two-factor learning model. The operant learning component would probably be more precisely described in this case as escape conditioning than as avoidance conditioning (Appel, 1964).

This conditioning method partly resembles those reported by Thorpe et al. (1964) and by Solyom and Miller (1967), who used "aversion relief" successfully with phobic patients, and by Lazarus (1959) with a 10-year-old boy afraid to sleep in his own bed. However, these cases differ from the present one, in that these patients' anxieties were associated with stimuli rather than with an operant (except in Solyom and Miller's case of Mr. B. M.), the only aversive stimulus used was an unconditioned one (electric shock), and operant conditioning of skilled behavior was not involved.

The use of aversive stimuli is usually held to be unsuitable in dealing with behaviors based on anxiety. Mowrer and Kluckhohn (1944) observed that if a subject has learned to make a particular avoidance act when in a state of anxiety, punishing that act may strengthen it by increasing the anxiety. Wolpe (1958, p. 116) described the imaginary case of a student fearful of speaking out in group discussion being forced to speak by the threat of a beating, but not benefiting because being driven by fear into the feared situation had if anything strengthened his fearful reactivity. For a similar reason, Jones (1961) referred to the punishment of responses mediated by a conditioned avoidance drive (such as anxiety) as being an undesirable technique even if effective. Schmidt (1964) found negative reinforcement to be the least effective method of modifying a highly anxious patient's verbal responses. Beech (1960) reported that the higher the patient's level of anxiety, the worse were the results of avoidance conditioning. Sloane et al. (1965) found that their neurotic subjects showed a heightened autonomic arousability and conditionability which seemed to impair their ability to learn volitionally to perform avoidance behavior, and suggested that therapy of the introverted neurotic patient should thus include alleviation of his anxiety or arousability. In Wilma's case anxiety was being offset by aversion relief, which thus tended to exempt her from the above warnings regarding aversive control.

According to Holland and Skinner (1961), it is poor technique to employ aversive stimuli in shaping skillful behavior because such stimuli elicit emotional responses which interfere with the development of all but comparatively simple behavior patterns. Presumably this applied less in Wilma's case because her learning of English speech was greatly facilitated by her possession of English language and Dutch speech, and again because her anxiety responses were being counteracted by aversion relief.

The outcome of Wilma's treatment was influenced by a variety of other factors less closely related to the formal conditioning program. Confined to the hospital, she was forced for the first time in her life to be dependent on English-speaking people outside her family. Although ambivalent about changing, she was increasingly motivated to secure her discharge by losing her mutism, and to begin life as a normal girl at last. While still in the hospital, she came to realize that only by speech could she deepen her relationships with a few preferred staff members. Pressure from her favorite counselor was probably crucial in her emitting the initial modicum of speech on which the conditioning program was based. Staff members made important contributions by reinforcing mutism less and less, and by encouraging and facilitating her avoidance of punishment, and this probably also strengthened her ties with them, as was observed in the studies of Lovaas et al. (1965, p. 99): "affectionate and other social behaviors towards adults increased after adults had been associated with shock reduction." However helpful or even necessary all these factors were, they were not sufficient to overcome her mutism without the formal conditioning program, as was clearly shown by the abrupt total standstills while the program was twice temporarily suspended. Only after seven months were these other influences able to sustain her progress. While it has been observed that stimulant drugs tend to facilitate conditioning (Franks, 1961), such an effect must have been negligible in this case, since Wilma received methamphetamine hydrochloride injections on only a relatively few occasions.

Elective mutism is probably not a single entity, but involves different causes in different cases (Reed, 1963). Apart from original intrafamilial factors, and the continuing influence of her passive aggressiveness, Wilma's case appears to have represented one major cause increasingly over the years: mutism as avoidance behavior when speech is too anxiety-provoking. This cause applied in the second of Reed's two groups of elective mutes, those who may have learned mutism as a "fear-reducing mechanism," and her personality more closely resembled those in that category (more tense and watchful, striving, and concerned about their condition). Her mutism was, however, more fixed and long-standing than in Reed's cases (or the vast majority of other reported cases), and her treatment had to include something in addition to the social reinforcements and nonreinforcements employed by Reed. The decisive additional measure involved physical punishment. It is properly held that punishment has only a very limited role to play in the psychiatric treatment of children (Alderton, 1967). In the circumstances of Wilma's case, however, it was considered to be justified: for years she had spoken only within her family circle, other forms of treatment tried had failed, and with the persistence of her mutism her social adjustment would have surely become increasingly deviant, and fixed as such. Significantly, neither the repeated use of punishment nor the loss of her mutism resulted in adverse emotional reactions or symptom substitutions.

Summary

Learning theory principles were decisively involved in the successful treatment of a case of elective mutism, long-standing and resistant to other measures. The patient was a girl, 12 years of age at the time of the formal conditioning program, which lasted seven months and involved progressive expansions in her use of speech, with failure to meet specific daily requirements resulting in an aversive injection the following morning. Her mutism was judged to reflect anxiety about speaking. It appeared that the daily renewed threat situation became a conditioned aversive stimulus, which her speech automatically terminated, resulting in both operant conditioning of her speech and counteraction of the anxiety by aversion relief.

References

Alderton, H. R. (1967), The role of punishment in the in-patient treatment of psychiatrically disturbed children. *Canad. Psychiat. Assn. J.,* 12:17–24.

Appel, J. B. (1964), Analysis of aversively motivated behavior. *Arch. Gen. Psychiat.,* 10:71–83.

Beech, H. R. (1960), The symptomatic treatment of writer's cramp. In: *Behaviour Therapy and the Neuroses,* ed. H. J. Eysenck. Oxford: Pergamon Press, pp. 349–372.

Delay, J. (1949), Sur les explorations pharmacodynamiques en psychiatrie: narco-analyse et choc amphétaminique. *Proc. Roy. Soc. Med.,* 42:491–496.

Elson, A., Pearson, C., Jones, C. D., & Schumacher, E. (1965), Follow-up study of childhood elective mutism. *Arch. Gen. Psychiat.,* 13:182–187.

Franks, C. M. (1961), Conditioning and abnormal behaviour. In: *Handbook of Abnormal Psychology,* ed. H. J. Eysenck. New York: Basic Books, pp. 457–487.

Holland, J. G. & Skinner, B. F. (1961), *The Analysis of Behavior.* New York: McGraw-Hill.

Houston, F. (1952), A preliminary investigation into abreaction comparing methedrine and sodium amytal with other methods. *J. Ment. Sci.* 98:707–710.

Jones, H. G. (1961), Applied abnormal psychology: the experimental approach. In: *Handbook of Abnormal Psychology,* ed. H. J. Eysenck. New York: Basic Books, pp. 764–781.

Lazarus, A. A. (1959), The elimination of children's phobias by deconditioning. In: *Experiments in Behaviour Therapy,* ed. H. J. Eysenck. New York: Macmillan, 1964, pp. 467–474.

Lovaas, O. I., Schaeffer, B., & Simmons, J. Q. (1965), Building social behavior in autistic children by use of electric shock. *J. Exp. Res. Pers.,* 1:99–109.

Mowrer, O. H. (1950), *Learning Theory and Personality Dynamics.* New York: Ronald Press.

— & Kluckhohn, C. (1944), Dynamic theory of personality. In: *Personality and the Behavior Disorders,* ed. J. McV. Hunt. New York: Ronald Press, 1:69–135.

Pustrom, E. & Speers, R. W. (1964), Elective mutism in children. *This Journal,* 3:287–297.

Reed, G. F. (1963), Elective mutism in children: a reappraisal. *J. Child. Psychol. Psychiat.,* 4:99–107.

Schmidt, E. (1964), A comparative evaluation of verbal conditioning and behaviour training in an individual case. *Behav. Res. Ther.,* 2:19–26.

Sloane, R. B., Davidson, P. O., Staples, F., & Payne, R. W. (1965), Experimental reward and punishment in neurosis. *Compreh. Psychiat.,* 6:388–395.

Solyom, L. & Miller, S. B. (1967), Reciprocal inhibition by aversion relief in the treatment of phobias. *Behav. Res. Ther.,* 5:313–324.

Straughan, J. H., Potter, W. K., Jr., & Hamilton, S. H., Jr. (1965), The behavioral treatment of an elective mute. *J. Child Psychol. Psychiat.,* 6:125–130.

Thorpe, J. G., Schmidt, E., Brown, P. T., & Castell, D. (1964), Aversion-relief therapy: a new method for general application. *Behav. Res. Ther.,* 2:71–82.

Wolpe, J. (1958), *Psychotherapy by Reciprocal Inhibition.* Stanford: Stanford University Press.

31. A Case for the Selective Reinforcement of Punishment

Donald M. Baer

Dr. Kushner has presented us with some intriguing examples of a relatively new technique applicable to clinical problems. He has been able to show good results with this technique. He has also cited similar recent work by other researchers in the field, much of which showed similar results. He has pointed to an extensive area of earlier research with animals using analogous techniques, out of which this human application was derived. Finally, he has been able to show that both the animal experiments and the recent human applications can be related to a common body of theory concerning the behavior of organisms in general.

By the usual standards of science, there ought to be delight and applause throughout the relevant clinical and research communities. Consider: a problem area of human suffering has been attacked, by bringing new ideas to it from what might be a closely related area of knowledge. The attack has proceeded in a responsible manner, first by repeated and intensive experimentation with laboratory animals; then, following promising results in that effort, by cautious applications to human cases typically not responding well to standard methods of treatment. The human applications have often been made in hospital settings under the scrutiny of concerned professionals, and when necessary have sacrificed good experimental design to the interests of the patient's best welfare. All of that, I suggest, is the essence of good and responsible science devoted to man's benefit. Had the technique in question been a vaccination to immunize us from cancer, there would indeed have been delight and applause. The delight would have been tempered by our standard scientific uneasiness about using a technique not yet completely understood, but that would simply have led to further research efforts in all relevant directions, and the applause, I think, would have been undiminished.

In this particular case, I wonder whether there will be that sort of celebration throughout the relevant communities, or whether uneasiness will be the prepotent response. Preliminary sorts of observations over the last few years suggest the latter to me. This case is different because the name of the technique is not *vaccination* but *punishment*.

Punishment is something that we may think we know a lot about, and none of it good. My own field of specialization is child development. In that

Reprinted from C. Neuringer and J. L. Michael (Eds.), *Behavior Modification in Clinical Psychology.* Copyright © 1970. By permission of Appleton-Century-Crofts, Educational Division, Meredith Corporation.

field, I am repeatedly jarred by statements of the form, "We know that punishing a child is worse than ineffective . . . " We know? My students are being taught that we *know* what we can demonstrate. They are probably happy with Dr. Kushner's report, because it is full of demonstrations and references to demonstrations with rather good consistency in what they show. I hope that my students are also uneasy about not possessing a complete understanding of punishment and its total effect on human behavior. However, their squirming should mean only that they wish I would be quiet soon so that they can politely return to the lab and try to answer some of the unanswered questions by demonstrations of their own. I mean to humor them in this ambition; I have only a few points to make here, and they are essentially moralistic rather than scientific points. Moralistic points are typically brief, perhaps because they require no experimental design.

I have suggested that we know what we can demonstrate. I have also suggested that we *think* we know that punishment is inherently a bad technique for accomplishing desirable behavioral changes. But Dr. Kushner's demonstrations and the others that he cites suggest the opposite: Punishment may be a very desirable technique indeed for accomplishing certain behavioral changes. If there is a moral point here, it is the one familiar to all scientists and practitioners alike: we had better get what we know in line with what we can demonstrate. That leads in a very straightforward way to a deduction: We had better continue a careful and extensive study of the punishment of human behavior. But if I read the feeling of the field correctly, there will be objections to continuing these demonstrations, as there have been objections in the past, and are today. It will be a shame if, consequently, the demonstrations are not pursued as extensively as our current curiosity and ignorance press us to do.

It will be even more of a shame if objections to such research on punishment are intrinsically confused in their own moral stance. Suppose, for example, that I show you a child, institutionalized as a retardate, who has over the years developed a very successful attention-compelling behavior—self-destruction. Suppose that in this case, the child pulls persistently at his ear and has finally come to the point where, if he is unrestrained, he will in fact literally rip it from his head. He has, let us say, half succeeded in this venture already. As a result, he wears a straightjacket throughout the hours of his existence, and he is so heavily tranquilized that he lies in a semi-stupor gazing vacantly at the ceiling. I suggest that he was taught this performance. He was reinforced for ear-tugging rather than for other, more desirable behaviors, because his caretakers were busy and could ignore acceptable behavior more easily than self-destructive behavior. Successively in their busy lives, they became used to his current self-destructive behavior, so that only when it was more self-destructive than usual would they consider that they must do something. Thereby, they reinforced intense self-destruction rather than mild self-destruction. Had they designed a shaping program to instruct the child in his own destruction, they could hardly have proceeded better. Note the systematic care with which they taught him to endure greater and greater pain in return for a few seconds of their attention.

Note that they used some of the cheapest reinforcers available to them: a little glancing at the child, a modest amount of vocal noise, and some brief laying on of hands. A moral onlooker to this process, if he understood it as such, might understandably display anger and indignation. Do we institutionalize our retarded children so that they may be taught, as cheaply as possible, to approach their own self-destruction; and do we then frustrate them on the brink of accomplishment in favor of the living death of 24-hour-per-day restraints or the half-living death of 24-hour-per-day stupor?

Certainly not by design. Yet it is strange how often it works to the same outcome, design or no design. No doubt we may escape the onlooker's moral indignation by pointing out that we meant well, and that we had no idea that response differentiation could be accomplished that easily with so simple a stimulus as human attentiveness, even in settings where attentiveness is rare. We may even point out that the whole indictment is, after all, only a hypothesis. (This last point is in fact a strong one, because the hypothesis is unlikely ever to be proven directly. I am unaware of any behavior therapist who would shape a child to pull his ear off his head, just to prove how easily it could be done by social influence in an institutional setting.)

However, we may not so easily escape the next moral trap. That is the one which becomes possible when our behavior therapist colleagues appear, apparatus in hand. They note the existence of self-destroyers in our institution, and wonder if they might not end that horror with some carefully applied aversive faradic controls. Some of us will be very interested until we discover that they mean electric shock. If we refuse *because* they mean electric shock, then I suggest that we have fallen thoroughly into the moral trap. In our professional wisdom, we have assigned people to institutional life, allowed them to be taught their own self-destruction, and confined them to a small hell in consequence. Can we now refuse that they endure a small number of painful episodes over a short span of sessions, hopefully designed to let them live the rest of their lives awake and untied?

My example is extreme. However, the behavior therapist is knocking at doors other than those of the institutions, and he is asking about behaviors other than those that are clearly self-destructive. Nevertheless, the moral formula (as best I can discern with training only in psychology) is much the same in any case. Is not a small number of brief painful experiences a reasonable exchange for escape from a life indefinitely distorted by durable maladjustment? It seems to me that this question changes only a little in its meaning, even when the form of maladjustment varies from the grave problems of self-destruction, drug addiction, and alcoholism to such quirks as excessive blinking. As many as twenty shocks over a few sessions may be greatly preferred to a lifetime of social handicap brought about by the fact that people think you look absurd blinking away like that—especially when they find themselves beginning to blink, too, and decide to keep away from you.

Am I arguing that a better life is an end which justifies a means to that end even as immoral as punishment? Clinical practice is too complicated, I believe, to allow even that simple formula to apply. *Not to rescue a person from an unhappy organization of his behavior is to punish him, in that it leaves him in a state of recurrent punishment.* The punishment may not be faradic, but apparently it hurts nonetheless. When the seventy-seventh girl that you have met starts edging away, staring strangely as you blink furiously on to new achievements in rate, then I think that in your misery you may ask your therapist some pressing questions. Among these should be the following:

1. Why won't you shock those blinks out of me? People hurt me when I blink at them; they do it every day and have done so for years; and either I turn into a hermit or they will keep hurting me the rest of my life.
2. All right, you're going to do it with positive methods instead. How long will it take?
3. All right, you're going after the real dynamics, not just the symptoms. How long will it take?

That question, *How long will it take?* is the morally critical question, in my opinion. For as time goes by while the therapist tries his hopefully more benevolent or more basic methods, the patient still undergoes punishment while he waits for a good outcome. In effect, the therapist has assigned the patient to a punishment condition from which he might have long since removed him. This robs that therapist of any *moral* superiority over another therapist who will assign the patient to shock punishment so that he may escape from social punishment. The basic questions would seem to be, which punishment is tougher, and which lasts longer? We have merely a bookkeeping problem here, not a moral one.

Is it really true that the therapist might have removed the patient from a socially punishing condition, by shocking his blinks out of him in a few brief sessions? Dr. Kushner's studies, and those of others, suggest that it may very well be true, at least sometimes. If we object to the study of punishment in humans, however, we will not find out much more about it. In particular, we will not find out when it is likely to work well and when it is not, and consequently we will be unable to do our bookkeeping. That is tantamount to saying that we will not find out when the process of therapy could be less punishing than it often is, because we object to research on punishment. More specifically, we would be saying that we will not find out how to make therapy less *socially* punishing than it often is, because we object to research on *shock* punishment.

One of the delights of moralistic argument, I am discovering, is the ease with which it can be extended in all directions. Let me now warn us all *against* punishment.

Punishment works, I submit. There is too much affirmative, careful demonstration to resist that conclusion. Consequently, punishers should succeed often in eliminating the behavior they mean to eliminate. That may reinforce them, which is to say, their rate of using punishment in the future, and in more diverse situations, will rise. Contributing to that tendency is the extreme simplicity of punishment technique and technology. Anyone with a hand to swing is equipped with a punishing device. The Sears-Roebuck farm catalog lists a number of inexpensive and reliable cattle prods. Furthermore, the punishment contingency is the essence of simplicity, compared to which positive reinforcement and its allied art of shaping looms as a formidable mystery indeed. Thus, it is possible that punishment could become the first and, woefully, the exclusive behavioral technique some carelessly trained persons might use. That would indeed be a tragic outcome. For one thing, punishment is painful, and the essence of my argument (and of everyone else's) is that we should have as little pain as we can. Thus, we want to use as little punishment as we can, not as much. To find out how to use one form of punishment so as to minimize other forms of punishment, and what the exchange relationships can be, we will have to study punishment; to study, we will have to use it. But to use punishment successfully is to subject oneself to an environmental event which may press one to use it again, and more than necessary. That, we shall have to watch with great care.

Furthermore, to apply punishment to another is to become discriminative for that punishment, very likely. Stimuli which are discriminative for punishment but for nothing else can acquire a punishing function themselves. If the person who applies punishment becomes himself a punishing stimulus for another, he should expect all the relevant behaviors: escape, avoidance, and removal with respect to that stimulus. One way to remove a social stimulus is to murder it. Clearly, anyone using punishment should look to his total stimulus function with great care. This care is very apparent in Kushner's studies, and even more apparent in those of Ivar Lovaas. Very limited punishment is combined with extensive positive reinforcement of other behaviors. In Lovaas' work particularly, positive reinforcement programs surpass "extensive" and approach "monumental." Probably, it is difficult to err in that direction.

Finally, it should be remembered that punishment is most effective as a behavior-removing technique. Some of the problems of clinical practice are exactly that, but they are typically combined with more extensive problems of behavior building (if a good and thorough outcome is to be achieved). Punishment is not an efficient technique of behavior building. In principle, it can be used. One can specify a behavior to be acquired, and punish all response other than that. The behavior may indeed be built up, but very often it will be acquired slowly, while the subject learns that whoever is programming the punishment would be a good stimulus to be rid of.

The fact that behavior which escapes punishment will increase is important to the design of punishment studies. If the therapist places himself in the position of programming punishment for the patient until the patient reports improvement, then the therapist should always consider that he may have conducted verbal conditioning rather than a therapeutic change in the patient's more critical behaviors. As long as the patient can avoid further punishment sessions simply by remarking that he no longer is impotent, or afraid of crowds, or depressed, or smoking, it remains possible that he will do just that—and only that. A considerable number of therapy studies seem to rely upon the patient's verbal report of his condition as the sole measurement of that condition. Verbal behavior responds to reinforcement, punishment, and extinction contingencies just as do other operant behaviors. The fact that the content of that verbal behavior appears to be a description of other behaviors does not remove it from sensitivity to such contingencies. This truism applies to any therapeutic technique, of course, but it may well have special urgency in punishment techniques.

In summary, then, it must be clear that I have not recommended punishment either as a way of life or as a way of psychotherapy. It is a technique of sharply limited applicability in the processes of behavioral change, but, as Kushner, Lovaas, and others show us, its applicability is well above zero, and its benefits may be great. To find out more thoroughly the extent to which this is true, we shall have to use punishment experimentally and carefully—but we shall have to use it. For it may be the case that we are now forcing some patients to endure much greater punishment than necessary, simply by declining to apply a smaller amount of punishment to them systematically and therapeutically.

Chapter Twelve

Ethical Issues

Several previous chapters of this book have mentioned ethical considerations in working with abnormal children, but this chapter focuses specifically on this topic.

Ethical Standards for Psychological Research

The American Psychological Association (APA) has become gravely concerned about ethical standards for psychological research, and in the July 1971 *APA Monitor* it published a detailed statement of ethical principles for consideration by all members of the APA. This proposed list of ethical principles was compiled by a committee of distinguished psychologists appointed by the APA. The list is concerned with the following issues: respect for the human subject and assumption of responsibility for his welfare; research involving physical or psychological stress; research involving the use of deception or the administration of drugs; and matters related to the invasion of privacy. The committee requested members of the APA to criticize the proposed principles and to suggest modifications to be incorporated in the final document that will eventually be used as the formal APA statement of what is permissible in psychological work with human beings.

The May 1972 issue of the *APA Monitor* proposed a revised statement of ethical principles incorporating suggestions received from the APA membership and requested further review and discussion. A summary of these proposed ethical principles follows:

1. Psychologists must observe stringent safeguards to protect the rights of human research subjects.
2. While the investigator should seek expert advice when there is any question about subjects' welfare, the final responsibility for following acceptable ethical practice always remains with the individual investigator.
3. The subject must be informed of all features of the research that might reasonably be expected to influence willingness to participate.
4. Openness and honesty should characterize the relationship between the psychologist and the research participant.
5. The investigator should respect the individual's freedom to refuse to be studied and to discontinue participation at any time.
6. There should be a clear and fair agreement between the investigator and

the subject, with the investigator being obligated to honor all promises and commitments.

7. Researchers should protect participants from physical discomfort, harm, danger, and all forms of mental stress. If the study involves any of these, the subject should be informed of that fact, and his voluntary consent to participate should be obtained.

8. Immediately following data collection, the subject should be given a complete explanation of the study, with full clarification of any misconceptions that may have arisen.

9. Where research procedures may result in undesirable consequences for the participant, the investigator has the responsibility for removing or correcting these consequences.

10. All information obtained from participants should be kept in complete confidence.

Hundreds of psychologists expressed their views on these principles to the APA committee, and some published their opinions and reactions in response to the originally proposed ethical principles. A major statement was published by Diana Baumrind (1971), who focused her comments mainly on misuse of trust that the subject places in the psychologist. She is highly critical of research enterprises that deceive, devalue, and manipulate subjects and violate their human rights. She states most emphatically that when the objectives and commitments of the investigator directly conflict with the well-being of the subject, the code of ethics should contain provisions that unequivocally protect the subject from the investigator. In this regard, Baumrind states, "Especially in the case of children, the subjects' rights not to be harmed or alienated from the power structure must supersede the rights of the investigator to know and to report."

Baumrind offers the following principles to indicate her position: "The researcher should hold himself responsible for the effects of his actions on subjects." Here she is very critical of the way college students have frequently been used as subjects in all sorts of psychological experiments that are alienating, degrading, frightening, and potentially harmful. "At this time and place, it is 'evil' for research psychologists in pursuit of professional objectives to contribute an iota to 'the attrition of human relationships in depersonalization and distrust,' and the research enterprise does not intrinsically require that they do so." No encounter between psychologist and subject should involve deceit, infliction of mental or physical discomfort, or be degrading to the subject in any way.

"Scientific ends, however laudable these may be, do not by themselves justify the use of means that in ordinary transactions would be regarded as reprehensible." In this regard, Baumrind is especially critical of the concept of "risk/benefit" discussed in the original APA proposal—that is, that the investigator must weigh the risk factor involved for the individual against the possible benefits for mankind and then decide whether to proceed with the experiment. To Baumrind, this approach is not acceptable. If there is possible risk to the individual, then the experiment should not be done unless it can be modified to eliminate the risk factor. According to Baumrind, "The investigator's problem in designing good research is to devise methods to achieve his research objectives that do not deceive, humiliate, or degrade his subjects."

The final principle put forth by Baumrind states: "A full disclosure of our professional code should be made public." She advocates publishing this ethical code in newspapers and magazines available to the general public. Moreover, a copy of the ethical code should be given to all subjects before obtaining their consent to participate in research.

Special Ethical Problems Concerning Children

Some of these principles, considered by both the APA committee and Baumrind, pose special problems in working with children. Particularly troublesome is the matter of "informed consent." At the adult level, this principle requires that the person be informed of such things as the purpose of the psychological assessment, nature of the psychological treatment involved, and possible consequences of participation in the psychologist's investigation before consenting to cooperate in these endeavors. Children, however, may not understand the meaning of information given to them, and are often in no position to consent or refuse to participate. This truly presents a dilemma. The commonly accepted notion is that parents should be informed and should give their consent if their children are to be tested, treated, or experimented with by psychologists.

Many of these issues involving psychological work with children are especially relevant to what transpires in school settings throughout the country, especially the psychological testing of children and placing the results in the official school records. Should IQ scores, answers to questions on personality inventories, responses to projective tests, and personal information obtained from school psychologists' interviews with children and parents become part of the child's school record? These records are certainly permanent, and if they contain private information about the child and his family, they could have important influences on a person's life long after the school system has any legitimate right to intrude on the individual's well-being.

While most would agree that school records should not remain open and available to interested parties throughout a person's adult life, there is considerable disagreement about who has the right to view information in a child's school record while he is enrolled in the school system. To give just one example, an interesting question is, "Should parents be able to obtain the IQ score for their child from his school record?" The controversy and wide-ranging disagreement that this question stimulates when presented for discussion by undergraduates in a child psychology course indicates that the answer is not an obvious and easy one.

Research Exemplifying High Ethical Standards

An excellent recent book, *The Humanization Processes* (Hamblin, Buckholdt, Ferritor, Kozloff, & Blackwell, 1971), devotes a section to questions of ethics. Since their studies used social and behavioral analyses of children who showed serious problem behaviors, they were very concerned that their work did not overstep certain ethical constraints. Before attempting to modify the response patterns of disturbed children, these investigators first obtained the "informed consent" of those legally responsible for the children. When working with psychotic children, this consent was obtained from parents; for work conducted in public schools, consent was obtained from teachers and school officials prior to the social scientists' initiating experimental manipulations of the children's responses and rewards.

Moreover, these investigators proceeded with their programs of habit modification only if they believed that the intended changes in behavior would result in long-range benefits for all involved parties, including parents, teachers, school officials, and especially the child subjects. In this regard, Hamblin and his colleagues emphasize the need for increased study of, and research devoted to, the long-term effects of the acquisition or non-acquisition of various skills and behavioral patterns in children.

In addition, these researchers state that the aim in their scientific work is to develop effective procedures for altering systems of social exchange between children and significant adults, and thus to modify behavior patterns but to do so with a minimum amount of discomfort to the participants. That is, in attempting to remedy a particular problem, they strive to select the procedure that will be least painful to those involved in the experimental manipulations.

A final and major point made by these authors is that in both conducting and publishing the results of experiments they must be careful to protect the privacy of their subjects. Although in their scientific reports it is often necessary to concern themselves with unfortunate behavior patterns and their consequences, they are especially careful to write in such a way that the people they have studied cannot be identified. That is, they try to ensure that their reports of findings will not result in parents or teachers punishing the children described. Similarly, if they observe parents, teachers, or school officials acting in some irresponsible or undesirable manner, they do not report this to higher authorities.

In other words, research conducted with the cooperation of these children and adults has the goal of making effective changes in systems of social exchange and kinds of behavior evidenced by their experimental subjects, but doing so without harming the participants. Such ethical considerations are relevant in any attempt to use principles and techniques of social and behavioral science to cope with human problems encountered in real-life settings.

Research Involving Questionable Ethical Practices

A recent incident provided a vivid example of the kind of research situations that have very important ethical implications. A doctoral candidate from a large Eastern university presented a colloquium for students and staff members in the Psychology Department at Brown University describing research on "learned helplessness" in children. This research constituted the basis for her dissertation in psychology. Essentially, the research project was concerned with effects of failure experiences on the later performance of elementary school children. In order to study this phenomenon, the research used two female experimenters, one known as the "success lady" and the other as the "failure lady." Some of the children in these experiments were placed into a problem-solving situation in which they were bound to fail; that is, the "failure lady" presented the unsuspecting child with block designs that could not possibly be made from the blocks given to him and then forced the child to struggle with this series of unsolvable tasks. The children were later placed into a similar situation, and the experimenters measured the extent to which the prior failure experience had a detrimental effect on the individual child's learning performance.

As one might suspect, forcing the child to fail and then confronting him with similar materials and tasks on another occasion resulted in marked negative effects on most children. What are the ethics of submitting innocent, naive, unsuspecting children to the devious manipulations of an experimenter who urges them to keep working at tasks that can lead only to frustration and failure? If you had a young child attending public school, would you allow him to be an experimental subject in the sessions conducted by the "failure lady"? When the person who presented the report of this research was asked about informed consent—that is, receiving approval to conduct the study—she stated that the teachers and school officials had given their approval for the research; further questioning revealed that parents had not been asked to give their approval nor had they been informed of the experiment that would manipulate the emotional and educational experiences of their children.

This critical analysis is not meant to imply that studies such as this should never be undertaken. We have not discussed the merits of such research and their eventual contribution to knowledge, perhaps even to improved methods of teaching. However, readers should be aware of some of the important ethical considerations that may eventually concern them directly as parents, teachers, or behavioral scientists.

The Issues

The three articles in this chapter discuss several of the issues we have mentioned. Two of them focus on how psychologists function in school settings and how information obtained from school children is used. The first paper, by Gilbert M. Trachtman, emphasizes issues such as confidentiality, privileged communication, and the invasion of privacy. The second paper, by Donald N. Bersoff, compares certain practices of school psychologists with Szasz's description of "institutional psychiatry." Specific issues discussed by Bersoff include the psychologist's role as an agent of the school system, the evaluation of children without informing them of the purposes of testing or possible uses of data obtained, and the dangers involved in labeling children. The final paper is a brief statement of important social issues; it is written by the distinguished child psychiatrist Robert Coles, who has been called "the most influential living psychiatrist in the U.S." Coles has dedicated his professional life to advancing the cause of all children who have been abused, neglected, and stifled as a result of their race, religion, or social class (see Coles, 1967). His views here, pointing to some small advances in recent years and stressing the many shameful conditions that still exist, seem a fitting note on which to conclude our discussion of ethical issues in abnormal child psychology.

References

Baumrind, D. Principles of ethical conduct in the treatment of subjects: Reaction to the draft report of the committee on ethical standards in psychological research. *American Psychologist*, 1971, **26**, 887–896.

Coles, R. *Children of crisis: A study of courage and fear*. Boston: Little, Brown, 1967.

Hamblin, R. L., Buckholdt, D., Ferritor, D., Kozloff, M., & Blackwell, L. *The humanization processes: A social, behavioral analysis of children's problems*. New York: Wiley-Interscience, 1971.

32. Pupils, Parents, Privacy, and the School Psychologist

Gilbert M. Trachtman

Pupil records, confidentiality, privileged communication, and invasion of privacy have been issues of great concern to educators and, most particularly, to pupil personnel specialists during the decade of the sixties. Legislation, legal rulings or court decisions, administrative regulations, and debate on these topics have frequently erupted out of the larger issues of civil rights and community control. In some instances, a particular conflict has been initiated by the political left; in some cases, by the political right. In some cases, the extreme left and extreme right have found themselves unwittingly allied against the establishment or status quo. This article attempts to review a selected handful of these cases and to discuss their implication for the educator, with particular reference to the practice of school psychology.

Clarification of Terms

It is necessary first to clarify terms, so that in any discussion we may speak to the same point. Terms such as privileged communication and confidentiality of records are sometimes used in the literature in different or overlapping contexts. Having failed to locate one definitive and ultimate authority for clarifying these terms, we offer instead some working definitions for the purpose of this discussion. The concept of confidentiality has been used to refer to the intimacy or privacy of communication between people at many different levels. It is possible to define at least four bands on the spectrum of confidentiality:

1. In the most general sense, confidentiality refers to the trust and faith we indicate when confiding in others.
2. Within our society, various subgroups develop codes and norms that make the behavior of group members more predictable. Thus, a member of a delinquent gang is free to share confidences with his pals because of the code prohibiting "squealing." In a more formal manner, and with loftier objectives, the 1952 Code of Ethics of the National Education Association requires teachers to respect the rights of students to have confidential

information about themselves withheld, except under certain specified conditions. Similarly, the ethical standards of the American Psychological Association (1968) state that "Information received in confidence is revealed only after most careful deliberation and when there is clear and imminent danger to an individual or to society, and then only to appropriate professional workers or public authorities [p. 358]." Thus, confidentiality at the professional level refers to the ethical responsibility of the psychologist or other professional not to disclose to a third party any private communications from a client. Information received in confidence may only be communicated to others with the informed consent of the client or under certain specified exceptional circumstances.

3. A particular aspect of confidentiality much in the spotlight in recent years has been the issue of school records, particularly the right of outside agencies to have access to records. Another controversy has focused on the availability of records to various personnel within the school; a third, and the most inflammatory, has been the right of parents to inspect the records of their children. This last issue has represented a unique problem within the area of confidentiality since parents, acting on behalf of a child who is a minor, in effect, represent the child or client and cannot therefore be considered third parties in the usual sense.

4. The next level at which we refer to confidentiality involves codification of behavior into written law. This is the concept of privileged communication which refers specifically to disclosure of information from the witness stand during legal proceedings. Privileged communication refers primarily to the legal protection afforded to the confidential relationship between two people, usually a professional person and a client. When a particular profession is granted privileged communication, members of that profession will not be compelled or even allowed to disclose information received from a client without the client's consent. The "privilege" referred to is therefore the legal privilege of the *client* to decide whether or not he will agree to the disclosure of information. While the wording of most laws usually grants privileged communication to a profession, the underlying purpose of the law is usually to protect the welfare of the client rather than the profession.

In this article, privileged communication refers to confidentiality existing by law; confidentiality relates to a broader spectrum of ethical standards, administrative regulations, and professional precedents in the absence of a specific statute.

Privileged Communication

The issue here may be somewhat confused by pointing out that in United States civil law the term "privileged communication" may also refer to oral or written statements that might ordinarily be libelous or slanderous by virtue of defaming a person's character. Under certain circumstances such statements may be accorded either absolute or qualified privilege, based on the philosophy that under these particular circumstances some statements may be of such social importance as to excuse their defamatory nature.

More generally, however, privileged communication refers to the protection of the confidential relationship between client and professional and is found in some form in the civil law of most nations today, most often as an exemption granted certain professional groups from testifying in courts of law about information entrusted to them by clients in the conduct of their professional relationships. While this general pattern exists in the United States, there are differences from state to state in the groups to whom exemption is granted and in the stringency of the law's provisions. Thus, some laws merely exempt certain professional persons from testifying, while others make the violation of a professional confidence a punishable crime.

The oldest and most clearly defined privilege in United States law is that granted in the attorney–client relationship. Privilege here has been extended to the advice given a client by his attorney, in some cases to the clerk or secretary of the attorney, and in some instances to prepared briefs or informal notes and memoranda made by the attorney. Although the first physician–patient privilege was established by New York State in 1828, it has since been granted in only about two-thirds of the states. The clergyman-penitent relationship has similarly been accorded privilege in about two-thirds of our states, but doubt has been expressed as to whether confidences entrusted to clergymen in the course of other relationships, such as marital counseling, are protected by privilege.

It is difficult for the law to define privileged communication for professional relationships where the profession itself lacks clear-cut legal definition. Many states have extended privilege to the psychologist-client relationship, and in some cases privilege has been tendered to optometrists, newspaper reporters, and police. Professional groups seeking to gain the legal protection of privilege should refer to the criteria proposed by Wigmore (1940), a leading authority on rules of evidence. Wigmore suggested that before granting privileged communication by statute, the following conditions should be fulfilled: (a) The communications must be offered with the expectation and understanding that they are not to be disclosed. (b) This element of confidentiality must be an essential element in maintaining a full and satisfactory relationship between the parties involved. (c) The relationship itself must be one which the community believes should be zealously fostered. (d) The injury to the relationship, if the communication were disclosed, must be greater than the benefits such disclosure would contribute to the correct disposal of litigation.

The individual psychologist should take the trouble to define his own status with regard to privileged communication. This must be accomplished locally, either through the good offices of a local or state professional association or directly through legal or governmental channels. The status of privilege for any individual professional varies with the profession, with the state, and even with the setting in which the individual functions. State statute is frequently definitive, but judicial precedent or legal opinion is just as often the only source of information. A few examples of this variability illustrate the point clearly. Specific judicial decisions have led to the general rule that there is no privilege in the absence of statute. Some courts, however, have ruled that communications made to one's physician are privileged even where there is no law granting such privilege.

Social workers in most states have not been granted privileged communication by law but have frequently appealed for this privilege in specific court cases. Privilege has sometimes been granted and sometimes been denied, occasionally within the same state.

In some cases, cities or states have adopted measures attempting to safeguard records in public agencies. Under such circumstances, the professional within an agency might gain privilege by virtue of his employment setting, which he does or does not receive by virtue of his profession alone. Thus, the status of the school psychologist varies from state to state in much the same way. Not only does every state vary with regard to local policy, but the school psychologist may be affected by two sets of statutes or precedents (one related to psychology, one to education), which in turn may be mutually supportive of privilege, mutually denying, or contradictory.

New York State, as an example, issues a school psychologist's certificate through the Education Department's Bureau of Teacher Education and Certification. This certificate is required for employment as a school psychologist. The provisions of this certificate do not include any recognition of a privileged communication status for school psychologists. The New York State Legislature has never defined the school records of children as being either public or confidential records. Regulations of the Commissioner of Education, however, which in New York State possess quasi-legislative status, have specified that records may be made available only to appropriate school personnel and, with parental consent, to appropriate personnel in cooperating agencies. Subsequent court decisions have agreed that mental health records of children are confidential except with the consent of the parent.

A school psychologist in New York State might thereby infer, on the basis of these Commissioner's Regulations and legal opinions, that despite the absence of legal statute specifically granting him privileged communication, he would be safe to assume such privilege in his professional functioning. Unless and until a court ruled otherwise, this would be a logical assumption.

To complicate the issue, however, New York State since 1957 has also issued a psychologist's certificate through the State Board of Examiners of Psychologists. It is now illegal in New York State for a person without this certificate to use the words "psychologist," "psychology," or "psychological" while offering or rendering services for remuneration to individuals, corporations, or the public, except in certain exempt settings such as public schools where the school psychology certificate is required instead. The law that, thus, essentially certified the private practice of psychology in New York State also placed the confidential relations and communications between a certified psychologist and his client "on the same basis as those provided by law between attorney and client."

This clearly, or relatively clearly, defines the privileged communication extended to the psychologist in private practice and his client. However, when a certified psychologist in New York State also possesses a school psychology certificate and works in the public school, does he infer the privileged communication implied by the Regulations of the Commissioner of Education, or does he assume the more certain privileged communication granted by the legislature? The opinion of the State Department's legal counsel is that the legally granted privilege applies to certified psychologists even when they work in schools. Other legal opinions vary, however, and this issue has not been tested in the courts.

In a recent review of privileged communication as it applies to psychologists, Shah (1969) points out that since most psychologist-client laws are based on the attorney-client relationship, it is difficult to generalize from precedents and interpretations based on the latter. There have, in fact, been relatively few actual court cases involving the psychologist-client privilege. Nevertheless, Shah offers the following generalizations as tentative interpretations:

1. A communication from a client may be considered privileged only if it was originally intended to be confidential.

2. Privilege must be claimed by the client or it may be considered waived.

3. The total communication is privileged on an all-or-none basis. Similarly, if several professionals have been consulted, privilege may be imposed upon all or none.

4. If the client is mentally incompetent or a minor, privilege is waived or asserted by the parent or guardian.

5. Privilege may also extend to others on the professional's team such as supervisors, associates, trainees, and secretaries.

6. A psychologist examining a client privately for an attorney or physician is serving as their agent and covered by any privilege afforded them.

7. As a safeguard to the community, most privileged communication laws require that physicians report certain communicable diseases, bullet or knife wounds, suicide attempts, abortions, or narcotic addiction. (Technically, these are not exceptions to privilege since the privilege relates only to disclosure during legal proceedings). Some privilege laws do include specific exceptions, such as homicide cases, where full disclosure is deemed socially more important. The privilege extended to attorneys excludes communications referring to planned crimes. This so-called "future crime" exception has not been included in several privilege laws written specifically for psychiatry or psychology, and its applicability to these professions is yet to be determined.

These generalizations may offer some useful guidelines for a general understanding of the concept of privileged communication. The relationship between professional ethics, legal statute, and judicial opinion, however, remains cloudy and relatively undefined. Ideally, existing statutes affecting professional functioning will have been written in consultation with professional associations and will therefore reinforce existing ethical principles bearing on the issue. The school psychologist functioning in sensitive areas with the joint support of a code of ethics and local statutes finds himself in an unusually fortunate situation. Where statute and ethic are in conflict,

the courts usually support the law, and the psychologist must make a personal decision in choosing to abide by the law or to defy the law on a question of ethical principle.

Most often the psychologist finds it impossible to locate any local statutes
or regulations pertinent to the issue of privileged communication. In the
absence of such guidelines, he should turn to his professional association
for assistance in defining ethical procedures and standards. Although it has
already been pointed out that theoretically there is no privilege in the
absence of statute, a number of exceptions to this general rule have also
been cited. It is reasonable to expect, therefore, that a psychologist pleading
the right of privileged communication in a professional relationship on the
basis of a recognized code of professional ethics stands at least a fair chance
of winning court approval for his stand. Again, however, individual differences among states are so great as to warrant further investigation of this
within local areas. Furthermore, in the absence of a privileged communication statute, each new plea for privilege must be presented on its own merits
since the courts have generally ruled that privilege cannot be created by
judicial decision.

Confidentiality

The preceding exposition of privileged communication provides a necessary framework within which to discuss some of the issues of confidentiality
that more often affect the school psychologist or other school personnel
in day-to-day functioning.

The psychologist in a particular school system rarely finds a statute defining areas of confidentiality, and often finds no clear-cut regulations in his
district. Where these regulations exist, he is bound by them, and should
he seek support from a state education department in opposing specific
regulations, he is most likely to learn that the local board of education is
empowered to establish such regulations in the absence of any contradicting
legislation or state commissioner's regulations. Where local regulations
exist, it is to be hoped that the school psychologist has some hand in shaping
them or, if they predate his arrival, in modifying them when warranted. Where
no regulations exist, the school psychologist may be well advised to join
with others on the staff in seeking to establish a formal confidentiality code
rather than waiting for the first "incident" to erupt before defining this issue.
In either instance, the school psychologist might seek guidance from the
ethical standards of psychologists and from patterns of behavior gradually
evolving out of privileged communication law. Principle 6 of the Ethics Code
(APA, 1968) stresses the importance of safeguarding information obtained
in the course of a professional relationship stating that "Such information
is not communicated to others unless certain important conditions are met
[p. 358]." Among the conditions which allow for revealing information
received in confidence are instances of "clear and imminent danger to an
individual or to society" (similar to the "future crime" exceptions in many

privilege laws). The psychologist may also ethically discuss confidential material "with persons clearly concerned with the case." Inherent in this proviso is the expectation that information is being shared only with others involved in a helping relationship to the client (i.e., teachers, remedial personnel) or to the psychologist (i.e., supervising psychologist) and that information is communicated in such a manner as to be of maximum value to other professional workers (i.e., nontechnical reports to teachers).

The psychologist on a school staff should be allowed discretion in withholding or communicating information received in confidence, and he can then base his behavior primarily on professional ethical standards. In some instances, an administrator or board of education has routinely demanded certain information considered confidential in nature from school psychologists and other staff members. In the absence of a higher statute or ruling, the psychologist may be bound to conform or leave his job. In such cases, while the psychologist may disclose required information without a breach of ethics, he should be aware of another ethical principle which states that the psychologist "defines for himself the nature and direction of his loyalties and responsibilities and keeps all parties concerned informed of these commitments [APA, 1968, p. 358]." Another clause under the same principle of client welfare requires that the psychologist accept confidential information from a client only after making certain that the client is fully aware "of the ways in which the information may be used [p. 358]."

When confidential information is requested by a third party outside the school, the ground rules should parallel the rules of privileged communication. The psychologist and, indeed, the school in general should refuse to release any information without authorization and should be obligated to supply information when authorized, with authorization for children, of course, coming from parents or guardians. In the absence of a privileged communication law, however, it seems a court may have the power to subpoena records and information which the school psychologist would otherwise consider confidential. There is some movement discernible in various parts of the country to reduce the access that outsiders have to school records. This movement is discussed more fully in the following section.

When parents have asked to inspect their children's school records, they have often been refused such access by the schools. This has resulted in litigation and rulings reviewed in the next section. If there is a trend here, it is toward increasing parent access to records.

A related but much more subtle issue is parental access to verbal communications made by a child in confidence to the psychologist. The psychologist is bound by the same ethical discretions described earlier in deciding whether or not to share this confidence with others on the school staff. While technically it might seem that parents should have the same access to such verbal communication as they do to the written record, this has not been clarified. There seems to be some sympathy for the psychologist having discretionary power to withhold confidential verbal communications from parents, even by those who would grant parents complete access to the written record.

Representative Cases

This section reviews a selected handful of instances in which rulings, legislation, or attempted legislation have focused on issues such as those discussed above.

Confidentiality of Records outside the School

In the absence of any protective statute, psychologists and other pupil personnel workers may find their records subpoenaed by a court or may find themselves ordered by their school administrator or board to release information to certain legal or governmental agencies. In some instances, existing law or ruling actually requires that information be supplied to third parties. Thus, for example, in Nassau County, New York, the Probation Department, in 1965, issued a School Court Probation Manual stating that pupil records must be made available to the Family Court or Probation Department without parental consent.

In New Jersey, Department of Education regulations stipulate that pupil records may be inspected by Selective Service, Federal Bureau of Investigation, and the United States Army and Navy, although the Board of Education is also allowed the discretion of withholding items of a confidential nature. In contrast, an attempt was made in the 1961 California Assembly to enact legislation restricting certified school personnel from disclosing information given to them in confidence by pupils. The attempt was unsuccessful, however. A proposed bill currently before the New York State Legislature would impose privilege upon "records or communications received from any pupil by psychologists, guidance personnel, social workers, and related personnel . . . . " Wisconsin, in 1967, passed a law granting privileged communication to college deans of men, women, and students and to school psychologists except in criminal cases (Wisconsin Statutes, Section 885.205). The bill originally included school counselors, but this was deleted by the legislature. Michigan law (Act 41, P.A. 1935) prohibits all professional school personnel from disclosing any confidential communications from students or any records in any civil or criminal court proceedings. Based on this statute, the State Department of Public Instruction has also issued corollary recommended procedures for confidential communications outside of court, advising the counselor that confidential information should be released only to others having a legitimate interest in the welfare of the student and only with consent.

Confidentiality of Records within the School

Communication of information about children within the school or among school personnel has rarely been a matter of legislative or judicial ruling, usually being considered a matter for internal professional judgment. Even here, however, great inconsistency can be noted. The attorney general of

Colorado, in a public communication to the commissioner of education, interpreting the so-called "Open Records Bill" states that the bill does not affect the use of records within a particular agency. A legal interpretation of the South Dakota pupil record code, however, states that the superintendent, principal, and counselor within a school system have complete access to pupil records. The Michigan Department of Public Instruction's suggested code for school counselors supports professional codes such as the APA Ethical Standards by suggesting that the counselor "give other school personnel such information and data . . . as they can use in the best interests of the client's welfare [p. 2]." One of the most forthright statements of respect for the psychologist's judgment has come from a school administrator. John Miller, Superintendent of Schools in Great Neck, New York, participating in a panel discussion on "Privileged Communication and the School Psychologist" (1959), differentiated sharply between the release of information in the interests of the child and the release of information in the interests of someone else such as a probation office, court, or police department. Differentiating further between objective data such as marks, test scores, or attendance records and more subjective data such as the interpretations and evaluations of psychologists and other personnel, he stated that the psychologist in his school system had the right to give him as much material as she thought he should have and to refuse to give him what he should not have. He charged the psychologist with responsibility for making such judgments based on the interests of the child and family and based on her judgment of the training and understanding of the other personnel involved.

Parental Inspection of Records

The right of parents to inspect school records became a formal issue in California when the legislature passed a law in 1959 giving parents the right to inspect a child's cumulative record. The law has been modified a number of times since, at one point leaving it to the school's judgment whether records should be shown. At the present time parents are entitled to examine the school records of their children.

In New York, a series of conflicts between parents and local school authorities, interspersed with legal opinions offered by the Law Division of the State Education Department and rulings by the Commissioner of Education, were finally climaxed by a 1961 court decision holding that parents were entitled to inspect the school records of their children (Van Allen v. McCleary; New York State, 2d, 501, January 20, 1961). The court pointed out that the Commissioner or legislature *could* issue contrary regulations binding on all schools in the state, but in the absence of such regulation, parents had the right of inspection.

This sequence of rulings and court decisions evoked a storm of response from professional groups, mostly in protest. Professional journals and associations used terms such as "serious threat," "irreparable damage," "grave alarm," and "grave damage," and it was predicted that school psychological reports would become "noncommittal, watered-down, and largely inconsequential formalities which will be of help to no one [Editorial, 1961]." These events have already been chronicled in great detail (Trachtman, 1963).

An Advisory Committee on Pupil Records (1961), appointed by the Commissioner of Education in New York State, and including the present author, then deliberated nine months and gave birth to a report which included a pioneering attempt to define the term "record." Final recommendations included the preparation of a manual on records, with a list of specified topics.

In retrospect, however, it seems that after nine months labor the Advisory Committee gave birth to a stillborn child. One year later a manual on pupil records was issued by the State Department of Education (1962). A thorough, comprehensive, well-documented manual, it dealt competently with all the topics suggested except for the one basic issue of clearly defining the term "record." Thus, instead of providing a definition of record which further clarified the Advisory Committee's attempt at definition, the manual offered a general and somewhat circular definition indicating that "any record relating to a pupil which is actually used by the school district in any manner, becomes a pupil record [p. 3]."

In Colorado, legislation on this topic has occurred quite recently. The so-called "Open Records Bill" (Colorado Revised Statutes 1963, Art. 2, Ch. 113) was enacted by legislative amendment in 1968 and permitted inspection of records by pupils, parents, or guardians, while simultaneously guaranteeing the confidentiality of such records from third parties including law enforcement personnel. A subsequent amendment in 1969 has apparently weakened the latter aspect of this bill.

Meanwhile, the battle by parents for free access to the records of their children continues. Despite the 1960 ruling by the Commissioner of Education in New York State and the 1961 court ruling, both defining school records as open to parent inspection, parents in some New York City schools have been denied access to records, and in at least one Manhattan school district a parent union has been formed and is now actively pursuing this issue.

Discussion

Before discussing these issues and their implication for the school psychologist, it is advisable that the author share his perceptions about the current state of affairs in public education, in this area of confidentiality. The people one chooses to quote are as good an indication as any. A statement made over 10 years ago by Friedenberg (1959) in a provocative textbook on adolescence seems to be still on target today. Freidenberg claimed that public school policies making pupil records available to outside agencies have made it dangerous for students to deal honestly either with the schools or with themselves. He expressed concern about the possible repercussions of such policies on the inner life and emotional dynamics of adolescents and stated:

> To argue that the school is obligated to provide the agencies of legitimate govern- ment with personal information about its students because it is itself a public agency, seems to me vicious nonsense. The school has indeed an obligation to society: to provide all the resources it can in support of the necessary intel- lectual and moral growth of future citizens. The record of the American school in this respect has been most seriously marred by the frequency with which it has willingly set its responsibility aside In urder to perform a minor chore for the community or for influential private groups, from the maintenance of athlotic spectacles to blood drives. But it might at least have drawn the line at serving as a police spy [p. 61].

Much more recently, Ira Glasser (1969), Associate Director of the New York Civil Liberties Union, wrote:

> There are only two public institutions in the United States which steadfastly deny that the Bill of Rights applies to them. One is the military and the other is the public schools. Both are compulsory. Taken together, they are the chief socializ- ing institutions of our society. Everyone goes through our schools. What they learn—not from what they are formally taught but from the way the institution is organized to treat them—is that authority is more important than freedom, order more precious than liberty, and discipline a higher value than individual expression. That is a lesson which is inappropriate to a free society—and certainly inappropriate to its schools [p. 190].

His article proceeds to document specific cases in which students have been denied procedural rights, in which school authorities have broken even their own regulations, and in which the Bill of Rights has been ignored. Other attorneys have described their inability to elicit specific rules or regula- tions from the Board of Education or Department of Welfare while defending a particular student or family.

Even more recently, the Russell Sage Foundation has released a report challenging the way pupil records are kept and used by most public schools in the United States. Announcing the publication of this report, Orville G. Brim, Jr., President of the Foundation, stated, "It is very difficult for you as a parent, to get information about your own child from school files. Yet those same school records frequently are opened to truant officers, the F.B.I., people in the social welfare field, to official bodies who are agents of the government [Anonymous, 1970, p. 49]."

The discussion to follow, then, stems from a frame of reference which perceives schools in general as being less actively concerned than they should about the welfare and protection of their pupils. No special case is made here for the poor, or disadvantaged, except to note that wherever such abuses take place, they will be heaped upon the poor a hundredfold.

Taking a somewhat oversimplified view of history, schools can be seen as one of many institutions organized by people banded together to form societies. As people found their societies becoming more complex, they also found that certain functions could be carried on most effectively by specialized groups. Thus, communities of people organized governing bodies, police and fire fighting units, sanitation agencies, health agencies, and, for the education of their children, schools. The schools, having been organized by parents to serve parental needs, should be responsive to the wishes of parents. The schools have no more intrinsic right to make decisions about children than do maids, baby sitters, or tutors hired by a parent. Although a parent may delegate more authority and responsibility to a tutor than to a baby sitter, and a group of parents might delegate even more authority to a school, the authority is delegated authority and subject to recall. The halting steps toward community control now being attempted in many regions are therefore seen as a healthy trend, even if some of the steps may be fumbling. We are now in a period where many parents are trying to reassume this responsibility for their children's education, where they are flexing their muscles, often without the prerequisite knowledge or experience in local government. After long years of frustration or denial, many parents have accepted assertive and vocal leadership without really examining it critically. Many excesses are perpetrated in the name of autonomy or local control. This *may* be a necessary stage of development, but at any rate, it is not the subject of this article. At the most basic philosophical level, one might contend, if we accept the idea of local responsibility, that the community has the right to destroy its school system if this is indeed its choice.

In other countries, and more recently in this country, as the institutions developed by people to serve people became more and more complex, they began, in many cases, to lose sight of their original mission. Eventually, the people hired other people to protect them from the institutions that were supposed to serve them. That, essentially, in an oversimplified way, is what the ombudsman is all about.

From these views, certain perceptions of the school psychologist's role seem to emerge naturally. Too often, school psychologists sound as if they see themselves protecting children from parents. In exceptional cases of parental neglect or abuse, there are laws which allow the state to intervene, and certainly all school personnel should be alert for such instances so that appropriate steps can be taken. Much more often, however, it is presumptuous of the school psychologist to come between parent and child in this manner. The psychologist is there, as is the school, to serve the parent. He should share his knowledge with parents freely and openly, offer advice if he has any, even try to convince the parents if he chooses, but he must keep in mind that he is a consultant and that the parent must reserve the right to ignore his advice. This means that records must be open to parents. They must have access to any information about their child which others have access to. Without this, a trusting relationship between parent and school is impossible. With a trusting relationship, few parents will ever demand the right to inspect the record, but will merely ask for interpretation of any material that could be useful to them. Where communities are in turmoil and reacting against the establishment, it is quite likely that the school psychologist will be perceived as part of the establishment which has not been helpful—particularly to minority group children. The school psychologist may be considered expendable in this community at this time. In fact, he may actually *be* expendable, but this is beside the point. The school psychologist is still ethically bound to communicate his best advice, but he should accept the right of parents to disregard his advice and to negate the value of his services—even mistakenly. Thus, if a special class placement seems the most appropriate recommendation, he must make this recommendation, even to a parent actively campaigning for the abolition of special classes. Even more important, for the psychologist working in ghetto or poverty areas, is the necessity to communicate information to parents who are not actively seeking or requesting it, since the activist minority in the ghetto frequently masks a large majority still unrelated to and unconnected with the schools.

Thus, it is possible not only to defend the right of parents to see records and the responsibility of the psychologist to cooperate with parents in this but to move one step farther. There are many different roles suggested for school psychologists. Every university has its own model to sell. It is suggested here that one function, common to all role definitions, could be for the school psychologist to serve as unofficial ombudsman. Accepting his responsibility to parents as paramount, the school psychologist would then view himself as protecting children from the school, wherever necessary.

This could be the beginning of a discussion, instead of the end. The points made have been raised, for further elaboration at another time, as a setting in which to offer conclusions about the rulings and laws cited earlier, and their implication for school psychology. For the school psychologist who writes speculative clinical reports in technical language, who rarely communicates with parents but is delighted to send copies of his reports to other agencies, many of the recent actions cited must be quite threatening. For the school psychologist who can see himself as an ombudsman, who sees himself as a helper of parents, and who sees the school as a service agency for parents, the movement toward parental inspection of records is certainly no threat, and he should be actively supporting those who are fighting to close the records to all outsiders.

Thus, for this observer, recent rulings and legislative actions do not seem to pose any major threat to the practice of school psychology as it should be practiced. One area still needing clarification is a definition of the term "records." In 1960, this author proposed a definition of records based on actual use, in which he urged that the record be defined

> as anything put in writing for others to see. Thus, anything I put in writing which anyone else could see, could also be inspected by the parent. Anything I put in writing which no one else could see, could not be inspected by the parent either. This would permit me to maintain personal notes which did not comprise part of the child's record but which I could use for storing tentative interpretations, speculations, test data and other material in raw form. The finished product, including scores, interpretations, conclusions and recommendations, would go on the record. Certain of our notes and data would be inviolate—we would be free to speculate and theorize. Our professional judgments and conclusions would be open to inspection [p. 5].

This definition was essentially adopted by the Advisory Committee on Pupil Records in its recommendations to the Commissioner but ignored by the Education Department in the manual on pupil records which it subsequently published.

Some such proviso should be allowed as very limited protection for the psychologist so that he can keep notes *for himself*. This much the psychologist, and other professionals, needs if he is to do his work competently. Beyond that, however, all of our efforts at protection should be focused on protection of children, not psychologists.

By and large, with occasional exceptions, the legislation and rulings cited in this article have tended to increase the protection afforded children—too little, very late, but at least in the right direction. If, on occasion, the comfortable functioning of the psychologist is interrupted, it may be that this is incidental and for the larger good. If the psychologist's functioning is directly and purposefully affected, this should be viewed as a symptom worth exploring—perhaps a sign of his failure to earn the trust of those he serves.

References

Advisory Committee on Pupil Records, State of New York. *Report of the Advisory Committee on Pupil Records, Report to the commisioner of education.* New York: State Education Department, 1961.

American Psychological Association. Ethical standards of psychologists. *American Psychologist,* 1968, **23,** 357–361.

Anonymous. School files held peril to privacy. *New York Times,* March 16, 1970.

Editorial. Privileged nature of psychological records. *Journal of Clinical Psychology,* 1961, **17,** 2.

Friedenberg, E. A. *The vanishing adolescent.* Boston: Beacon Press, 1959.

Glasser, I. Schools for scandal—the Bill of Rights and public education. *Phi Delta Kappan,* 1969, **41,** 190–194.

Privileged communication and the school psychologist. Workshop conducted by New York State Teacher's Association, Great Neck, New York, October 2, 1959.

Shah, S. Privileged communications, confidentiality, and privacy. *Professional Psychology,* 1969, **1,** 56–69.

State Education Department, New York. *Manual on pupil records.* Albany, N.Y.: Author, 1962.

Trachtman, G. M. Editorial: From the pen of the president. *Nassau County Psychological Association Newsletter,* 1960, **8,** 5.

Trachtman, G. M. The school psychologist and confidentiality of records. In M. G. Gottsegen & G. B. Gottsegen (Eds.), *Professional school psychology.* Vol. 2. New York: Grune & Stratton, 1963.

Wigmore, J. H. *A treatise on the Anglo-American system of evidence in trials at common law.* (23rd ed.) Vol. 8. Boston: Little, Brown, 1940.

33. School Psychology as "Institutional Psychiatry"

Donald N. Bersoff

In a recent and provocative book, Thomas Szasz (1970) differentiates between what he calls institutional psychiatry and contractual psychiatry. Institutional psychiatry is characterized by the fact

> that the institutional psychiatrist is a bureaucratic employee, paid for his services by a private or public organization [p. xxiii]

and not by the client he is asked to see. Further,

> the institutional psychiatrist imposes himself on his 'patients' who do not pay him, do not want to be his patients, and are not free to reject his 'help' ... [p. xxiii].

This mode of operation is contrasted to contractual psychiatry wherein the patient actively seeks help from a private entrepreneur and is free to reject it if he wishes.

Szasz discusses the dangers inherent in the practice of institutional psychiatry and sees it as a totally abusive system whose most important characteristics are force and fraud. In many ways, there are close analogies between the current practices of school psychologists and those of the institutional psychiatrists. These similarities may be helpful to detail and discuss.

Who Is the Client?

The major similarity is that, like the psychiatrist hired by a state hospital or the Veteran's Administration, the school psychologist is an employee of the institution which hires him and to which he thus has primary responsibility. This arrangement can be implicit or stated. For example, in one manual concerning internship training in school psychology, it is stated that one of the goals of such training is

> to develop an understanding that the goals of the school psychologist are the same as those of the school and its professional staff [State Department of Education, 1969, p. 32].

From *Professional Psychology*, 1971, **2**, 266–270. Copyright 1971 by the American Psychological Association and reproduced by permission.

Later on, in delineating the function of the school psychologist, the manual states,

> The primary function of the school psychologist shall be the intensive, individual psychological study of children referred to him because of learning and/or adjustment problems [p. 66].

On the one hand, then, it is quite clear that the school psychologist is an agent of the school system working along with other professionals to further the aims of the institution. At the same time, it is also made quite clear that the major function of the psychologist is to evaluate children. Thus, the putative client is the child and ostensibly the psychologist works to help him with academic or behavioral deficiencies. Yet, the psychologist is carefully instructed to remember that such help must be within the goals of the school. Interesting questions arise as a result. What does the school psychologist do when what might benefit the child he has been referred is at variance with the stated goals of the school administration? What happens when a principal or superintendent requests that certain decisions about class placement be tendered about a child because it is in the best interests of the school system that such changes be effected? These and all other "who is the client" issues must apparently be resolved, under the present system, in favor of the psychologist's institutional employer.

Who Is Being Helped?

Although the psychologist and those who have referred the child to him see this referral in terms of a "This is being done to help you" attitude, it is often forgotten that the child is an involuntary participant of any evaluation or modification procedure. The psychologist may explain to the child why he is being tested, but his permission is rarely asked before an intelligence or other test is administered. Even this explanation to the child is hardly ever honest. One can only imagine a school psychologist saying to a child, "You are being evaluated today because your teacher finds you a highly disturbing individual and seeks to have you removed from her class. My job is to see if that is possible. If you do not behave on the tests I am about to give you within certain acceptable limits of intelligence and/or emotional indicators, you will be transferred to an adjustment class or be excluded from school, the choice of which depends on how deviant you are from these norms." While that is essentially the real reason for testing, it is more likely that the child hears some brief speech about how this testing session will be very beneficial to him because it will aid in securing more information that will eventually lead to helping him. Thus, to use Fulkerson's phrase (1965), for almost all children evaluated by a school psychologist, the testing situation is characterized by a high degree of "response uncertainty" wherein the child does not know the nature of the testing instruments, the purpose of testing, or the use to which the information he provides may be put. Thus we have an involuntary client almost completely in the dark about why he is there, being tested by someone whose primary responsibility is not to him. Any resistance to this procedure by the child (or his parents) is not viewed, however, as being evoked by this situation but is more likely to seen as either (or a combination of) lack of motivation, passive-aggressivity, internally stimulated anxiety, evasion, or paranoid suspicious-ness.

Not only does the child run the danger of being placed in a situation where he is asked to reveal information about himself, though he does not know how the information will be used, but only infrequently is he likely to come out of this situation without some damaging label. Szasz likens psychological testing to the water ordeal used in witch finding. If an alleged witch, completely restrained by ropes and dumped into deep water, floated, she was guilty; if she sank, she was innocent. In either case, she was dead. And, like the witch, the child referred for testing by a teacher or principal usually ends up in the same position; though not dead he is tagged and labeled, if not for life then for the academic portion of it. The fact of referral leads to a bias to uncover pathology or exceptionality, especially when additional special education units and subsequent financial support from the state for these units depend on children to fill the classes. The danger of a formal connection between school psychology and special education has been discussed elsewhere (Bersoff, in press), and it is the issue of labeling that is more germane here. But, when school psychologists are specifically seen as employees of a school system (and indirectly, part of Divisions of Special Education), they are more likely to abet the goals of those institutions than to serve the interests of the child.

Is Labeling Helpful?

Nowhere is this more apparent than in the labeling of children as neurologically handicapped. If there is a myth of mental illness as Szasz suggests, there is also the myth of brain damage in children. Certainly, organic intracranial diseases do exist in children; some children have demonstrable tumors or suffer the sequela of anoxia, meningitis or toxicity. But, by and large, for the vast majority of children designated as neurologically handicapped there is no primary evidence. At least when a child is labeled as educably retarded there is some reasonably reliable and valid primary evidence, by virtue of an IQ score, that retardation exists. However, the diagnosis of brain damage in children is usually made on the basis of secondary evidence at best—subtest scatter on intelligence tests, rotations on tests of visual-motor perception, scores on supposed tests of "psycholinguistic ability," mixed laterality, etc. While a medical examination is almost always an inherent part of the evaluation process, the physician also usually arrives at his diagnosis on the basis of secondary evidence (sometimes because the school psychologist's report tells him so). An EEG may be required but in at least one state, while the EEG is mandatory, it need not be positive for the child to be considered as neurologically handicapped. Thus, the institutional school psychologist, working in concert with an institutional physician, has the power to label someone as something for which there is no direct evidence and, on the basis of that label, have the child removed from his regular classroom without his permission and to a class with other children also so labeled against their will.

This might not be considered the same kind of force and fraud associated with institutional psychiatry if the labeling itself were not so destructive and the special class placement, in reality, helpful. But labeling is destructive and there is little substantiated evidence that placement in a class for brain-damaged children accomplishes the stated goals of increased academic functioning.

As to the first point, it has been found that people are increasingly rejected, not on the basis of described symptoms (on a continuum of "normal" to "paranoid schizophrenia") but rather on the basis of the kind of treatment received (on a continuum from none to incarceration in a mental hospital). Thus, a person with schizophrenic symptoms, but not labeled as such and described as not receiving any help whatsoever, was seen as normal, but a normal person, but not so labeled and described as having been in a mental institution, was seen as severely disturbed (Phillips, 1963). One could hypothesize the same phenomenon existing in a school setting. Children who may have symptoms consonant with "neurological handicap" or "emotional disturbance" may be seen as significantly more "normal" if allowed to remain in a regular classroom than if transferred to special classes with titles denoting the exceptionality. Seen as "ill," these children would be more likely rejected by the larger school society and increasingly isolated. Admittedly, however, while the specific hypothesis is plausible, it needs to be tested with the appropriate population.

As to the second point, concerning the efficacy of special class placement of those designated as neurologically handicapped, the evidence is muddy at best. Recent investigations (Cruickshank, 1961; Cruickshank, Paul, & Junkala, 1969; DeLozier, 1966; Gage, 1969; Towne & Joiner, 1968; and some unpublished studies[1]) cast doubt, at least, on the assumption that such classes lead to improved academic achievement and subsequent successful return to regular classes. Thus, like involuntary incarceration into a mental hospital by an institutional psychiatrist, involuntary placement into a "special class" rarely benefits those whom it is overtly, explicitly, and allegedly designed to help. In most cases, those aided are those directly related to the dominant institution—the teachers, the principals, and the superintendents (and the school psychologist whose presence and salary are now justified).

School psychologists rarely go into the profession because they actively seek to become oppressive agents of the "institution." They enter the field, most say, to "help children." But, as this article has sought to indicate,

[1]See Ankey, Fiscus, & Kabler, 1970, and Wroblewski, 1970. Both studies were performed in partial fulfillment of the requirements during an internship in school psychology, Ohio State University.

in many of their functions—labeling children as retarded, disturbed, or brain-damaged; testing children without their permission and without giving full knowledge of the possible consequences of testing; or removing the child from regular classrooms to potentially damaging (or at the best, inconsequential) special classes—school psychologists are very much like the institutional psychiatrist who acts on the basis of force and fraud, and against the best interest of his client, the individual child.

References

Ankey, R. F., Fiscus, E. D., & Kabler, M. L. An evaluation of the programs for learning disability students in the Franklin County Schools. Unpublished manuscript, Ohio State University, 1970.

Bersoff, D. N. School psychology and state divisions of special education: A suggestion for change. *Journal of School Psychology* 1971, in press.

Cruickshank, W. M. *A training method for hyperactive children*. Syracuse: Syracuse University Press, 1961.

Cruickshank, W. M., Paul, J. L., & Junkala, J. B. *Misfits in the public schools*. Syracuse: Syracuse University Press, 1969.

DeLozier, R. C. A study of the needs of neurologically handicapped children as related to an appropriate educational program. (Unpublished doctoral dissertation, University of Utah.) Ann Arbor, Mich.: University Microfilms, 1966. No. 66–10, 125.

Fulkerson, S. C. Some implications of the new cognitive theory for projective tests. *Journal of Consulting Psychology,* 1965, **29,**191–197.

Gage, S. A study to predict the influence of several factors in determining future success of neurologically handicapped students. Unpublished Master's thesis, Ohio State University, 1969.

Phillips, D. L. Rejection: A possible consequence of seeking help for mental disorders. *American Sociological Review,* 1963, **28,** 963–972.

State Department of Education. *Internship program in school psychology.* Columbus, Ohio: State Department of Education, 1969.

Szasz, T. *The manufacture of madness.* New York: Harper & Row, 1970.

Towne, R. C., & Joiner, L. M. Some negative implications of special placement for children with learning disabilities. *Journal of Special Education,* 1968, **2,** 217–222.

Wrobiewski, C. A study to investigate achievement gains of learning disabled students under three different treatments. Unpublished manuscript, Ohio State University, 1970.

34. Social Issues and the Child Psychiatrist

Robert Coles

Those of us who went to medical school in the 1950s and took our psychiatric residencies during that decade heard very little, if anything, about "social psychiatry." Even the "public health" taught to medical students and young doctors was apt to be highly theoretical, and all too conveniently and ironically removed from the concrete social and economic realities that plague millions of families—and many of them, of course, live right next door to some of this nation's leading medical centers. I have in mind the endless "cycles" we learned—to be honest, memorized for a test and forgot —in the particular "public health" course I took; cycles that had to do with parasites, some of which we knew were problems in far-off Africa or Asia, some of which we did *not* know to be around in abundance just a few blocks away from our fine, imposing hospital and medical school. No effort was made to connect those cycles (worm to animal to man—and on and on) to the lives people live, here or abroad; the extreme poverty, the joblessness, the rural shacks or urban slums, the domination and exploitation of millions and millions of uneducated, malnourished men and women on this planet by the powers that be—rich landowners, generals and their well paid and kept troops, dictators of one sort or another, and not least, giant corporations who own oil wells all over the world, obtain minerals and other raw materials from every continent, and in essence take away wealth from already poor nations so that rich ones can become even richer.

Now, what does that sorry state of affairs have to do with the training of child psychiatrists? Those are political and economic matters, one can hear it said. Our problems are "inner" ones; that is to say, we are concerned with children whose fears and anxieties get out of hand, in response to (we have all learned from Freud) the particular and various ways those children were brought up by their parents. In this regard, I remember all too well an experience I had when a second-year resident in child psychiatry. I had been treating a young black child for what was then called a "learning phobia." Yes, I had taken a "family history," and yes, the mother was being seen by a social worker. (There was no father, only a confusing succession of men visitors, some of whom stayed a few weeks, some a few months.) But the social worker wanted to "analyze" the mother, not find out how (and why) she had come North in the first place—and lost her husband, who died of tuberculosis. I was determined to find out what was going on between the mother and her only son that could account for the "acting

From *Child Psychiatry and Human Development*, 1971, **2**, 67–69. Copyright 1971 by Behavioral Publications, Inc. Reproduced by permission.

out" the boy demonstrated, not to mention his lethargy and stubbornness with his teachers, his refusal to pay them any respect, his defiance of them—all women, I had found out, and no doubt "mother surrogates" or "substitutes" or whatever.

Meanwhile (the year was 1957) I had given no thought to the color of the child's teachers, or to the possibility that I ought to look into what was happening between the child and them—and I mean happening *on its own merits*, apart from some spillover ("transference") from mother to teacher. At the very end of "treatment" (I was going into the air force) the boy apparently (I only now realize) decided to stop putting up with my ignorance, my thoughtlessness. He asked me to come visit his neighborhood. He was the second black child to ask me to do that, but still I didn't stop and ask why. True, I knew that racial prejudice was no stranger to the United States; and if I had been quizzed, I might even have come up with some other explanations than the ones I did find to explain the child's request that I come meet his friends, see their homes, get to know where and how they lived. I might have told my "supervisor" that this child was born in a rural shack in the South, had been poorly fed, had seen relatives and neighbors die young, including his own father, had been made afraid of white people from his earliest years, had learned that white people all the time threaten, insult, and humiliate black people, had come North with a confused, saddened, grieving, frightened mother, who had for months tried to find work —only to give up and throw herself and her daughters and son at the mercy of those men, those oedipal interlopers, I had heard about in my office—those equally frustrated and burdened men who live in ghettos where the unemployment rate can be something like 30 percent; that is right, *30 percent*.

There is a psychological issue, such an unemployment rate. No matter how categorical we get, no matter how we try to bury our heads in sand of our own making, there is no doubt that the forced migration of blacks and whites to our cities from regions like Appalachia or the rural South and the economic conditions in the cities encountered by those millions of citizens (similar things are now going on all over the world) are for the parents and children involved profoundly "inner" events, events of the mind, events that critically, decisively even, affect "human development." The boy I was treating was afraid of his white teachers, and with good reason. In recent years I have worked with those teachers as well as with boys like the one I have been mentioning, and I know full well how afraid such teachers are, in turn, of their pupils. And if there is, unquestionably, an idiosyncratic "factor" in all that fear, based upon the "private" or "personal" experiences that children and teachers have had, there is certainly something else at work, powerfully at work: the influence of a nation's history, its social traditions, its political and economic "structure," its distribution of power and wealth, on the child's mind—specifically on his or her unconscious and conscious assumptions, hopes, fears, anxieties.

No doubt today (1972) most young child psychiatrists would have no trouble agreeing with what I have just insisted upon, though some of the journals and the agenda of certain professional meetings still make it hard to say that those same young psychiatrists don't have to deal all the time with the narrowness and ideological rigidity of their teachers. Nor will it do if we all accept "social psychiatry" for the poor, but forget to apply what such a point of view means for us, the upper-middle-class child psychiatrists who so predominantly see in our offices children from much the same background as our own. Years ago (1958) Redlich and Hollingshead (*Social Class and Mental Illness*) pointed out how persistently we are at the mercy, so to speak, of the way we live—our position in the society we belong to. Whom we see, whom we child psychiatrists seek out, whom we feel comfortable talking with, whom we are quickly prone to dismiss, find uncongenial, think of as "difficult" if not "hopeless" or "untreatable"—all of those "facts," those daily psychotherapeutic "events," have to do with dozens and dozens of experiences we have gone through as we have grown up here, not there, under such and such set of circumstances rather than any number of other possible ones.

It is about time that some of our more theory-prone colleagues—who seem always willing to mull over and endlessly refine the various abstractions that have become at the very least tenets, *laws* even, rather than tentative formulations—began to think about childhood as something more than a highly private experience between a mother, a father, and a couple of "siblings," or as a matter of "cognitive structures" gradually and inevitably developing and asserting themselves. Both Freud and Piaget never meant to isolate the psychological phenomena they described so shrewdly and influentially from the larger social and economic currents of life that relentlessly affect the way a child grows, the values that a child comes to have, the inclinations and habits of mind such a boy or girl develops. There have been times in my work when I have heard children speak what I have just written down. Common sense it is, *their* common sense spoken to me. I am sure they have given me credit for having a bit of common sense myself; but maybe they have also suspected (known unconsciously?) that even as they have their moments (and longer) of blindness, people like me can also manage to overlook things that are painful, unsettling, embarrassing—and shaming.

Chapter Thirteen

Conclusions

The 1970s challenge us in many areas of abnormal child psychology, as we have seen. Problems of diagnosis and classification of childhood disorders are still the source of considerable disagreement; no completely adequate diagnostic scheme has yet been formulated. While there have been noteworthy advances during the past quarter century, as described by Eisenberg, let us hope that the next decade will witness much greater progress on many fronts of the struggle against social forces contributing to psychopathology in children. If Albee's advice and recommendations are heeded, there will be major changes in the models guiding the treatment of disturbed individuals as well as in the kinds of people who will deliver the services. The move would be away from a "mental disease" model with medical personnel treating emotional illnesses and toward a "psychosocial learning" model with non-professionals being trained to provide the reeducation that seems to be the fundamental need of the majority of those who suffer from personal and social maladjustment in contemporary society.

Interactions between parent and child have been described as crucially important determinants of childhood psychopathology. While this book has emphasized the effects of parents on their children, it should not be overlooked that children also affect their parents. An abnormal child—especially one whose deviance takes the form of extreme withdrawal or constant irritability—can influence his parents to behave much differently than they would toward a more normal child. In other words, family relations should not be viewed solely as a one-way street, with parents being seen as having negative effects on their children.

These particular issues are intimately related to the heredity versus environment, or nature versus nurture, controversy that was emphasized in the chapters discussing racial inheritance of intelligence and possible influences of deprived social conditions on the educational attainments of poor children. Obviously, there are no universally accepted answers; some experts recommend the continued study of inherited differences, while others maintain that this is a waste of time since it will never be possible to resolve the heredity versus environment controversy.

The issues related to various types of childhood pathology again revealed considerable disagreement on the relative importance of constitutional (hereditary) versus social (environmental) factors, but the disagreement varies from one type of problem behavior to another. For example, few people attribute childhood neurosis to biological determinants; it is largely accepted that such neuroses (for example, school phobia) usually result from disturbed parent-child relations. Whether one takes the psychodynamic approach (and attributes the neurotic behavior to unresolved conflicts in Freudian psychosexual stages of development) or the learning theory approach (and attributes it to specific learning of maladaptive behaviors), it is agreed that the malfunctioning results from interpersonal experiences.

In the area of juvenile delirquency there is somewhat more disagreement about the relative roles of co.istitutional, psychological, and social factors. While some theorists or investigators emphasize inherited physical characteristics such as body-build, others are mainly concerned about social class differences and still others focus on personality traits. With the present state of knowledge in this field, it seems best to remain open to the possible influences of all of these factors, especially operating in combinations, as suggested by the biopsychosocial theory described in this book.

While there may be lack of unanimity regarding the causes of delinquency, all agree that delinquents of all varieties are difficult to treat therapeutically. It must be stressed that motivation for change is a fundamental prerequisite for successful psychotherapy; if the client or patient does not want to alter his personality or behavior and feels no need for therapeutic help, then conventional psychotherapy is bound to fail. In our discussion of juvenile delinquency, we described some innovative treatment approaches that have been relatively more successful in motivating delinquents to modify their behavior in socially healthy directions.

Probably the most controversial aspect of childhood psychopathology is childhood psychosis. Here the heredity versus environment controversy has clearly divided theorists (and therapists) into opposing camps; some, like Bettelheim, maintain that infantile autism results from traumatic interactions between mother and child during the first years of life; others, like Rimland, postulate that biological impairment present from birth causes this most serious of childhood disorders. Not only do many of the world's leading experts disagree about the causes of this form of child psychopathology, but until recently there has been indiscriminate use of terms referring to sometimes similar and sometimes different phenomena: one man's "childhood schizophrenia" is another's "infantile autism" and yet another's "symbiotic psychosis of childhood." This book has shown the current progress in diagnostic techniques, with Rimland and others carefully spelling out the specific criteria that differentiate seemingly similar forms of childhood psychosis.

Returning to the role of mother-child relations, major changes have occurred in the thinking of professionals who work with psychotic children and their families. Only a decade or so ago, the mother was viewed as the evil force lurking behind every psychotic child, and "cure" could be attained only by removing the child from the mother's negative influence; mother and child were treated separately—the child was usually institutionalized in a psychodynamically oriented treatment center and the mother was seen by a psychiatrist or psychiatric social worker for individual psychotherapy.

What a far cry from the approach advocated today by clinical investigators like Schopler and Reichler, who view parents as co-therapists helping their own psychotic children to overcome developmental defects believed to result more from organic inadequacies in the child than from psychological disturbance in the family.

While biological aspects seem to receive most of the current emphasis in theorizing about psychotic children, recently the need for far-ranging social changes has been stressed in regard to attitudes toward and treatment of the mentally retarded. Albee and others have pointed out that only a small portion of retardates are biologically damaged and/or physically incapacitated, while the vast majority are physically healthy and could lead relatively normal lives if our society took a different attitude toward them.

Locking up retardates in the kinds of state institutions that exist today has been criticized as the wrong treatment approach. It will be interesting in the years ahead to see just how many of today's proposed innovations will actually come to fruition. Of course, with our current national priorities, we may make great strides toward learning how to maintain life on distant planets while merely continuing to pack the bodies a little closer in our "human warehouses" here on earth.

At this point in the history of psychology, there are few conclusive answers to the many perplexing questions concerning various approaches to treatment of disturbed children. The lack of agreement between psychodynamically oriented clinicians and experimentally oriented behaviorists is particularly evident when psychotherapy and behavior therapy are compared. However, perhaps the future will witness a synthesis of these two currently disparate therapies, forming an approach known as "psychodynamic behavior therapy," which may be more powerful and effective, yet more tolerant, than either of its antecedents.

The most controversial issues in the area of treatment are probably the administration of drugs to hyperkinetic children and the use of punishment to control the behavior of severely disturbed children. Influential, well-informed people speak on behalf of either side of the argument on both issues. Some recognized authorities maintain that medication serves a vital role in treating disturbed children, especially those with hyperkinesis and various forms of learning disabilities, while others liken this treatment to placing defenseless children in straitjackets. The same is true with the application of aversive stimuli (such as isolation, electric shock, or a slap in the face): some psychologists, psychiatrists, and educators expound the long-range virtues of such treatment, while others see this merely as professionally sanctioned child abuse.

The final issues in this book were also largely ethical, discussing the rights of children, especially in the school systems where the invasion of children's privacy has received little attention. The closing paper by Coles emphasized neglected social issues that have affected the welfare of children in the recent past. Thus, this book has presented the many important issues we have left unresolved far too long and the almost overwhelming number of critical problems that await solutions in the field of childhood psychopathology.

Name Index

Subject Index